BEYOND THE ASYLUM

Studies of the Weatherhead East Asian Institute, Columbia University

The Studies of the Weatherhead East Asian Institute of Columbia University were inaugurated in 1962 to bring to a wider public the results of significant new research on modern and contemporary East Asia.

BEYOND THE ASYLUM

MENTAL ILLNESS IN FRENCH COLONIAL VIETNAM

Claire E. Edington

CORNELL UNIVERSITY PRESS
Ithaca and London

Cornell University Press gratefully acknowledges the role of the Association for Asian Studies First Book Subvention Program for its support of this book.

First published 2019 by Cornell University Press

Library of Congress Cataloging-in-Publication Data

Names: Edington, Claire, 1984– author.
Title: Beyond the asylum : mental illness in French
   colonial Vietnam / Claire Edington.
Description: Ithaca [New York] : Cornell University Press,
   2019. | Series: Studies of the Weatherhead East Asian
   Institute, Columbia University | Includes bibliographical
   references and index.
Identifiers: LCCN 2018041940 (print) | LCCN 2018047923
   (ebook) | ISBN 9781501733956 (epub/mobi) |
   ISBN 9781501733949 (pdf) | ISBN 9781501733932(cloth)
Subjects: LCSH: Mental illness—Social aspects—Vietnam—
   History. | Mentally ill—Care—Vietnam—History. |
   Mentally ill—Vietnam—Social conditions. |
   Psychiatry—Vietnam—History. | Psychiatric hospitals—
   Vietnam—History.
Classification: LCC RC451.V5 (ebook) | LCC RC451.V5
   E35 2019 (print) | DDC 362.2/109597—dc23
LC record available at https://lccn.loc.gov/2018041940

For Dan

What are these pavilions on the side of the road,
Enquires the voyager who goes joyfully
Towards the mountains or the sea, to enjoy the best
Of holidays while putting worries to the side?

That they appear elegant with their vaulted flowers,
Their green foliage mounting high towards the skies,
Their grassy patios for the pleasure of eyes,
And over there, in the distance, the mellow beauty of the setting sun.
Do not judge them too much, friend, on appearance,
All while maintaining a full pardon:
Those "afflicted by god" serving at the house,
Those who know the worst of Gehenna,
Fighting without respite against their loss of reason,
Knowledge, Kindness will not ease their pain.

Pélissier, Administrator of Civil Services, Saigon, January 7, 1945
Dedicated to Dr. Baccialone, director of the Psychiatric Hospital of
Biên Hòa, and his "devoted collaborators"

Contents

ILLUSTRATIONS

Acknowledgments

This book, ten years in the making, would not have been possible without the support of a breathtaking number of individuals. I first thank Susan Pedersen and Ronald Bayer, whose intellectual energy and capaciousness, patience, and generosity model the very best qualities of what it means to be a teacher and mentor. Each challenged me every step of the way while also encouraging me to develop my own voice and trust my instincts as a historian. At Columbia University, I also thank Kim Hopper, David Rosner, James Colgrove, Jennifer Hirsch, Constance Nathanson, Emmanuelle Saada, and Kavita Sivaramakrishnan who all took me seriously and provided valuable forms of insight and support. Among those who shaped this book's early development, special thanks are owed to Eric Jennings, Sarah Ghabrial, Aimee Genell, Maria John, Charlotte Legg, Sarah Cook Runcie, Toby Harper, Mari Webel, and David Wright, and especially Jessica Pearson for being such a trusty reader and loyal companion throughout our years in New York City. Laurence Monnais, whose foundational work on the history of colonial medicine in Indochina made this book possible in the first place, encouraged me from the beginning to push my research in new directions. For her enthusiasm and support, I owe a huge debt of gratitude. Michele Thompson generously helped me to navigate the precolonial landscape of Vietnamese medical theories and practices as I was finishing the book. Hans Pols—my esteemed collaborator and favorite partner in crime—worked with me to better understand the relationship between French Indochina and the Dutch East Indies and the broader regional and transimperial context of this story. James Goodyear first ignited my curiosity about the world of tropical medicine and empire. I hope this book makes him proud.

Among those scholars of Vietnam, I would like to express my deepest appreciation to Erik Harms, Hue Tam Ho Tai, Mitch Aso, Caroline Herbelin, Thuy Linh Nguyen, Jason Picard, Christina Firpo, Michael Vann, Kathryn Edwards, Olga Dror, Ivan Small, Allen Tran, and especially Haydon Cherry, Charles Keith, and Martina Nguyen for taking me under their collective wing. Christopher Goscha, Peter Zinoman, and Richard Keller each played a crucial role in shaping my thinking about this topic long before they offered their comments as reviewers of the manuscript. Thank you for helping me to transform this book into a more rigorous, impactful, and interesting story. Phuong Nguyen and Vivienne Le provided not only tireless instruction in the Vietnamese language but also perceptive insights into the tender labor of translation, across both languages and cultures. Huyen Pham, for providing critical research assistance in Hanoi during the latter stages of the book, thank you for your resourcefulness and bright energy.

This book would not have been possible without the generous support provided by the National Institutes of Health predoctoral training program in Gender, Sexuality and Health; the Weatherhead East Asian Institute at Columbia University; the Alliance Program for Doctoral Mobility at Columbia University (with special thanks to Henri Bergeron at Sciences Po); the D. Kim Foundation; research grants provided by the University of Massachusetts, Boston, and the University of California, San Diego; and Harvard University's Mahindra Humanities Center, as well as various travel awards made possible by the Mellon Foundation, Columbia's Mailman School of Public Health, the Vietnamese Studies Group, and the French Colonial Historical Society.

I am also immensely grateful for the invaluable assistance provided by librarians and archivists across three continents. In Vietnam, I thank the staffs of the archives at National Archives Center No. 1 (Hanoi), National Archives Center No. 2 (Ho Chi Minh City), and the National Archives of Cambodia in Phnom Penh. For providing essential logistical support during many research trips to Vietnam, I owe a huge debt to Le Minh Giang and his team at Hanoi Medical University, especially Hang Thu Dang. I also thank the staffs of the New York Academy of Medicine (NYAM), the Archives Nationales de France in Aix-en-Provence, the Bibliothèque Interuniversitaire de Médecine in Paris, and the Centre de Documentation de l'Institut de Médecine Tropicale de la Service de Santé des Armées in Marseille (PHARO).

In my travels I have extended my family circle, for which I am profoundly grateful. In Hanoi, an especially heartfelt thank you is owed to Asia Nguyen Cooper and Giles Cooper, Phong and Hue Nguyen, and Jenny and Lasse Melgaard, all of whom offered me a home away from home. At the University of Massachusetts, Boston, Josh Reid, Abigail Balbale, Olivia Weisser, Conevery Bolton Valencius, and David Hunt helped me in ways that were more important to me than they knew.

In my new home at the University of California, San Diego, I have encountered a brilliant and supportive set of colleagues. I especially thank my treasured writing buddies—Lilly Irani, Paloma Checa-Gismero, Todd Henry, and Saiba Varma—for alternately focusing and distracting my attention when I needed it the most. Cathy Gere has also been an incredible source of support and sanity throughout this whole process and, moreover, has become a dear friend. Andrew Scull's work on the social history of madness inspired this project long before we became colleagues and coteachers at UCSD. I continue to learn from him. I am fortunate to have received thoughtful feedback from many of my colleagues, both near and far, who read all or parts of the manuscript: Daniel Navon, Simeon Man, Wendy Matsumura, Jessica Graham, Abbie Miyabi, Matthew Vitz, Saiba Varma, Jin Kyung-Lee, Cathy Gere, David Hunt, Andrew Scull, Charles Keith, Diana Kim, Sarah Milov, Hans Pols, and Laurence Monnais.

To my editor at Cornell University Press, Emily Andrew, and her entire staff, thank you for holding my hand throughout this process, just as promised. I would also like to acknowledge Ross Yelsey at the Weatherhead East Asian Institute for his professionalism and for moving things along so smoothly from start to finish. Portions of chapter 3 were previously published as a 2016 article in *Comparative Studies in Society and History*, "Building Psychiatric Expertise Across Southeast Asia: Study Trips, Site Visits and Therapeutic Labor in French Indochina and the Dutch East Indies, 1898–1937," with Hans Pols (58[3]: 636–663). Portions of chapter 4 were previously published in another article, also in *Comparative Studies in Society and History*, entitled "Going In and Getting Out of the Colonial Asylum: Families and Psychiatric Care in French Indochina" (55 [3]: 725–755).

Finally, thank you to my friends who have lived with me (and this project) for many years: Rachel Rosenberg, Rachel Barker, Morgan Heck, Matthew Spooner, Mary Spooner, Emilie Adams, Sarah Milov, Kyrill Kunakhovich, and Jeffrey Lenowitz. To my family, no words can express my gratitude. Thank you, Billie, for inspiring me with your creativity and for expressing your love and support in ways that only a little sister knows how to do. I'll see you at the finish line. For my mother and father, none of this would have been possible without you. Thank you for the GP. My parents-in-law, Simone and Larry Navon, my brother-in-law Joshua, and of course Jimby, for embracing me as their own from the very beginning. Last of all, this book is dedicated to Daniel Navon, who has followed me all over the world for the last ten years and at countless points offered insights that significantly reshaped the story told in this book. With tireless affection and boundless support, he has also fundamentally altered the story of my life, making it more beautiful than I ever thought possible.

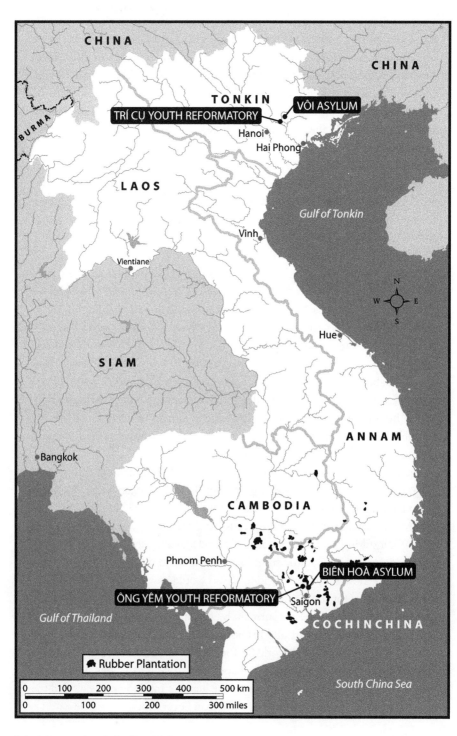

CHINA

CHINA

TONKIN

TRÍ CỤ YOUTH REFORMATORY · VÔI ASYLUM

Hanoi

Hai Phong

LAOS

Gulf of Tonkin

Vinh

Vientiane

SIAM

Hue

ANNAM

Bangkok

CAMBODIA

Phnom Penh

BIÊN HOÀ ASYLUM

ÔNG YÊM YOUTH REFORMATORY · Saigon

Gulf of Thailand

COCHINCHINA

🌳 Rubber Plantation

| 0 | 100 | 200 | 300 | 400 | 500 km |
| 0 | | 100 | | 200 | 300 miles |

South China Sea

Colonial possessions in Southeast Asia

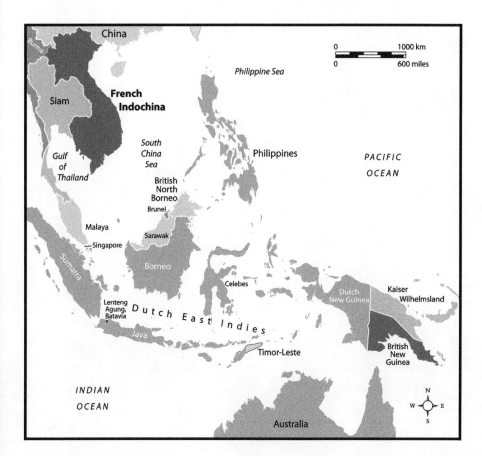

French Indochina

BEYOND THE ASYLUM

Introduction

Writing the Social History of Psychiatry in French Colonial Vietnam

In December of 1920, Sau was admitted to the Biên Hòa asylum outside Saigon, a year after the asylum first opened its doors. Sau was thirty years old and worked as a security attendant at a large commercial house in the city center. Charged with multiple counts of assault, theft, and vagrancy, Sau came to the attention of colonial authorities like many others who were eventually sent to the asylum: as a threat to public security. Once confined, Sau was diagnosed with delirium, characterized by violent episodes brought on by heavy drinking. Six months later, he had improved to the point that the presiding psychiatrist recommended his release, but only under the condition that his family exercise strict surveillance. Sau's family had long petitioned the colonial government for his release, as many other children, parents, and spouses of asylum patients would do throughout the interwar years. Two years later, in June of 1923, Sau found himself once again at the asylum, this time after committing murder. A doctor charged with providing an expert opinion in the case found Sau to be irresponsible by reason of insanity and recommended his confinement. Yet he used Sau's case to warn of a broader pattern in which "the existence of these individuals is a vast cycle where prison and asylum alternate with phases of liberty when they commit minor offences, misdemeanors and crimes which lead to a new confinement."[1]

Sau's case file is one among hundreds of patient case files preserved in the colonial archives of both Vietnam and France. These files include detailed notes on clinical diagnoses and treatment regimes, as well as the entrance and exit certificates of patients who often traveled across a vast territory, from the Mekong Delta to the highlands of Laos. They contain the handwritten correspondence of family members and asylum directors as well as the paperwork generated from other branches of the colonial administration: expert medical opinions formulated as part of court trials, registration cards for prostitutes, the photos and fingerprints of juvenile delinquents sent to youth reformatories, police reports for crimes ranging from petty theft to aggravated murder, and the labor contracts of plantation workers discharged from their employment on neighboring rubber plantations.

These documents serve as powerful reminders that patients occupied other social roles that shaped their experiences both inside and outside psychiatric institutions. They also underscore the extraordinary movements of patients, many of whom seemed to cycle endlessly in and out of asylums and between hospitals, prisons, poor houses, pagodas, and family homes. Taken together, these individual patient itineraries challenge our notion of the colonial asylum as a closed setting where patients rarely left, run by experts who enjoyed broad and unquestioned authority. Instead, they reveal how ideas about what it meant to be abnormal, as well as normal enough to return to social life, were debated between colonial authorities and the public throughout the early decades of twentieth century. For individuals like Sau, what it meant to find oneself on the inside or outside of the colonial asylum often shifted with the changing fortunes of individual households, the prerogatives of colonial administrators, and the professional ambitions of psychiatric experts.

This book is a social history of psychiatry and mental illness in French Indochina. I focus on the region that is now known as Vietnam during a period of major transformation under French colonial rule, from shortly before the official foundation of the Indochinese Union in 1887 through the beginning of the Second World War, when the French grip on the colony came undone. In the late nineteenth century, French observers, newly arrived to Indochina, remarked on what they believed to be a striking absence of mental illness among the indigenous population. Those few believed to be mentally ill were thought to suffer from more chronic forms of dementia or senility and did not pose any serious public danger. Why then did the French decide to build an asylum that opened in 1919, and how did demands for confinement grow so quickly that psychiatrists were no longer able to keep up? Explaining this remarkable shift is one of the central tasks of this book.

Specifically, I trace the kinds of social arrangements that allowed for the identification and transformation of mental illness into a problem of colonial governance. From the late nineteenth century, new kinds of pressures taxed those social bonds on which the care of the mentally ill traditionally depended, while the movements of people from north to south, from country to city, posed unprecedented challenges to the efforts of colonial policing. With the onset of the economic depression in the early 1930s, families found it increasingly difficult to care for their own, and the burden of care for the sick and indigent fell increasingly upon the colonial government. On the one hand, this is a story of the institutionalization of mental illness in Indochina under French rule. On the other hand, even as French psychiatrists enjoyed a widened jurisdiction, they came to rely more than ever on the participation of the Vietnamese public. I argue that the way "abnormal" individuals came to circulate throughout the colony reveals the emergence of new networks of institutions and people that tied the structures of Vietnamese private and public life together with those of the French colonial state. This history of psychiatry is therefore intended as more than a history of a medical category or field of professional practice. Rather, it is the story of a society's transformation as told through the experiences of those at its margins.

In the following pages I set out to revise our understanding of psychiatry in the colonies by first separating the history of psychiatry from the history of confinement.[2] The story of the creation and expansion of colonial asylums does not sufficiently answer the question of how and why people were placed in these institutions (and why they left) and how medical experts were continuously drawn into broader networks of care and economy. By "getting out of the asylum," I therefore mean to shift our focus from the asylum itself to its relationship with the world beyond its walls. Historians have emphasized psychiatry's contribution to a colonial discourse about race and how it figured within a wider biopolitics of colonial rule.[3] Yet the social histories of the asylums themselves and how they functioned within local colonial political systems remain little explored. This book adopts a wider perspective that takes us past this narrow focus on experts and discourses. Instead, it looks beyond the asylum to ask what the history of psychiatry can tell us about the local dynamics of colonial rule. In particular, I propose that we think about the power of the colonial state to confine abnormal individuals as dependent on a wide range of social actors, including Vietnamese families and French prosecutors, whose own strategies for managing mental illness at times intersected with, and at others diverged from, the agendas of colonial experts. Such a perspective forces greater attention to the role of ordinary people in shaping knowledge production and enacting forms of social control in the community.

Getting Out of the Asylum

The asylum was, in many ways, a unique kind of colonial institution. As both hospital and prison it brought together naturalist explanations of disease with social judgments about individual behavior. It has therefore served as the natural point of departure for scholars who have sought to examine and critique the close links between medicine and power in colonial settings. This research agenda is largely indebted to Frantz Fanon, who in his 1959 work *A Dying Colonialism* described the clinic and medical knowledge as spaces of colonial violence and called for resistance against imperialism and the sickness it generated. In his writings, Fanon (who was himself a psychiatrist, born in Martinique but trained in France) argued that psychiatry, by insisting on the overdetermined inferiority of the colonized, worked to justify and facilitate the brutal use of state power. Rather than locate the origins of Algerian violence in the inherent features of the North African mind, Fanon insisted that the violence of colonialism actually engendered madness and savagery among the colonized. He therefore called for violent action as a necessary and reciprocal step in the development of revolutionary consciousness and the liberation of colonial society.[4]

This perspective continues to frame much of the historical literature in which the colonial experience is often presented as essentially a dialectical relationship between colonizer and colonized. The importance of wider social frameworks is dwarfed in favor of explanations that focus on the repressive dynamics of colonization: in terms of coercion and resistance, surveillance and evasion. Historians of medicine, for example, tend to organize their studies around the question of what is specifically *colonial* about colonial medicine; answers to this question typically focus on the role of expert discourses and practices in both legitimizing and maintaining colonial rule. For instance, historians of psychiatry have emphasized how the mind became a critical field for shaping scientific ideas about race and difference throughout the early twentieth century in ways that set the development of psychiatry in the colonies apart from that of psychiatry in the metropole.[5] More recently, scholars have come to consider the field's development from wider perspectives: in the context of the growth of international scientific networks, as a forum for colonial debates over the obligations associated with the civilizing mission, and how knowledge of the "native mind" served as a guide for colonial policymakers. From this growing body of research, spanning India and the Pacific, East Africa and the Maghreb, a portrait emerges of a profession whose science became less a tool for social control per se than an important means for underwriting the ideologies and structures of colonial power.[6] Yet even as scholars have widened the scope for inquiry, the asylum continues to take center stage, both as a symbol of colonial hegemony and as the site where the limits of this hegemony were tested, whether because of cultural misunderstandings, lack of resources, or active forms of resistance within the asylum itself.

Historians have therefore come to describe asylums as sites where experts never exercised more than an incomplete grasp over the production of knowledge.[7] These works demonstrate that the lessons of Michel Foucault's *Madness and Civilization* do not travel easily from Europe to the colonies, where considerations of race played a critical role in shaping colonial medical discourse and where colonial states continued to exercise violent forms of repression even as they incorporated new disciplinary forms of control. And yet, while careful to emphasize the limits of psychiatric authority in colonial settings, scholars have largely stopped short of interrogating what the limits of expert authority can reveal about the social histories of the places under consideration and, in particular, the role of ordinary people in shaping these histories outside a strictly European psychiatric sphere of control. As a result, they often miss the ways in which hybrid forms of power and knowledge were produced in spaces where experts continued to exert their influence yet were also forced to engage with local understandings and practices around insanity. By considering the limits placed on colonial psychiatrists through a process of daily negotiation and exchange, in this book we see something more than just the shortcomings of a hegemonic European science. Instead we see how the arrival of French psychiatry interacted with long-standing local beliefs and practices surrounding mental illness, and the ways in which Vietnamese families and communities used or rejected these new institutions to their strategic advantage.

This perspective draws on recent works in the history of psychiatry in North America, and Britain in particular, that have begun to look much more closely at the dynamic between informal patterns of family care in the community and formal medical treatment in institutions. The examination of linkages between the family and the asylum, and increasingly the crucial intermediary role of friends, neighbors, and community members, has provided scholars with an invaluable opportunity to reexamine assumptions about the social role of asylums in the nineteenth century.[8] These accounts situate the asylum within a wider social context to reveal the kinds of exchanges that shaped the construction of the category of the "insane" person and that worked to both constrain and enable the daily exercise of institutional regimes. David Wright, for instance, argues that the confinement of the insane, as well as their discharge and reintegration into the community, resulted from the participation of a diverse array of social actors—not, for example, as a "consequence of a professionalizing psychiatric elite but rather as a strategic response of households to the stresses of social change or economic depression."[9] As Joseph Melling writes, this emphasis in current research on the detailed reconstruction of the social and cultural contexts of psychiatric treatment has enabled us to explore a "micro-politics of care" that shows bargaining among different actors who had unequal power resources and capacities but who could nevertheless exert some degree of choice if not control over their environment.[10]

These works bring critical attention to the role of extrainstitutional care and insist on the fluidity of the boundaries between asylum and the community rather than a Great Confinement. Yet they remain restricted to nineteenth-century histories of psychiatry in North America and Western Europe.[11] In the colonial literature, references to local actors and indigenous understandings of mental illness are used primarily to frame discussions around the cultural relativity of diagnostic categories, yet families rarely figure in the literature as key participants in the colonial psychiatric system as it developed.[12] Given the well-documented practices of family caregiving in psychiatric settings in Vietnam and across the globe, such an omission from the historical literature risks missing an important part of the picture. In settings as diverse as India, Senegal, Cameroon, Papua New Guinea and Japan, families escort patients to the doctor's office, pay regular visits, and even stay with patients throughout the course of their hospitalization.[13] They assist doctors by feeding patients, performing domestic duties, carrying out simple nursing tasks such as the administration of medication, and providing vital forms of emotional support. More fundamentally, the ability of families to recognize distress and to filter communication between doctor and patient means they have the unique capacity to shape the way expert psychiatric knowledge is produced and how patients are treated. In colonial Vietnam, families not only were key participants in the colonial psychiatric system—they actively shaped the development of that system.[14]

We therefore need to revise our thinking about the totalizing reach of colonial asylums (and their limits) by paying closer attention to those more hybrid forms of accommodation and dependency that extended out into the community. In the following chapters, I set out to trace a kind of colonial "micropolitics" of psychiatric care in order to insist on the historic permeability of the boundaries between asylum and community.[15] By micropolitics,

I mean those everyday exchanges between French experts, colonial authorities, and Vietnamese families that resulted not only in small erosions in the authority of colonial psychiatrists but also, and more significantly, in the emergence of a new, more diffuse kind of psychiatric power. This power tied the authority of European science, backed by a repressive colonial state, together with the social norms of local communities that prescribed the bounds of the conduct of individuals, as well as the obligations and duties of families charged with their care. I locate this micropolitics of psychiatric care within a dense web of interconnections among families, neighbors, colonial officials, and doctors that greatly expanded opportunities for the identification and policing of the mentally ill in colonial Vietnamese society. These connections also ignited controversies over what counts as mental illness, what should be done about it, and who exactly should be responsible for providing care.

In the following chapters, I work to uncover a kind of middle ground where Vietnamese subjects succeeded in limiting the authority of French psychiatric experts in the colony even as they helped to expand colonial psychiatry's overall power and scope. As a result, colonial psychiatrists, unable to impose a single logic, were forced out of necessity to adopt more flexible relationships with the families of their patients and were thereby pulled into alternative forms of evaluation. Families, meanwhile, motivated by their own concerns about the preservation of social order and the integrity of kinship networks, sought or challenged the authority of colonial psychiatrists as they saw fit. I understand Vietnamese families as agents who, in the context of psychiatric care, pursued their own strategies of negotiation, collaboration, and, at times, subversion of colonial rules and practices. Armed with a different set of cultural beliefs and healing traditions, they nevertheless engaged with professional French psychiatrists to find common space for thinking about and discussing mental illness. Families, in their letters to asylum directors, worked to alternatively inform and challenge the coding of certain social behaviors as "deviant" and to influence notions about what counted as psychiatric knowledge and formed the basis for decisions about confining and releasing patients. In the context of psychiatry, the act of designating an individual as abnormal did not solely represent the pervasive power of the state.

It is important to underscore that these exchanges did not occur between equal partners but among colonial actors with vastly different levels of access to power and resources, not least of whom were the patients themselves. Yet in debating the suitability of individuals for social life, experts and laypeople came to pursue their own strategies in ways that do not neatly adhere to more traditional narratives of colonial repression and resistance. Not all French colonial officials agreed on whether to confine certain patients, and the desires of families to take care of the mentally ill at home often clashed with the wishes of their neighbors. Some families pleaded for the release of family members from the asylum, while others actually challenged the refusal of colonial doctors to exercise the power of confinement. Remarkably, these discussions largely occurred during the 1920s and 1930s, a period of high political drama in Vietnam marked by prison revolts and the birth of an anticolonial nationalist movement. Historians of Vietnam have tended to focus on the violence and economic oppression that characterized the expansion of French imperialism in the region. As a result, there remains little written on the social history of the region. Instead, the dominant narrative is of crisis and conflict, and it centers on the political forces that would bring Ho Chi Minh to power and eventually wrest control from the French in 1954.[16]

By contrast, this book tells a different kind of story about how ordinary people used colonial institutions for their own ends. It shows how Vietnamese subjects interacted with colonial experts in ways that helped specify the conditions under which the state could remove individuals from society, both for their own sake and for the sake of others. Debates revolved around the mental health of the patients but also the capacity of the families to assume their care upon release and the asylum itself as the most appropriate site for treatment and rehabilitation. Indigenous agency did not always imply resistance to the colonial state and, in those instances where the strategies of households and French psychiatrists aligned, could actually serve to greatly strengthen state efforts to police the mentally ill. In this social history of psychiatry, the more quotidian struggles of everyday life take center stage, as French authorities drew on the power of local norms and networks, as well as the force of law and punishment, to manage mental illness in the colony. These efforts resulted in outright confrontation in some cases and uneven forms of cooperation in others both within and outside the colonial bureaucracy. Vietnamese who resisted the institutional confinement of family members pursued other forms of treatment and surveillance in the community that, while perhaps more familiar, were no less stigmatizing and restrictive to the personal freedom of the mentally ill.

By bringing the participation of the Vietnamese public and the importance of noninstitutional settings into view, the following chapters emphasize that the possibilities for the identification and social control of the mentally ill in colonial Vietnam did not diminish but rather multiplied and deepened. The legal recognition of mental illness in Vietnam long predated the arrival of French asylums, and the medicalization of deviance took place not only in the pages of patient case files but also in the context of popular Vietnamese scientific journals. How these two different systems of addressing mental illness came together to intensify attention on the poor, sick, and socially marginal held important implications for the lives of patients and their families and the policing of colonial society more generally. That is the focus of this book.

Setting the Stage

The story of the birth of the colonial asylum is told against the backdrop of the deep transformation of Vietnamese society under French colonial rule. At the moment the book opens in the 1880s, the consolidation of French rule in the form of the Indochinese Union—comprising the protectorates of Tonkin, Annam, and Cambodia and the southern colony of Cochinchina— was nearly complete after a series of bloody wars and revolts. A pacified Laos was later added in 1893. Because of the unevenness of conquest (Cochinchina and Cambodia, for instance, had been seized by the French first in the 1860s) and the different forms of administration that characterized territory, each incorporating varying levels of French colonial and imperial Vietnamese influence, the development of the colony as a whole was asymmetrical. Whereas the South's integration into the global economy was speeded by the formation of a rice export industry in the Mekong Delta, in the North modernization advanced more slowly. This began to change at the turn of the century with the passage of the Law of 13 April 1900, which required that all French colonies balance their own budgets and use public debt to finance public expenditures. This mandate for financial independence transformed the colonial state into a truly modern "fiscal state" with the power to maximize economic growth and revenue generation using new coercive mechanisms.[17] Governor-General Paul Doumer invested state funds in public works projects like roads, railroads, and waterways, built on the backs of conscripted Vietnamese labor, to promote colonial development. In addition to establishing state monopolies on the production and sale of opium, salt, and alcohol, Doumer introduced new taxation measures in order to widen the colony's revenue base and break traditional village autonomy over land ownership. The gradual commercialization of agriculture, coupled with the pressures of rural overpopulation, eventually forced farmers off their land and spurred migration to coastal cities and the large rubber plantations of southern Cochinchina.[18] Urban centers like Hanoi, Haiphong, and Saigon became magnets for huge swells of displaced people who came under the thumb of the colonial police force but who also required new forms of charity assistance and access to basic health care. That many of the asylum's patients were originally picked up on vagrancy charges far from home reveals the extent to which heightened mobility and expanding networks of expertise and surveillance made these populations newly visible.

Imperial Connections

This book pursues two intersecting chronologies: the global development of French psychiatry and the history of the local confrontation of two medical systems within colonial Vietnam. French colonial psychiatry did not look the same everywhere; the fact that different parts of the French empire had different relationships with the metropole undoubtedly shaped the production of knowledge about psychiatric illness, as well as the political stakes attached to this knowledge. For instance, while Algeria's proximity to France provoked questions about the mental capacity of local peoples and their possibilities of assimilation into French society, these questions were always much less pressing in Indochina, a source of relatively few migrants to the metropole.

Psychiatrists in the two colonies also adopted different kinds of discourses around race and mental health. Whereas the Muslim population of North Africa was often characterized as inherently violent and impulsive, the Vietnamese, at first, were thought to be at limited risk of mental illness, and their disorders were generally characterized as more of a "psychic weakening" than true agitation. The Algiers School of French Psychiatry, which opened in 1925, promoted a biological model of ethnic psychological difference that reflected the hardening of racial lines in interwar Algeria and contributed significantly to the intensification of colonial violence against North African populations.[19] While no equivalent school operated in Indochina, Vietnamese patients continued to be described as *dégénéré* long after the diagnostic designation had fallen out of favor in the metropole, and French psychiatrists characterized the indigenous mentality as superstitious and therefore particularly susceptible to "ideas of grandeur" and "mystical delusions." Even as doctors insisted on the similarities between Vietnamese and French populations as the basis for importing psychiatric knowledge from the metropole— itself a striking departure from the posture of the Algiers School—they nevertheless did so on the basis of notions of a fundamental distinction between the races.

One aim of this book is therefore to offer an in-depth look at French colonial psychiatry from an alternative vantage, Southeast Asia, as a counterpoint to the dominant North Africa story. Indeed, while Algeria has received much more scholarly attention, it was Indochina that in the 1930s earned the praise of international onlookers for having made the most "serious efforts" at psychiatric assistance in all the empire.[20] Even in Tunisia, where Antoine Porot's clinic opened to much acclaim in 1911, innovations arose but in the context of the treatment of European patients. While considered a crucible for colonial mental health reform, Algeria did not adopt a more comprehensive system targeting indigenous communities for another two decades. Furthermore, psychiatrists in Indochina were well aware of what was happening at home in France, in other parts of the French empire, and in the neighboring colonies of other empires. Exchanges among psychiatric experts over the classification of disease, diagnostic tools, and treatment practices took place in the pages of French medical journals and the meetings of international organizations, as well as study trips to the colonial asylums in the Dutch East Indies as described in chapter 3. From these activities a new global, and specifically regional, dialogue about mental health emerged that forms an important part of this story.

Colonial psychiatry in Indochina appeared at a time when the principles of modern French psychiatry, founded on the asylum-based model of care through confinement, were being questioned and reassessed. Violent press campaigns against asylums exposed the poor condition of patients and threw the discipline into crisis. At the turn of the twentieth century, "alienists" started to refashion themselves as "psychiatrists" in order to gain greater legitimacy from other scientific disciplines. They aligned themselves most closely with neurology, embracing a biological model that traced the origins of madness to the "form of a cerebral lesion, a hereditary defect in the nervous system or a racially determined organization of the brain structure."[21] This model held sway much longer in France than in other parts of Europe, particularly Germany, where fields like psychoanalysis, which assume a psychogenic rather than organic origin of mental illness, gained greater traction. In the colonies, the belief in a determinism, not only of organs but also of the transmission of mental problems across generations, helped to explain the racial inferiority of colonized peoples in increasingly scientistic ways.

For European psychiatrists who witnessed the failure of reformers to remake the asylum at home, the development of colonial mental health programs was seen as a key location for therapeutic innovation and professional revitalization. In Indochina, colonial psychiatrists actively participated in a growing international movement that rejected long-term institutional care in favor of mental hygiene and open psychiatric services.[22] The 30 July 1930 law, which formalized and extended the colony's psychiatric assistance program, contained a number of important innovations, including the introduction of open services into French law for the first time.[23] As Richard Keller has argued in his work on French North Africa, colonial psychiatrists saw themselves as medical pioneers, capable not only of modernizing colonial space and rejuvenating their science but also of exposing the limitations and dangers of the indigenous mind and thereby protecting social order in the colonies.[24] Colonial asylums may have emerged as "spaces of experimentation," to borrow Keller's term, but the nature of this experimentation varied with the unique social and political environments within which these institutions operated.[25] Another aim of this book is therefore to examine the ways that the history of French psychiatry intersected with the history of local exchanges between Vietnamese and French medical systems, itself embedded in the dynamics of French imperial expansion in the region.

Local Encounters

This history of imperial expansion dates from the sixteenth century, when the first French traders and Catholic missionaries arrived in Southeast Asia. However, it would not be until the early nineteenth century that the persecution of Catholic missionaries and their converts would, in the words of historians Pierre Brocheux and Daniel Hémery, "mesh with imperialism, nationalist sentiment and economic considerations to impel intervention in the Mekong Delta."[26] French naval commanders stationed in the South China Sea launched a series of attacks beginning in 1858. As the conquest of the region proceeded in piecemeal fashion, of paramount concern to the French navy was the protection of troops from tropical diseases such as yellow fever, cholera, and smallpox. Haphazard attempts to control epidemics proved largely futile, and it was only in 1890 that a dedicated colonial health service as separate from the military, the Service de Santé des Colonies, was created.

The ensuing expansion of a health infrastructure in Indochina, a core aspect of France's "civilizing mission," targeted both indigenous communities and Europeans, who were starting to settle in greater numbers.[27] Under the motto "Vaccinate, Record, Disinfect," the Assistance Médicale Indigène (AMI) was introduced in 1905 by Governor-General Paul Beau. Organized around a network of hospitals in the major urban areas in northern Tonkin and southern Cochinchina, the AMI also emphasized campaigns against the colony's major epidemic and endemic diseases, including mobile vaccination units and public health education. Between 1912 and 1914, the AMI doubled its budget, which resulted in both a physical expansion and a growing specialization of health facilities. These activities were further strengthened by the introduction of French public health laws and the 1902 opening of the Hanoi School of Medicine, which trained local Vietnamese "auxiliary doctors" (*médecins auxiliaires*), who nevertheless remained subordinate to French physicians. The creation of the first overseas Pasteur Institute in Saigon in 1891 also contributed to basic scientific research in the colony and the development of vaccinations. It was not until after World War I, however, that a health policy tailored to the needs of the colony took shape as French officials sought to rationalize colonial development and promote the ruralization of the health system. The rise in numbers of patient consultations—from 678,494 in 1907 to close to 14 million in 1937—reflected the steady evolution in the demand for hospital care among the Vietnamese population.[28] It also signaled the increasing difficulty of families to care for their own, as colonial doctors complained about the numbers of destitute and hungry showing up at their door. With hospital pavilions dedicated to the mentally ill stretched to capacity and amid growing international pressures to act, local officials in Indochina began in 1897 to seriously debate the merits of establishing an asylum, and in 1912, the colonial administration granted authorization to move forward.

After many delays the Biên Hòa asylum would finally open its doors outside Saigon in January 1919. A second asylum, Vôi, opened in Bắc Giang province near the colonial capital of Hanoi in 1934. Unlike British asylums in India, Indochina's mental hospitals treated European and indigenous patients in the same facility.[29] Patients were segregated into different pavilions according to their race, gender, and severity of symptoms, which ranged from chronic forms of dementia to more acute forms of psychosis. Asylums in French colonial Vietnam were organized as large agricultural colonies, where patients would work the land on the path to healing and eventual liberation. These colonies offered a model of rehabilitation that connected strategies of social reform through labor across the imperial world. For colonial psychiatrists, agricultural colonies seemed to offer a modern conception of psychiatric care that promised not only "cerebral hygiene" and discipline through physical labor but also, in simulating the appearance of freedom, a kind of moral reeducation. These therapeutic and disciplinary goals came to merge with more pragmatic concerns: with nearly a third of asylum patients participating in agricultural work, the program also offset major financial costs to the institution. Annual asylum reports reveal the ways in which colonial psychiatrists framed the therapeutic and economic imperatives for labor and how they came to articulate a vision of psychiatric care that blurred the distinctions between patients and laborers, between institutional order and the organization of social life beyond the asylum.

While annual reports from the Biên Hòa and Vôi asylums provide one picture of daily life at the asylum, deeper frustrations voiced in the personal correspondence of asylum directors and the minutes of oversight commissions provide an alternative and richer view. At every turn, asylum administrators were beset with the challenges of failed surveillance and interpersonal violence produced by patient overcrowding, diminishing budgets, and problems with staff recruitment and retention. From within the colonial administration too, psychiatrists faced threats to their professional authority as prosecutors and prison officials questioned the basis of their "medical-legal" opinions offered during the course of criminal trials. These myriad challenges exposed the pressure points of these institutions, particularly their financial vulnerability during the economic depression of the early 1930s. The challenges only deepened their dependency on crucial forms of extrainstitutional support. Asylum administrators understood the need to cast some out in order to make room for new, more serious cases, which increased their reliance on ancillary hospital networks, the cooperation of other colonial bureaucrats, and the willingness of families to provide care in the community. By the mid-1930s, psychiatrists began to look for expanded markets for their expertise, turning their attention to the social question of crime prevention, and they worked hard to forge alliances with colonial experts in child welfare, law, and education to reform the juvenile delinquency establishment.

Asylum directors could not and did not operate in isolation. Their reliance on the public to not only present patients for treatment but also take care of patients upon their return home meant they were continually forced to negotiate the terms of patient entry and release. Moreover, psychiatrists did not come to Indochina finding a blank slate, devoid of any local expertise or ways of coping with madness. Rather, they encountered forms of care in the community that predated French occupation and that would play an important role in the expansion of the formal asylum system throughout the interwar years. In fact, the practice of traditional medicine would be explicitly promoted, while also circumscribed, by the colonial administration during the interwar period. What exactly defines "traditional Vietnamese medicine" is a topic of continuing debate, particularly in terms of what distinguishes "southern," or Vietnamese, medicine (thuốc nam) in relation to that of its northern Chinese neighbors (thuốc bắc). China remains a critical reference point to this day for what makes something Vietnamese, from family and kinship structures to civil administration, educational systems, and, most important for the purposes of this study, health beliefs. Indeed, as Michele Thompson notes, the tributary relationship between China and Vietnam

resulted in the "regular and formal exchange of medical texts, materia med-
ica, and medical practitioners" over several centuries. These exchanges were
well documented by missionaries and navy medical officers who traveled
widely throughout Vietnam and christened for the first time the particular
confluence of traditions that seemed to characterize local medical practices,
a distinctive *médecine Sino-Annamite*.[30]

The syncretic nature of Vietnamese traditional medicine is clearly evident in understandings about mental illness in Vietnam today, which bear
the marks of several philosophical and epistemic systems: Buddhism, Confucianism, Taoism, and Western biomedicine. Naturalistic or folk medicine,
supernatural or animistic beliefs, and metaphysical explanations or Chinese
hot/cold theory also play important roles.[31] The particular influence of traditional Chinese medicine can be seen in the holistic notion of physical and
mental health: emotional states are closely tied to physical disturbances and
vice versa. This blurring of psychological and physical health is underscored
by the Vietnamese term for psychiatry, or *tâm thần*, in which *tâm* refers to the
heart/soul while *thần* refers to the spirit /soul. Whereas Western biomedicine defines health as the absence of illness, in Vietnamese culture health
is achieved by the continual maintenance of balance between external and
internal, physical and moral forces. This holistic or integrative notion of
health does not fit neatly within the particular mind-body dichotomy found
in Western conceptions.[32]

Throughout the early twentieth century, Vietnamese families called on
a diverse range of treatment options—from herbal remedies to spirit possession to institutionalized care—in order to meet the needs of individual
patients.[33] Families sought the care of both local and foreign experts, but they
also asked for advice on home remedies in the pages of popular medical journals that emerged in the 1920s and 1930s as part of Vietnam's vibrant press
culture. This pluralist approach to mental illness is a hallmark of Vietnamese
medicine more generally, which stresses the natural and supernatural causes
of disease and incorporates outside influences including Western biomedicine.[34] Yet even when French doctors and Vietnamese families broadly agreed
about the presence of mental illness that required treatment, especially for
those patients suffering from more severe disorders, important differences
emerged when it came to interpreting the origins of the affliction and what
should be done about it. The cultural content of mental illness itself—how
symptoms of psychiatric distress were experienced and expressed by patients
and how they were interpreted by those closest to them—also posed serious
challenges for colonial doctors who insisted on diagnosing disorders based
on classification schemes developed in France. In this study of psychiatry

during the colonial period, I am less interested in making arguments about the cultural relativity of mental disorders than in examining how physicians, bureaucrats, patients, and their families all sought to make their claims of mental health and illness intelligible to each other. Furthermore, I argue that much of the psychiatric decision making during this period was guided less by the diagnosis of specific disorders than by finding the cheapest and most efficient way of managing abnormal individuals. Definitions of cure and recovery in the files of patients reveal the strong pragmatic and financial considerations that often guided the course of treatment.

On Method: Looking Inside Out

Each chapter of this book examines the relationship between the asylum and the community from a different point of view. Starting with the French legal definition of the *aliéné*, or insane person, the book gradually expands its focus from the discourse around mental illness to the daily practices of asylum itself and then on to the interactions of the institution with the complex social world outside its doors. In this way, the book progresses as a series of concentric circles radiating outward from the asylum, considering the history of mental illness in colonial Vietnam from multiple and widening perspectives. At the same time, the book is organized roughly chronologically so as to give readers a sense of the profound changes occurring within Vietnamese society, as well as global shifts in psychiatric knowledge and colonial policy, that characterized the late nineteenth through early twentieth centuries.

The case files of patients who cycled in and out of colonial asylums, sometimes multiple times over a period of years, present a unique life history of some of the most marginalized people in Vietnamese society. It is because their scope reaches beyond the purely clinical that patient case files are such rich yet problematic sources for historians of psychiatry. They tell an official history of madness through the eyes of the clinician, leaving patient voices mostly absent. They inevitably reflect inherent biases of culture and class, and the form of the case file itself shifts over time as practices of data collection and modes of psychiatric classification change. These concerns are particularly magnified in the history of colonial psychiatry, which features even greater imbalances in the doctor-patient relationship and the framing of diagnoses across vast cultural divides. Over the last two decades, the use of patient case files as historical sources has begun to shift as historians of medicine have started to ask new questions about the experience of patients in asylums and the social histories of the institutions themselves. The presumed

weaknesses of case files have been transformed into real advantages for critical historical analysis. Yet the reading of colonial asylum archives continues
to reflect the powerful and, at times, stultifying role that an almost exclusive
focus on race and colonial oppression has played in framing the kinds of
questions that are asked of case files. Historians of colonial psychiatry tend
to approach patient files as a series of discursive representations that helped
to consolidate racialized notions of the "other." They also search the files
for forms of patient protest, whether in the content of their delusions or in
forms of disobedience within the asylum.[35]

In this book I propose what at first might appear to be a counterintuitive
approach to the study of colonial asylum archives. Here I read patient case
files for what they can tell us about life outside the asylum as much as the
life inside its walls. By looking inside out, I use these files in order to uncover
the experience of confinement and the pressures on those entrusted with
patient care, to track the movements of patients in and out of the asylums,
and to reveal the dynamics of social life outside these institutions. Letters
from the parents, spouses, children, and other relatives of patients in asylums, for instance, can reveal a number of facets about Vietnamese life under
French colonialism that have not yet received sustained scholarly attention:
the practices and expectations for caregiving in the community, the forms of
dependence and survival that guided the decision making of households, and
the ways in which indigenous understandings of mental illness helped shape
diagnostic practices and informed the process of confinement and release.[36]
Patient case files allow us to uncover some of the texture of daily life in
French colonial Vietnam—those emotional ties and everyday pressures that
resulted in new strategies and forms of accommodation within and between
families, communities, and the French colonial state throughout the early
twentieth century.[37]

Reading patient case files alongside advice columns in popular Vietnamese scientific journals, homegrown novels, and local translations of foreign
medical texts allows us to see just how far ideas about psychiatry and mental
illness traveled outside the colonial asylum and to what extent they resisted
the racist impulses of colonial psychiatry. Reversing notions of racial inferiority, some local authors instead cast mental illness as a marker of civilization; it stood as visible proof that the Vietnamese too struggled to keep up
with the fast pace of modern life. Readers learned that mental illness was
not an inevitable or immutable condition but one that individuals could and
should take steps to rationally manage. It even provided a new language with
which to register critiques of colonial society: the avarice of Vietnamese
elites, the erosion of traditional gender norms, the superstitious practices of

rural villagers, the romantic idealism of young women, and the plight of the urban poor wrought by the destructive forces of French colonization.

To look beyond the asylum therefore means to situate the development of colonial psychiatry within both local exchanges between laypeople and experts and the transnational movements of people and knowledge. The numbers of asylum patients pale in comparison with those of patients confined in prisons throughout the colonial period. But once we understand the asylum as a node in a larger network of disciplinary practices and institutions, we begin to get a sense of the reach of psychiatric norms into daily life and the range of the different kinds of actors—doctors and prosecutors, parents and neighbors—who all participated in deciding the fate of the mentally ill. Debates over whether patients were ready to reintegrate back into society and the kind of care they would receive therefore reveal more than just the limits of expert authority in colonial settings. Instead, the movement of psychiatric patients in and out of asylums offers new insight into the social history of Vietnam, the history of French imperialism, and the colonial history of medicine.

Note on Terminology

My decision to focus on the colonial territories that would become the polity now recognized as Vietnam—Tonkin, Annam, and Cochinchina—means that my use of the terms "Vietnam" and "Vietnamese" in this study is anachronistic. These identifications, themselves contingent and contested during the colonial period, map uneasily onto the borders and identities of the places and actors discussed in this book. Without a more perfect alternative, I realize that some nuance is inescapably lost. At various points throughout the text I also refer to "Indochina" and "indigenous" populations. I understand these terms as colonial constructs used (sometimes pejoratively) by French bureaucrats and doctors to make sense of their wider social world. In addition, because the question of translation—not only across languages but across cultures—plays such a prominent role in this book, I have decided to provide the original French or Vietnamese terms in parentheses, and in their original diacritics, when appropriate.[38]

I also wish to clarify that my use of the term "mental illness" in the pages that follow refers to an individual's loss of social competence—manifested in extreme or otherwise abnormal behavior—that prompted their families and neighbors, or state authorities, to seek their removal from public life and delivery into the hands of experts. The historical instability of mental illness as a concept—its layered and varied meanings, and especially its emergence as a pathology that requires insitutionalization—is precisely what this book sets out to uncover. Patient case files most often refer to patients as *aliéné*, derived from the French term *aliénation mentale*, or the state of being alienated or estranged from one's true rational self. Throughout the 1930s, patients were increasingly referred to by terms that denoted a more specific psychiatric diagnosis. In Vietnamese newspapers and the medical press, common terms like *điên* and *cuồng* were used alongside French terminology to identify different broad categories of mental disorders. My use of the word "insane" or "lunatic" (or any one of a number of broad diagnostic terms) in this book represents a literal translation from the original text and does not purport to mean that these patients were actually mentally ill; it indicates only how the French understood and expressed the need for confinement and how Vietnamese families and communities understood and made use of these terms to pursue their own strategies. Whenever possible, I allow patients to tell their side of the story.

CHAPTER 1

A Background to Confinement

The Legal Category of the "Insane" Person in French Indochina

By the early 1880s, doctors at Chợ Quán Hospital had their hands full. Patients suffering from syphilis, tuberculosis, and dysentery showed up at the hospital's doors without entry tickets while a number of criminals and vagrants in varying states of mental distress arrived by police escort. They included Nhut, arrested for attacking a European police agent with a saber in the throes of a nervous breakdown. There was also Bich, later diagnosed with epilepsy, who had threatened the life of both his sister and his brother's father-in-law, succeeding only in cutting off three of his fingers. Some patients clearly seemed disturbed but did not present a dangerous threat. With no prospect of recovery, they were eventually returned to their families, who promised to provide vigilant oversight. One woman, Nhuan, arrived at the behest of her husband following an excited outburst that had since faded into a quiet sadness after her hospitalization. Others seemed to have no family connections. One Chinese patient, blind in one eye, deaf and mute, entered the hospital in the summer of 1879 after he was found wandering in the streets. His doctor noted a diagnosis of "idiocy" in his case file and deemed him "incurable." With no home to return to, the patient became an employee at the hospital, where he was kept out of trouble by preparing meals for other patients.[1] Louis Lorion, a young French naval doctor who briefly worked at Chợ Quán, later noted that the hospital's facilities, especially those for violent mentally ill patients, left "a lot to be desired, at least during the time when I was in service at that establishment."[2]

Chợ Quán Hospital first opened in 1864 in the growing colonial capital of Saigon. Intended as the centerpiece of French efforts to highlight the benefits of modern medicine, it was also the first hospital created for the exclusive treatment of indigenous patients (*hôpital indigène*). Despite early enthusiasm, the hospital quickly fell into disrepair due to shaky construction and the damage caused by periodic flooding. By the time Lorion arrived, it had undergone some significant reforms initiated by the French navy, which had assumed control over the hospital's operations. It now occupied two main buildings, and its staff consisted of two military physicians on loan from the navy, including Lorion, two French civilian nurses, and a group of Indochinese nurses, whose inclusion represented an innovation at the time.[3] The hospital nevertheless continued to suffer from a chronic lack of funding due to the absence of any official health care policy in the colony. By the spring of 1882, amid a flurry of requests for admittances, the hospital's director announced that he would no longer accept any new patients suspected of mental illness, the cabins dedicated to their care "now being completely occupied."[4]

Upon his return home to France and civilian life, Lorion published a study in 1887 entitled *Criminalité et médecine judiciaire en Cochinchine* in which he insisted on the remarkable rarity of mental illness in the colony. This was not a surprise, Lorion explained, given the state of development of indigenous society as well as the moral characteristics of its people, whom he described as "fickle, occasionally hardworking, very patient, easygoing."[5] Hundreds of years of rule under arbitrary and ancient governments had left the local population (or "Annamites," Lorion's preferred term) with only a "mediocre" taste for politics, and the kinds of "big problems which impassion the Occidentals" left them "completely indifferent." While not "fatalist like the Arabs," Lorion wrote, the Annamites nevertheless approached life with an extreme stoicism, accepting good fortune with the bad. This insight applied even more strongly to the Cambodians, a "degenerate people whose apathy has become proverbial in Indochina" and who, alongside the ethnic Moi people, occupied "the lowest rung in the ladder of civilization."[6] These observations helped to explain the idiosyncratic nature of crime in the colony, distinguished by few violent episodes or crimes of passion. In Lorion's estimation, because of fundamental differences driving "yellow" and "white" forms of criminality, importing modern penal methods from France to Cochinchina would be of little use. Unfamiliar with the violent passions of European life, the local population proved "more vegetative than intellectual" and therefore seemed at little risk for mental illness. The notion that the Annamite was too patient and apathetic to be truly susceptible to mental illness not only contributed to racist justifications for colonial rule but also informed the expectations and judgments of colonial administrators, who insisted for years that there was no need for an asylum. These conclusions increasingly contradicted those of doctors and hospital directors, who made it clear in their official communications that things looked more dire from the front lines. While Lorion insisted he had met only a small handful of mentally ill individuals during his time in the colony, hospital records hint at a different picture that had slowly started to emerge before the turn of the century.[7]

In the thirty years following the publication of Lorion's study, French colonial rule in the region further consolidated with the introduction of a racially stratified legal and taxation system, the expansion of the plantation economy, and the development of new networks of hospitals and prisons. This chapter follows the birth of the colony's first asylum set against this backdrop of the increasing penetration of French institutions into Vietnamese society. Specifically, it traces the emergence of the "insane" person—or, to use the French term, *aliéné*—as an official category of personhood deserving of legal protections and entitled to state-provided services. In just a few decades, colonial officials moved from claiming there was very little legal basis or practical need for an asylum in Indochina to achieving one of the more comprehensive mental health care systems in the French empire. Here I use the debates over extending France's famous 1838 asylum law to Indochina as a way of tracking shifting understandings about the pervasiveness of mental illness in the colony, among indigenous and European populations alike, and what should be done about it. A combination of local developments and international pressures would eventually transform perceptions about the problem of the mentally ill into a problem of colonial governance for the first time.

Debates over whether to extend the French asylum law of 1838 reveal how initial attempts to square Vietnamese with French styles of jurisprudence eventually gave way to more pressing questions about the nature of mental illness in the colony and the subsequent need for an asylum. By the turn of the century, the notion that the colonial state would bear the burden of providing care for the sick and indigent who, abandoned by their families, poured into the colony's rapidly growing cities, began to come into view. The networks of caregiving and policing that developed to target this floating population in the 1910s and 1920s served as a kind of "surface of emergence" for mental illness as a visible, largely urban, social problem.[8] Whether or not a person legally qualified as insane, his or her social and medical designation as someone who was mentally ill nevertheless taxed colonial resources in ways that could no longer be ignored. The opening of the colony's first asylum in 1919 inaugurated a new phase, which witnessed attempts to translate the French legal concept of insanity to a vastly different social and institutional context. The promulgation of comprehensive asylum legislation in 1930, which drew on the principles of the 1838 French asylum law but updated and adapted them in important ways, signaled just how dramatically the conversation about mental illness in the colony had changed. This chapter therefore examines the colonial career of the legal concept of the aliéné and how it channeled broader debates about the role and responsibility of the colonial state, the need for new kinds of knowledge and new mechanisms of social control, and ideas about Indochina as a distinctive kind of place.

Chinese Borrowings and Local Medicines

In the late nineteenth century, the popular belief among colonial administrators like Lorion that local populations did not in fact suffer from violent forms of mental illness, therefore failing to meet the French legal definition of insanity that required state intervention, took hold. Instead, the colonial government relied on local forms of care in the community that predated French occupation but that would nevertheless play an important role in the eventual establishment of the formal asylum system. These therapeutic practices reflect the deep, yet uneven, penetration of Chinese culture in Vietnamese society over several centuries.[9] For instance, the Vietnamese word for "crazy," điên, takes its root from the Chinese word dian, which translates as "upside down." Like Chinese physicians, the Vietnamese tended to attribute madness to either external disruptions (such as wind or ghosts) or internal imbalances (produced by somatic or mental processes or both) that produced abnormal states of qi, or vital energy. In writings dating from the fourteenth century, Lê Hữu Trác (or Lãn Ông as he is more commonly known), warned of the pathological effects of uncontrolled emotions, noting for instance, "A joy too lively [agitation, overstimulation] leads to a dispersion of wind (khí)."[10] Just like wind in nature, wind in the body was thought to accelerate and disrupt normal functioning. He also cautioned that overwork and stress might lead to a weakening of the liver and of the lungs, prompting the "three spirits (hồn)" and "seven vital fluids (phách)" to vacate the body and allow "nightmares and sensory hallucinations" to enter.[11] In this analysis, which borrowed heavily from Chinese models, strong emotions produce both mental and physical effects and may themselves result from physical changes emanating from both within and outside the body.

Southern Medicine

Discussion of treatments for "frights," "obsessive" thoughts, anger, jealousy, and anxiety in traditional Vietnamese medical texts reflects not only Chinese influence but also the prized use of indigenous herbal remedies. Tuệ Tĩnh, one of the two titans of traditional Vietnamese medicine alongside Lãn Ông, described the uses and modes of preparation for over six hundred species of flora in his famous "Miraculous Drugs of the South" ("Nam Dược Thần Hiệu").[12] For Tuệ Tĩnh, whose Buddhist philosophy assumed a close relationship between humans and their physical environment, the key to good health lay in the use of *locally* derived cures—hence the now famous adage "Use southern medicine to treat southern people." Although originally written for a Chinese audience, the text was eventually published in Vietnam in 1761 where it became an indispensable guide for how to treat common ailments, including conditions that resembled madness. These remedies, typically of a yin, or cool, thermal nature, promised to address the yang symptoms associated with madness by "dissipating heat, draining fire and extinguishing wind." They included Job's tears (otherwise known as coix seed or Chinese pearl barley), described as a "little sweet" and used for the elimination of "wind, humidity and heat." "Spicy, sour and bitter" chives were thought to "lower qi, relieve pain in the region of the heart, staunch bleeding, support men's sexual energy and dissipate heat." Because of the close ties between physical and mental health, it made sense that the same remedies could cure different kinds of ailments. Remedies derived from "animals with scales" had a salty flavor and promised not only to promote the circulation of blood and prevent allergic reactions but also to "ward off evil spirits" and "stop convulsions, forest fevers and children's frights." Tuệ Tĩnh recommended roasting them "until golden" in order to use them.[13]

Remedies with calming powers for reducing mental agitation included the dried flowers of *ích mẫu thảo* (honeyweed or Siberian motherwort, used in Europe since at least the seventeenth century), *nghể chàm* (Japanese indigo, which held therapeutic powers beyond dyeing clothes), and *mạch môn đông*, a sweet, slightly bitter herb that promised to clear heat and soothe irritability.[14] Tuệ Tĩnh also recommended the use of *thủy xương bồ*, or sweet flag, an herbaceous perennial plant that grows in water, for its powers to cure "rheumatism, calm thoughts and emotions, and evil thoughts," as well as to mitigate "uncontrolled rage."[15] He instructs his readers how to prepare the sweet flag: once its leaves "rise above the rocks [of a stream] to a length of nine nodes [of the plant] and one inch, take a bamboo knife and peel off the outer skin. Crush it; then either roast it until dry or soak it in rice water and dry it in the sun." Gustave Dumoutier, in his 1887 study of Vietnamese pharmacy practices, confirms the popularity of sweet flag for its therapeutic properties as well as its mystical powers in protecting the home from the influence of evil spirits when it was suspended above the door the fifth day of the fifth month. In fact, the plant is still widely used as a medicine in Asia today. It is rich in *beta asterone*, a potential candidate for the development of drugs to manage cognitive impairment associated with conditions such as Alzheimer's disease. Texts dating from the nineteenth century cite other local remedies, including *thạch hộc* from the orchid family, found in the rocky formations of upper Tonkin, used to fight pain and "frights." The root of *Glycyrhiza glabra*, also known colloquially as licorice (*cam thảo*), as well as aloe (*lô hội*) were also commonly prescribed treatments for insanity. Multiple sources reference the use of dehydrated silkworms to treat epilepsy and the reliance on cures derived from the traces of human excrement.[16]

In their everyday lives, individuals most likely drew on a range of influences to make sense of madness in their families and communities: Chinese notions of *qi* alongside homegrown "southern medicine," with its emphasis on local pharmacopeia, as well as the work of indigenous healers such as fortune-tellers and spirit mediums, Buddhist monks and Taoist priests.[17] Understandings of psychiatric health and illness in Vietnam, especially in rural areas, are often linked to beliefs about the deep relationships between the living and the dead. Many trace mental illness to divine retribution for a prior sin, such as offending one's ancestors, attributing it to the work of those gods, genies, and divine creatures that populate Sino-Annamite mythology. Mental illness implies not only a condemnation of the individual but also an indictment of the honor of the family as a whole, who is charged with the duty of caregiving. Because of their otherworldly origins, only a medium is deemed capable of ridding the body of those evil spirits (known as *ma quỷ*) intent on exacting revenge. The aim of exorcising rituals is to relieve families and their patients from personal suffering and to return patients to their normal social lives.[18] These practices will be discussed at greater length in chapters 4 and 5. What is important here is that what looked like madness in Chinese society probably also closely resembled what looked like madness from the perspective of the Nguyễn imperial court in Hue. It therefore seemed reasonable to impose the same kinds of legal regulations.

Madness in the Gia Long Code

In 1812, the Nguyễn emperor issued the Gia Long Code (*Bộ luật Gia Long*) in order to resuscitate Confucianism after thirty years of rebellion, sweeping away earlier legal provisions that protected the rights and status of women and introducing new taxes and compulsory military service. The promulgation of a common law also aimed at centralizing authority across a vast territory that stretched from the Red River Delta in the north to the Mekong Delta in the south, from the cosmopolitan trading ports of low-lying coastal cities to the ethnic minority communities of the highlands. Given the tremendous cultural and geographic diversity, as well as the prized autonomy of Vietnamese village life, this was not an easy task. Neither strictly nor evenly applied, the law rather served as a kind of flexible framework that village authorities selectively imposed in ways that seemed consistent with local customs.[19]

The Gia Long Code faithfully replicated many elements of Qing Chinese law that from as early as 1669 had recognized madness as a protected category requiring a specific and modified set of legal responsibilities.[20] It ordered that the mentally ill person who committed murder must pay 12.42 ounces of silver as punishment to cover the funeral costs for the family of the victim. This was the exact same penalty (to the cent!) that a Chinese offender was expected to pay. Perhaps even more noteworthy was the emphasis on the *prevention* of crime and, in particular, the responsibility of families to mitigate the potential danger of someone recognized as suffering from madness. For example, Article 261 of the Gia Long Code required that not only must the family officially declare the mentally ill individual to the relevant local authorities, but they must also confine and chain the person at home, in a solitary chamber, and exercise the appropriate oversight.[21] This followed from a 1689 Qing law that first introduced preventive confinement and later specified the use of chains in 1732. Just like a Qing law introduced in 1766, the Gia Long Code ordered local magistrates to provide chains and locks to families. Households without a secure room would have to entrust their mad relatives to the country jail.[22]

The Gia Long Code also carefully detailed the responsibilities and penalties for family, neighbors, or guardians if fault was determined on their part for the crimes and offenses committed by those entrusted to their care, following either from the failure to disclose the existence of a mad person in the home or from poor surveillance. Magistrates too were punished for failing to take proper measures once an individual's madness was declared. Punishment for letting a mad person commit murder brought one hundred strokes of a heavy stick; for those who let a mad person commit suicide, a penalty of eighty strokes was imposed. The Qing Code of 1732 detailed the exact same punishments. Families, neighbors, magistrates, and even prison guards were, in this way, physically punished for the crimes of the mentally ill person (who remained untouched).[23]

Viewed more and more as a permanent threat that required continuous and vigilant oversight, mad people faced ever harsher forms of punishment in eighteenth-century China. The Gia Long Code reflected the increasingly punitive nature of Qing law, for both the mentally ill and their families.[24] It specified that even if an individual's symptoms had disappeared, families could not release him from his chains until the completion of a full investigation, including testimonials from the chief of the family and their neighbors. Liberation without following the proper procedures would result in punishment. Furthermore, in the event the individual committed murder, besides the atonement specified by the regulation, she was to be chained in perpetuity, with no prospect of release even in the event her condition improved. Killing two or more people resulted in death by hanging, thereby marking the limits of the special protections for the mentally ill.[25]

The success of these prevention efforts remains difficult to assess in the absence of available local records. Even so, it is reasonable to believe that in nineteenth-century Vietnam, as in China, many families decided not to make declarations of madness to the authorities.[26] So long as no insane relative got into trouble, one could safely escape punishment. For households without the appropriate facilities and who therefore faced the prospect of entrusting their family members to the country jail for *several years even after they had recovered,* the risk may have seemed well worth it. This is especially true for families whose experience with madness more closely resembled that of a chronic, manageable condition rather than the official view of madness as essentially violent and unpredictable. Perhaps this is why Lorion claimed there was no mental illness in the colony; patients were simply guarded at home, out of practical and economic necessity given the punitive legal structure, and therefore rendered largely invisible to French colonial officials.

The borrowing of Qing law reveals some important aspects about the history of madness in precolonial Vietnam. First, it shows the emergence of madness as its own legal category that carried its own punishments, particularly in terms of the failure of families to prevent violent crimes. The introduction of madness as a legal category may have helped to consolidate official views of what madness itself looked like—dangerous and homicidal, forcing a confrontation with the state—but it also opened a widening gulf for how people understood and accommodated most forms of madness within their home and their community: as bizarre behavior that could be tolerated and even treated through home remedies and ritualistic healing. Second and more important, the law officially designated the family and community as the primary sites for surveillance and caregiving. Indeed, it was only in the absence of a sufficiently equipped household that the state was expected to take over the responsibility for confinement. In making this designation, the law affirmed the nuclear family—composed of parents, children, and occasionally other relatives—as the primary unit for social organization and site of caregiving.[27] It also made sense to expand the task of surveillance to extended family and neighbors, given the close proximity of social relations that characterized rural Vietnamese life, as exemplified by the custom of shared land use and the internal management of village affairs by a council of local notables. This reliance of the state on family and communal resources would persist long into the period of colonization, even as colonial bureaucrats struggled to revise and update local laws according to French legal conventions and the Western medical view of madness as a mental illness.

Attempting Reform

The first colonial regulations to address mental illness date to an October 1883 decree in Cochinchina that created a system of provisional oversight for the care of the mentally ill among the native population. This decree appeared as part of a sweeping overhaul of the legal system: the French penal code replaced the Gia Long Code in March 1880, and the French civil code was promulgated three years later. A curious hybrid that recast Vietnamese law in French legal language, the 1883 decree followed local precedent in specifying the judicial procedures by which families could gain guardianship of an individual judged to suffer from mental illness. The decree followed the Gia Long Code by providing the legal basis for parents or spouse to initiate a formal inquiry into the designation of an individual as insane and in need of official oversight. The individual would then acquire the same functional legal status as that of a minor and be entrusted to the care of a guardian referred to as a *trưởng tộc* who would exercise his functions under the authority of a village notable. The patient's family would cover all necessary costs and assume responsibility for his or her surveillance, which often meant placing the individual under lock and key.[28]

The 1883 decree also expanded the scope for demands to include those initiated not only by family members but also by the colonial prosecutor's office. The indigenous tribunal would then solicit advice from the family, in some instances to order an investigation into a specific case, and afterwards offer a judgment of what the French termed an *interdiction* that could be subject to appeal. The interdiction would take effect on the same day that the judgment was rendered, and the decision would be posted, within ten days, in the chambers of the tribunal and the town hall to broadcast the individual's changed legal status to the public. An interdiction, according to the French Napoleonic Code, refers to a prohibition made against a person's exercising civil rights for himself or herself, validated by a judgment of a civil court. In the context of mental health, it denotes the legal certification of an individual as insane and incapable of managing his or her own affairs.[29] Interdiction represented the extreme end of a continuum in nineteenth-century French legal culture that withheld the full exercise of rights from the insane, married women, children and criminals, and, later, colonial subjects in the empire. Lacking the capacity for rational judgment and autonomy, these *incapables* instead required tutelage (or removal from society altogether) while others— namely, adult men—freely exercised their full liberties. Indeed, the discourse on the supposed limits of the mental capacity of native populations was mobilized by colonial officials throughout the empire as an important justification for their continued subject status.

In many ways, the wording of the 1883 law reflected the heterogeneity of Indochina's legal landscape writ large. Perhaps most striking for its lack of uniformity, colonial law in Indochina can best be described as the superimposition of different legal traditions that reflected at once the formal division of the population according to race and the uneven expansion of colonial power in the region throughout the nineteenth century. In particular, as Peter Zinoman writes, a "fundamental distinction" in the degree of application of French laws emerged between areas governed directly as colonies—including Cochinchina in the south and most of Laos—and those ruled indirectly as protectorates, including Annam, Cambodia, Luang Prabang, and Tonkin, which comprises much of what is today northern Vietnam. Of all the territories, Cochinchina, the first territory in Indochina to be conquered by the French in 1859, most closely resembled the French model, with all subjects, French and native, subject to French criminal law by the 1880s. Colonial officials in the protectorates, meanwhile, relied much more heavily on native administrative structures in order to govern.[30] In general, the Gia Long Code continued to regulate local customs such as family affairs, marriage, and property succession.

French legal reformers often criticized the code as typical of uncivilized societies, as unduly obsessed with punishment. Republican-minded critics, for instance, complained that the 1883 decree, and the Vietnamese legal precedent on which it was based, addressed mental illness only to the extent of removing individuals from society or punishing them for their crimes and exacting penalties against their families for failing to fulfill their responsibilities as caregivers. It said nothing about the need to provide patients with any guarantees of protection, nor did it prescribe the confinement of the mentally ill under the surveillance of certified experts.[31] Rather, the law stood as confirmation of a long-standing customary practice that it now sought to regulate.[32] Some French officials therefore began to suggest an alternative, namely, the promulgation of the June 30, 1838, asylum law from France.

The French 1838 asylum law represents a hallmark moment in the history of modern psychiatry.[33] It was the first law to establish the incapacity of the aliéné to exercise his or her full political rights and to impose the mechanisms for his or her removal from society. Most important, the law was founded on the idea that certain mental disorders were susceptible to improvement under the guidance of medical experts. The pioneers of modern French psychiatry, Philippe Pinel and Jean-Etienne Esquirol, campaigned for a system of state-supported asylums based on the understanding that therapy for insanity required the removal of individuals from their habitual milieu. By insisting on a brand of institution-based therapy that required the isolation of patients and their oversight by specialists, Pinel and Esquirol worked successfully to gain state sponsorship of the psychiatric profession.[34] The 1838 law mandated the creation of a nationwide network of asylums staffed by full-time medical doctors. It also served as a training facility for future specialists. Critics of the law (of which there were many) cited the risk of arbitrary confinement, arguing that the sanctions contained in the 1838 law inadequately protected patients from the abuse of being shut away in the asylum without just cause. These attacks followed a number of scandals regarding the suspicious detentions of political dissidents. Furthermore, by allowing recourse to the judiciary only after the internment order had been made, the law of 1838 seemed to violate the fundamental French legal principle of the judiciary as the sole guarantor of individual liberty.[35]

Even as criticisms of the law intensified at the end of the nineteenth century in the metropole, some colonial officials nevertheless recommended its extension to Cochinchina in 1897. The fact that the possibility was raised by the prosecutor's office, rather than the health service, reflects the extent to which mental illness remained a problem of social order and legal jurisprudence. As M. E. Assaud, the prosecutor-general underscored in his request to the governor-general, the regularization of confinement proved urgent not only in terms of securing the "goal of legality" but also in terms of "avoiding complaints. . . . This lacuna in our local legislation must be filled as soon as possible."[36] It would be another ten years before the proposal gained some traction. In 1907 the governor-general of Indochina wrote a number of high-ranking bureaucrats in the colonial administration to ask for their opinions on whether to extend the law. For members of the health service increasingly frustrated by the crowded conditions of their hospitals, the project represented a welcome investment. The local director of the health service in Tonkin, for instance, noted the recent rise in the numbers of mentally ill, among both indigenous and European patients alike, and underscored the need for services dedicated specifically to their care.[37] The mayor of Haiphong, a large port city south of Hanoi, also endorsed the plan but expressed concerns over extending the provisions of the law to indigenous populations and the dangers of racial mixing within the asylum.[38] And of course, there was the conundrum that even if the 1838 law happened to be promulgated, there would be no asylum to receive patients!

The question of whether or not to introduce the law was never just an abstract exercise in legal thinking. For many it represented an expensive commitment to a large infrastructure project. Until the state granted formal approval to measures that would require Vietnamese villages to contribute funds toward public assistance, the colonial administration would be burdened with covering the entire costs of care.[39] Moreover, the 1838 asylum law itself appeared not only antiquated but also exceedingly complex and had become the object of "many recriminations" in the metropole. Taking advantage of the law to detain problematic family members—a well-documented form of abuse in France—would almost certainly occur in Indochina as well.[40] As a result, the system would depend on various "Prefects, Presidents, Prosecutors and Mayors" to visit these establishments and provide important (and expensive) forms of oversight. Hanoi's mayor cautioned that if a similar system for indigenous populations should be instituted in Indochina, "we will see to which dangers we would have exposed a population inclined to exercise vengeance and reprisals."[41] Others such as Morel, the resident superior of Tonkin, simply found the law "untimely."[42]

Given these considerable challenges, as the mayor of Hanoi pointed out, it remained to be decided if the promulgation of the 1838 law was necessary at all. First, he posed the following question: Are there, in fact, aliénés in Tonkin? In crafting his response, he relied on the formal definition of *aliéné* from a French legal dictionary, even citing the actual page number. He wrote, "We give the name *aliéné* to a person whose reason is perverted, totally or in part, but at the point at which the use of his liberty becomes an incessant danger, either for public security and order or for his own personal safety, or for his fortune, and for whom measures are taken, in the general interest of the police for public order and security and the protection of the interests of the aliéné during the period of confinement." According to this definition, no cases meriting the designation of aliéné existed in Tonkin. Here he adopted Lorion's view that the indigenous peoples of Indochina did not suffer from acute forms of mental illness, only those more chronic forms of dementia or imbecility. Simply lacking the full use of their mental faculties, they did not pose a serious threat to the safety of their community.[43]

Dangerous forms of mental illness carrying the legal requirement of confinement therefore did not seem to apply. Rather than introduce new technologies of confinement, legislation was simply needed to regulate proper forms of surveillance in the community. Among white settlers, the mayor of Hanoi reported few cases of dementia (which he was careful to distinguish from true madness) in the city's European-only hospitals. Most were military personnel who comprised the majority of a small but growing white population in the colony.[44] These patients would eventually be sent back to France, where they would encounter a "more comfortable and hygienic setting for recuperation" than the tropical climate of Indochina. In any event, the small numbers of European settlers meant that the establishment of asylums for their care would be of little practical use while the Vietnamese population traditionally "cares for and guards its own sick." Given the apparent absence of any dangerous forms of mental illness, among either the indigenous or European populations, as well as the high costs attached to the project, the mayor opposed the promulgation of the 1838 law on both ideological and practical grounds. He applied the narrow legal test of the aliéné—casting only those who were the most gravely ill and socially disruptive as deserving of the designation—in order to make an argument *against* the further expansion of state infrastructure.[45] In this way, any notion that the development of asylums was marked by a voracious confinement did not hold fast during this early period, as many colonial officials assumed an essentially conservative posture vis-à-vis the care of the mentally ill.

While many municipal and regional authorities resisted efforts to turn mental illness into a problem of colonial governance, others signaled the dangers of maintaining the status quo. Outrey, the lieutenant governor of Cochinchina, voiced his enthusiastic support of bringing the 1838 French asylum law to Indochina: "The promulgation of this law seems indispensable. Indeed it frequently happens that the Administration is obligated to confine those individuals seized by a 'furious madness,' whom it is not

possible to allow to circulate freely without also compromising public security. But this practice, which is necessary, is nevertheless illegal, in the actual
state of local regulations because it violates the principle of individual liberty
and is not authorized in any text." The asylum law was therefore essential,
he concluded, both in the interest of the colonial administration, which was
"insufficiently armed" against those suffering from mental illness, as well as
in the interests of the patients themselves, "who, in the future, can no longer be confined without the achievement of many formalities with the aim
of wrapping their confinement in all the necessary guarantees for the safe-
guarding of their personal interest."[46] The invocation of "individual liberty"
also hints at how the language of republicanism inflected debates over the
creation of a colonial asylum.[47]

In Tonkin, piecemeal legal remedies had long been implemented in order
to circumvent the creation of a more robust and costly system. A December 1891 law, for instance, charged the mayors of various municipalities in
Tonkin with taking the necessary steps against the insane who might "compromise public morality, the security of people or the conservation of property."[48] Until the early twentieth century, this was the only legislation that
assumed state responsibility for insanity in Tonkin and applied exclusively to
urban areas. When in 1908, colonial officials discussed extending the hybrid
decree of 1883 from Cochinchina to Tonkin, Hanoi's mayor lent his support
to the measure. In his view, the reliance on families to provide care would
obviate the need for an asylum. The resident superior of Tonkin agreed that
local laws and customs could continue to provide sufficient forms of surveillance and protection so long as the "demented" remained relatively harmless. At the point he did become dangerous, "that is to say when he becomes
an *aliéné* in the proper sense of the term," he would be directed to the Hôpital Indigène.[49] Focusing on these kinds of makeshift measures would, in the
words of Hanoi's mayor, "save a lot of money," sparing municipal budgets
while also sufficiently protecting patients.[50]

Not to overly burden local budgets in order to address what seemed to
be a minor and easily managed problem remained the paramount concern.
Most mentally ill therefore remained at home, with only the most violent
patients sent to hospitals, where special pavilions were dedicated to their
care. However, it quickly became apparent among medical officials, especially those working in the south, that these measures were wholly inadequate. In May 1882, at the Chợ Quán Hospital in Saigon, where we started
this chapter, the director expressed frustration that his demands for the next
year's budget to include the construction of four new cabins, essentially doubling the protopsychiatric service, had fallen on deaf ears. With the service

already at full capacity, he clearly anticipated future growth. Indeed, this complaint surfaced amid a rush of inquiries about the possibility of admitting new patients. The mayor of Saigon, for instance, wrote to ask about the transfer of a female patient into the hospital's care from her police cell, which he described as an "inhumane" stopgap measure.[51] The availability of nurses proved a pressing issue, with at least one patient given up to the Central Prison in Saigon because the hospital simply did not have the means to contain a "raving lunatic"(fou furieux).[52] Unsurprisingly, those doctors, particularly those working in urban areas, who experienced firsthand the challenges of working with this patient population tended to worry more over the implications of doing nothing.

Notwithstanding widespread resistance to the formal implementation of the 1838 asylum law, colonial doctors continued to look to the law as their implicit model for professional practice. Yet without the establishment of formal legal regulations and the mechanisms to enforce them, confusion remained. The question of whether hospital directors were required to accept all patients for whom admission was demanded, either by public authorities or by colonial subjects, generated significant anxiety, especially given the constraints of space and resources. Furthermore, without a sufficient number of European doctors to certify the presence of mental illness as an essential part of the normal confinement process, hospital directors were often forced to rely instead on the testimony of the patients' "families, neighbors, and village authorities."[53]

First Proposals for an Asylum

Repatriation to France offered one possible solution to the growing gap between patient demands and available expertise. This policy had been adopted for European populations, at least informally, for many years. In 1880 the governor-general took the first steps to care for European patients in Indochina when he agreed to build a pavilion dedicated to the care of the mentally ill at the military hospital in Saigon.[54] These hospital beds provided temporary relief for patients until they could be repatriated to France. Doctors favored repatriation for Europeans for whom the unfamiliar exposure to intense heat, as well as more familiar struggles with alcohol abuse and the distance from home, manifested in the onset of various nervous disorders.[55] This argument emerged out of widespread beliefs about the difficulties of whites to adapt to tropical climates, most clearly expressed in a medical condition known as neurasthenia, which will be discussed at greater length in chapter 5. In an interesting move, variations on this argument would later be used to protest against exporting Vietnamese patients from northern Tonkin to the Biên Hòa asylum in Cochinchina on account of differences in climate.[56] Concerns about the exposure of European patients to contagious disease in major hospitals also helped to consolidate colonial opinion in favor of repatriation.[57] The alternative—to keep European patients in Indochina for treatment—raised difficult questions about the responsibility of the colonial state to care for mentally ill patients indefinitely, especially without the necessary specialists and resources at hand.[58]

At first, discussions to formalize repatriation included the possibility of sending all mentally ill populations, both indigenous and European, civilian and military, to France. This proposal was soon abandoned. In 1902, at the August session of the Colonial Council, an advisory body that included both French and Vietnamese representatives based in Saigon, a special committee charged with examining the issue expressed their concerns over repatriation of indigenous populations. They cautioned that indigenous patients would be hospitalized with "1,200 to 1,300 other French patients and forced to endure a different climate and diet to which they were not habituated." Besides the onerous costs of patient transport, the idea of "sending a mad person 4,000 leagues in order to try to recover his sanity" itself seemed crazy.[59] A few months later in November of 1902, the colonial administration signed a contract with the St. Pierre Asylum in Marseille formalizing an agreement to receive French patients from Indochina.[60] The contract stipulated that patients would be admitted and cared for at a rate of two francs per day. For indigent European patients, the colonial administration of Cochinchina agreed to reimburse all costs—treatment, transportation, etc.—incurred by the French government. This represented a new and more burdensome arrangement for the colonial administration, which had previously relied on the patients' department of origin and funds of public assistance in the metropole to cover the costs of their hospitalization in France.[61] Sending patients to France was therefore an expensive proposition.

Of all Europeans ever repatriated, most came from the military, which constituted the majority of the white population in Indochina until the early twentieth century. In the ten years following the formalization of the agreement with the St. Pierre asylum, 209 patients were sent back to France, including 177 military officers and 32 civilians. Vietnamese members of the military were also eligible for repatriation. From 1900 to 1905, 94 cases from the European military were repatriated to France as well as 14 Vietnamese cases.[62]

A parallel, racially divided, system soon developed. While European patients would return to France, the indigenous population, as well as any foreign nationals of Asian descent, would remain in Indochina as part of a plan endorsed by the Colonial Council. The council voted in 1903 to establish an asylum that would service the entirety of the colony in order to concentrate resources rather than spread them thin across multiple institutions.[63] Cochinchina would support half the costs of the establishment while the other colonial territories would split the remainder of the costs, prorated by the number of their inhabitants and the number of days of hospitalization incurred by patients from each region. An official decree would set the daily rate of patient care. Because of the project's high price tag, the lieutenant governor of Cochinchina wrote to his northern counterpart in Tonkin in the fall of 1903 to ask if he would help share in the financing of the asylum. The resident superior of Tonkin in turn asked those French provincial chiefs under his jurisdiction for their opinions about the need for the asylum. Their varied responses reveal to what extent mental illness had emerged as a problem of colonial governance by the early twentieth century.

The View from the Provinces

Most provincial chiefs reported a low incidence of mental illness and therefore downplayed the need for an asylum. The chief of Yên Bái province confidently registered a grand total of zero cases.[64] One official hypothesized that the rarity of more "tragic" or violent forms of madness in his region could perhaps be attributed to the low rates of alcoholism.[65] Those individuals designated as mentally ill were largely considered "inoffensive," marked by a kind of "softening of the brain." As a result, they did little to threaten public security and did not merit the designation of aliéné. In the words of the chief of Bắc Giang province, "They rarely leave the village of their birth, live off the compassion of others . . . . As a result there is very little urgency to adopt the project of constructing a centralized asylum for the insane." He remarked that funds would be better spent in the establishment of a leper colony in Tonkin, maternity wards, and schools in Hanoi for the training of mobile vaccination teams and, above all, the education of indigenous midwives.[66]

Others saw value in asylum care but objected to the plan for one centralizing institution, which would require patients to travel across vast distances. The chief of Truyên Duang province, for instance, worried about sending patients from Tonkin to Cochinchina because of the change in climate as well as the difficulties of negotiating with navigation companies who, he anticipated, would refuse passage to the insane.[67] The pitfalls of separating patients from their families also caused some anxiety. Because of the spiritual basis of Vietnamese beliefs about mental illness, including the "special prayers and sacrifices performed on behalf of the patient," most colonial administrators believed that families would be unwilling to give up their own. Simply put, "they refuse to believe that our doctors can cure them."[68] Many feared that removing patients from their families would not only make the colonial administration appear inhumane but also prove politically unwise, especially for those who had "not yet given any worry to the administration."[69] It also undoubtedly meant that the colonial government could not count on families to support the cost of confinement.[70] Finally, there was the negative effect of separation on the patient's possibility of rehabilitation to consider. The provincial chief of Sơn Tây, for instance, argued against "pull[ing] the insane away from their natural milieu where there is still a chance for recovery, for there they can more easily reclaim their consciousness of themselves and the world around them than in an agglomeration where melancholy and desperation could not but aggravate their mental state."[71] Given these concerns over family reactions, reinforced by the costs and difficulties of transport, many provincial chiefs recommended the creation of several asylums rather than one centralized asylum far away. The notion that Tonkin should undertake a similar project of its own was a constant refrain.

Not surprisingly those provincial chiefs who perceived a greater problem of mental illness within their own jurisdiction were more likely than not to support the establishment of an asylum.[72] The reasons for favoring the project proved equally diverse. Many tended to agree that insanity was quite rare in Tonkin, though they supported the project on both practical and humanitarian grounds. It would relieve pressure on the administration from the demands of those families who *insisted* the state take responsibility for a troubled family member but then had little recourse beyond sending the patient to the ill-equipped Indigenous Hospital in Hanoi.[73] While some invoked the language of humanity to voice their opposition to the project, in terms of the emotional difficulty of separating patients from their families, others would use the same language in support of the asylum, in terms of protecting patients from wrongful and often brutal treatment at home. Emphasizing the horrors of home care not only reinforced colonial notions about the backwardness of Vietnamese practices but was also an easy and effective way of pushing for the creation of new, more modern, institutions. The chief of Ninh Bình province declared the construction of the asylum to be of the "highest humanitarian and moral order." He noted that, at best, the mentally ill were tended to by their family members and at worst, especially if they were dangerous, would become the objects of repulsion and brutal violence, including enclosure in cages.[74] Such a practice proved "disastrous for the moral education of the people."[75] Moral lessons waited not just in witnessing the poor treatment of the insane but also in observing "the sad spectacle of their demise," another benefit of removing patients to the asylum.[76] Others floated the possibility that cures among mentally ill at hospitals would over time dissipate "ignorance and popular loathing" of mental illness and the popular notion of the asylum as a place of last resort.[77]

In general, colonial officials in Tonkin agreed that the creation of an asylum could be very useful both from a humanitarian point of view and from the perspective of maintaining order. However, the argument that the institution must be established locally won the day. While it would come with a "high price," wrote the resident superior of Tonkin in his letter to the lieutenant governor of Cochinchina, "at least it would have the advantage of not offending the morals and beliefs of the *indigènes* by removing their family members to far-flung regions of the colony." As a result, he relayed the bad news that it would be "impossible" for the local budget of Tonkin to support the project of an insane asylum in Cochinchina.[78] This decision would delay the project for a colonial asylum for years to come.

At the turn of the twentieth century, one could say that colonial policy around mental illness represented more of a social action than a medical one, with recourse to the hospital used to segregate and confine rather than to diagnose and treat. The continued reliance on family resources to support the care of the mentally ill in the community appeared to many French colonial officials as a more humane and less onerous alternative than insisting on the separation and confinement of the mentally ill in specialized institutions. Nevertheless, the lack of experts and more comprehensive regulations placed pressure on what resources did exist for the hospital treatment of the mentally ill in the colony, especially on those doctors charged with their care. It would take a combination of local developments and international pressures to transform perceptions about the problem of the mentally ill as a problem of colonial governance and to recommence the search for a more permanent solution.

The Ground Shifts

Even as the initial inquiry into the creation of an asylum stalled, Indochina's colonial administration, including its health service and hospital network, continued to expand throughout the late nineteenth and early twentieth centuries.[79] In 1892, the French law mandating that any person practicing medicine had to have a doctorate in medicine was applied to Cochinchina. Shortly thereafter, in 1897, a general budget for Indochina was created that included provisions for the creation of a health care director for each territory. A law passed the following year, in January 1898, established a preliminary plan regarding the classification of hospitals, the conditions of admittance, and their general functioning. In 1902, the French public health law entered into effect throughout Indochina, and the Hanoi School of Medicine opened its doors for the purposes of training "auxiliary" doctors, a term used to designate local physicians who remained subordinate to their French counterparts. In 1905 the Indigenous Medical Assistance Program (Assistance Médicale Indigène, or AMI) was established. The first of its kind in a French territory (along with that of French West Africa), the AMI oversaw a vast health care program including both preventive and treatment programs and the creation of a basic hospital network. The service formed an integral part of France's broader civilizing mission by providing free health care in facilities funded by various local, provincial, and municipal budgets. Earning the approval of the local population formed one of the early explicit goals of the expansion of the colonial medical service.

The following year witnessed the first wave of construction under the purview of the AMI. By 1908, Indochina was home to 153 medical institutions, both publicly and privately financed, including 5 major hospitals. Much of this expansion occurred in Saigon, Hue, Hanoi, and other large urban centers and led to major disparities in access to medical care as compared to rural regions. This was especially true for Cambodia and Laos, which had to make do with a loose network of makeshift and poorly supported hospitals.[80] These new hospitals, however, soon became overcrowded, with colonial officials reading demands for services as evidence of increasingly favorable public opinion toward Western medical practices. In 1908, the Indigenous Hospital of Hanoi reportedly housed one hundred patients per room instead of ten, its theoretical capacity. Because of overcrowding, it became clear that Indochina's facilities would have to, in the words of Laurence Monnais, "build, rebuild and specialize: to build to respond to a growing demand, to rebuild to combat the weather damage that caused a tremendous strain on limited budgets, and to specialize to make the capital a recognized center of French medicine and a showcase for its scientific expansion."[81]

This push for the specialization of Indochina's health services occurred as strains on the meager resources dedicated to mental illness in the colony continued to grow. The picture that emerges from contemporary accounts is that of an improvised and incomplete system, premised on sending only the most acutely ill patients to generalized services in hospitals if those were available. Those patients who posed a more serious risk to public security were destined for prison cells or, whenever possible, immobilization in a cot at a hospital.[82] In October 1904, François Rodier, the lieutenant governor of Cochinchina, wrote to the various heads of provinces under his authority about the growing numbers of patients at Chợ Quán Hospital in Saigon suffering from mental illness and other incurable diseases such as paralytic beriberi and chronic bronchitis. Over a nine-year period, between 1902 and 1910, Chợ Quán received a total of 209 mentally ill patients or an average of 23.2 per year, diagnosed with a range of mental and neurological disorders including epilepsy, paralysis, hysteria, monomania, "mental troubles," and idiocy.[83] In 1907, concerns over patient crowding resulted in plans for an isolation wing for the mentally ill. Composed of ten cabins, to be placed in the most distant wing of the hospital, the new pavilion would allow the hospital staff to keep the insane under observation without disturbing the other patients.[84]

In order to "put an end to this state of affairs," which "detours the hospital from its true destination," Rodier commissioned a new study for the creation of an asylum. While waiting for its eventual approval and construction, he stressed that the mentally ill could no longer remain hospitalized at Chợ Quán. Those currently under treatment were to be returned to their village of origin and placed under the guard and surveillance of the local notables. Provincial chiefs were charged with taking the necessary steps to protect patients upon their return as well as to ward off any danger they might present to public security. Medical care would be provided by the provincial doctor or, in his absence, by the "nurse-vaccinators" trained at the École Pratique de Médecine currently housed within the hospital's walls.[85] Most patients therefore returned home after a period of isolation at Chợ Quán. Meanwhile, members of the Colonial Council continued to stress the need for an asylum, arguing "day by day cases of 'furious madness' become more numerous and constitute a public danger against which administrative and judicial authorities are presently disarmed."[86]

In Tonkin, colonial administrators met with similar challenges over what to do with mentally ill patients who were too sick or violent to be taken care of at home. The Indigenous, Hanoi, and Quảng Yên Hospitals were all filled to capacity. Only Hanoi Hospital possessed the facilities dedicated specifically to the care of the mentally ill, which even then consisted only of three cells.[87] Between 1906 and 1910, the Indigenous Hospital in Haiphong received a total of twenty-two mental patients, which it housed in common rooms or, in the event they became agitated, isolated in "disciplinary rooms" typically reserved for sick criminals. By 1916, the hospital still lacked the facilities to accommodate all of its mentally ill patients, making it effectively impossible to isolate them from the rest of the patient population. As a result, the commander of the indigenous police force in Haiphong complained that the colonial government was reduced to returning patients to the surveillance of their families and villages, a surveillance that was necessarily "illusory" given the nature of "indigenous constructions that were not suitable for the isolation of individuals." He quoted the words of a local notable, or *lý trưởng*, from the village of Lực Hành, located in the suburban zone outside Haiphong, who observed, "not without reason, that in not keeping individuals constantly bound hand and foot there is little possibility of preventing them from evading when the desire strikes them."[88]

It was not just the ease of escape that worried colonial officials. Individuals whose families did not possess the resources or willingness to provide care would reportedly be cast off, and

> abandoned to their sad destiny, chased from the village, they become errant, without shelter, a raggedy and dirty specter from which one would turn away and who live off begging and theft, given over to the malicious curiosity of crowds until his death comes or, by chance, stopped by the police, he is brought to the asylum. There he is, without civil status, inscribed under the designation of "X" and this is how we have among our lodgers a dozen Xs.[89]

At the turn of the century, what to do about those found wandering the streets, given over to a life of begging or theft, posed a major challenge to urban policing. The mentally ill counted among the rapidly growing number of beggars, juvenile delinquents, prostitutes, and other undesirables who were drawn to new urban centers in colonial Indochina. This "floating population"—in the words of one French colonial administrator—many of whom proved too weak or sick to make a living, relied on the generosity of privately funded night refuges and poorhouses for temporary shelter and relief.[90] Hospitals were unable to open their doors to all those in need because, as the governor-general grimly put it, "hunger does not constitute an illness."[91] Meanwhile the police force was kept busy in a frustrated attempt to ferry vagrants just outside the city lines, only the next day to find them back exactly where they had first removed them, "at the market, beside the banks of the little lake, in front of the post office, basically everywhere where they should not be."[92] The criminalization of vagrancy also meant that the poor and unemployed crowded municipal and provincial jails, where they constituted a significant proportion of the incarcerated population, second only to thieves and murderers.[93]

The growth in vagrancy in the north can be attributed to periodic subsistence crises that hit the region in 1906 and again in 1915–17.[94] The increase

in the price of rice, following a series of natural disasters, meant that
many left home in search of work or aid. This was not a new phenomenon. Crop failures and famines, typhoons and floods had compelled people to abandon their villages since well before the arrival of the French.
The violence of colonial conquest, however, accompanied by the decline
of rice production and its transport, left rural populations newly vulnerable.[95] They tended to head for the cities, where, as the resident of superior
of Tonkin remarked, the colonial administration is "obligated, in effect,
to close its eyes and tolerate their presence."[96] The attitude here is one of
sour resignation, and he goes on to encourage the colonial administration
to simply wait out periods of hardship and guard against abuses of colonial beneficence by an inveterate and lazy public. Others spoke matter-of-
factly about the profound changes happening within Vietnamese society
as a consequence of urbanization. For some French observers, city life,
characterized by an atomization of existence, seemed to stand in strong
contradistinction to the ethic of collective solidarity that had traditionally guided Vietnamese social life.[97] As the governor-general of Indochina
pointed out in a 1921 letter on Hanoi's vagrant population, "In the big
city, everyone lives for themselves; one has enough worries to not also
take on those of one's neighbor; egoism is de rigueur, altruism is a matter
of public administration."[98] The implication here was that responsibility
for social assistance had perceptibly shifted from families and communes
to the colonial administration, at least in urban areas. In this way, the use
of the designation "X" mentioned above worked to describe a new kind
of colonial subject—the anonymous, rootless individual separated from
his or her family and increasingly dependent on colonial resources. Still,
as Van Nguyen Marshall has argued, despite the rhetoric of the civilizing
mission, French efforts to alleviate poverty in the colony were always partial and ad hoc at best, defined in terms of charity relief rather than true
social welfare and always as a form of social control.[99]

With shelters stretched to capacity and poverty deepening in the colony,
how to cope with the vagrancy problem would become even more pressing
after World War I. New regulations were devised that worked to increasingly
criminalize the poor. As one colonial official put it in 1927, the simple act
of "begging [became] . . . a crime following the creation of the Thai-Ha-Ap
poorhouse" in Hanoi, which effectively became an auxiliary of the prison
system.[100] According to the new regulations, no longer could indigent persons enter or leave the poorhouse on their own accord but instead fell under
the discretion of a judge who would decide the length of their stay. This did
little to solve the problem as beggars continued to cycle in and out of the

poorhouse, careful to provide different names upon each reentry.[101] Those apprehended and eventually sent to the asylum tended to come to the attention of colonial officials as beggars or vagrants first, and only later, as new kinds of institutions and legal mechanisms emerged, did they become identified and sorted as a distinct population that required distinct forms of care and control. In this way, the networks of caregiving and policing that developed around vagrancy in the 1910s and 1920s became a kind of "surface of emergence" for mental illness as a largely urban, social problem.

Renewed Push for Reforms

It was in the context of these debates about state responsibility toward the indigent and infirm that French officials in Indochina continually revisited the question of creating an asylum. The first serious discussions date from 1907 and again in 1908.[102] In 1910, Governor-General Antony Klobukowski opened an October session of the Conseil Supérieur de l'Indochine by expressing his vote in favor of the foundation of an asylum in Cochinchina. Two days later, the vice president of the Colonial Council, himself a doctor, submitted a report that highlighted the poor conditions of care for the mentally ill and echoed the urgent need for an asylum. He spoke of a recent visit to Chợ Quán Hospital, where,

> like me, gentlemen, you had before your eyes a poor devil, a veritable wreck of a human, a victim of a tenacious atavism or one of those diseases which throws a profound obscurity into the human brain. He was chained at the heart of a cell which today we no longer even give to the worst criminals: he does not receive any light of day—the only thing that could give him a bit of joy, to awaken those gentle sensations among the miserable—only that which comes through a thick door, pierced by a window and only opened from time to time, is all that he can think about. A life this miserable, in our time, can only continue if it is ignored. To know, that is to condemn. Does our colony not have the obligation to create, without delay, an establishment where the right to light, the right to a means of existence [la vie matérielle], since these disinherited are refused those moral and intellectual pleasures by fate and by nature.[103]

Here we see one of the earliest articulations of the mentally ill person in Indochina as a person deserving of protections and of a colonial state obligated to provide him or her with a minimum level of care and comfort. While the aliéné as a legal category of personhood would not be formally introduced into colonial law for another six years, it had nevertheless expanded beyond its earlier framing as a violent threat to be protected against.

Given the mounting pressures on the colony's hospital system, colonial doctors and administrators pushed for a more complete and statistically accurate account of mental illness in the colony. In general, mental illness among Annamite populations continued to be perceived as quite rare, at least as compared with European populations in the metropole. The medical inspector for Indochina, Dr. Rangé, offered this explanation in a 1912 report on the state of mental illness in the colony to the twenty-second meeting of the Congress of French and Francophone Alienists and Neurologists in Tunis: "The Asian populations of our Indochina colony still ignore almost all of occidental civilization, impassive, indifferent to questions about the future which impassion us, opposing a conservative quietude of mental equilibration to the incessant agitation of the European, still unscathed, at least for the time being, but for the defects and degeneration engendered by alcohol intoxication, these populations will supply rare subjects for the alienist."[104] This language typifies much of official characterizations of life in the colony as colorless and monotone, deprived of any real activity or ambition among its largely rural, farming population. Accordingly, the disorders of those found to be mentally ill generally represented more of a "psychic weakening" than true agitation.

While some attributed the relative lack of mental illness in the colony to the unique aspects of the Vietnamese personality, others offered another kind of explanation: they stressed that the perceived rarity of mental illness in Indochina was "certainly much more *apparent* than *real*," especially given the lack of reliable statistics.[105] Indeed, doctors and other colonial officials often complained about the imprecise basis for understanding mental illness in the colony. Even Rangé underscored this in his own report:

> It is difficult to give a statistic indicating the percentage of mental illness in the population. Even in urban centers, families only rarely bring themselves to a European doctor; the sorcerer only is consulted, and often the *dément* is relegated to a corner, if he is inoffensive, and enclosed in a cage made of bamboo if he is dangerous. It is only by chance that we are informed of his existence. The figures . . . given by the chief doctors of the provinces are not comparable with each other. Some note only those cases that they themselves observed at the hospital, while others note all those cases which have been signaled by the notables without proceeding with a verification. Given these conditions, the most wise and prudent thing to do would be to not

come to any sort of generalization and instead simply report the cases as signaled province by province.[106]

The diagnostic procedures upon which assessments were based were often riddled with errors including imprecise and vague allusions to patients with "mental troubles," "mental alienation," and "idiocy."

In a 1913 article published in the Paris-based journal *Annales d'hygiene colonial et de médecine coloniales,* Henri Reboul, a physician and director of public health in Indochina, also complained about the poor quality of mental health statistics. On the basis of his own personal documentation and information gathered from local authorities, Reboul determined that while the incidence of mental illness might be low, the absolute number of mentally ill guarded in their villages remained elevated. He guessed, on average, one hundred mentally ill for every six million inhabitants of Annam, all the while admitting this was probably a conservative estimate. Most of his mentally patients at the main hospital in Hue arrived at the behest of the police, not their families. The service's two cabins often operated at full capacity, forcing him to house mentally ill patients alongside those criminals who required hospitalization. Reboul remained convinced that once a regular hospital service for the mentally ill was put in place and run in satisfactory conditions, families would learn to entrust their patients under the surveillance of experts and "we will discover a whole other site of local pathology which until now has remained totally unrecognized."[107] In this way, Reboul attributed the apparent rarity of mental illness among indigenous patients to the low visibility of mental illness in the colony, a product of the prejudices of families as well as the lack of services that could capture patients in official statistics as the basis for policymaking.

Both of these texts demonstrate the networks of psychiatric expertise that were beginning to connect metropole with colony and specialists throughout the empire. The 1912 meeting in Tunis where Rangé presented his report marked an important turning point in discussions about the need to put into place comprehensive psychiatric services in all of France's colonial possessions. This meeting centered on broad discussions about the content of the civilizing mission as well as the role and responsibility of French doctors in improving the health and living conditions of colonial subjects. For psychiatrists, developing mental health services in the colonies represented an important opportunity to revive their profession, whose reputation had fallen into serious disrepair at the turn of the century. The failure of efforts to reform the asylum system at home, coupled with therapeutic inefficacy, opened French psychiatry up to intense criticism from both the state and popular media as Germany pulled ahead as the European center of psychiatric innovation. In particular, the meeting signaled French concerns about falling behind other European powers that had made more progress in implementing psychiatric services in their empires.[108]

Reboul, alongside Emmanuel Régis, a professor of psychiatry in France, authored the meeting's final report in which they underscored that colonization "created not only rights, but also imperative duties," on the part of the colonizers, including the "duty of medical assistance to those in need."[109] Their report recommended the organization of a service of psychiatric assistance in different colonial outposts according to certain common principles but with room for adaptation to local conditions. They called for a two-tier system that would consist of a service for patients suffering from acute or more short-term forms of mental illnesses and asylums for those with chronic or incurable conditions.[110] They also recommended the organization of medical training in the colonies and the creation of a corps of specialists. Inspiration was sought in the works of other colonial powers, especially the Dutch in the East Indies, who had built one of the most comprehensive asylum systems in the colonial world, thereby significantly outpacing French efforts. Throughout the early 1900s, French doctors took a series of study trips to Java, commissioned by the colonial government with the goal of gathering texts related to legal regulations and asylum design including documentary photographs.[111]

Following this seminal meeting, Indochina's government authorized the construction of an asylum that same year and dedicated funds to its construction in 1914.[112] This coincided with the doubling of the AMI's budget between 1912 and 1914.[113] The credit necessary for the project was fixed at 90,000,000 piasters, but the newly formed Assistance Aux Aliénés received only a fraction (100,000 piasters) for the construction of the asylum. The arrival of World War I delayed the construction project. It was another four and a half years before the Biên Hòa asylum welcomed its first patients outside Saigon, in January 1919.[114]

1918 Asylum Law

In November of 1918, in anticipation of the Biên Hòa asylum's grand opening early the following year, a new law established the provisions for the asylum's functioning and oversight. It marked the first attempt to formally regulate institutionalized psychiatric care and to legally designate the aliéné as an official category of person in the colony. While colonial officials continued to use terms such as *dément* and *fou* to describe what appeared to them as mental illness, the term *aliéné* was invested with a specific legal meaning in terms of the protections accorded patients and guarantees of care they would receive upon confinement. The decree contained certain general dispositions that reproduced, in part, aspects of the 1838 French asylum law and adapted them to the administrative vocabulary of the colony. Others were discarded because of the "irreducible differences that exist between the metropolitan and Indochinese social milieux."[115] The November 1918 law fixed the provisions for the administrative oversight of the asylum, mechanisms for the entrance and exit of patients, and the internal functioning of the asylum, including the type of work that would eventually be demanded of patients.[116] These measures were applied only to the indigenous population of Indochina, with repatriation continuing to guide official policy for European patients.[117] The law, however, remained silent on important points about the civil capacity of those admitted to Biên Hòa and the administration of their property once they were confined. Furthermore, the law failed to distinguish between the "special ethnic characteristics and dissimilar juridical norms" that prevailed among the various groups of patients.[118]

As the governor-general of Indochina would later emphasize, the law constituted only an initial step in the search for a definitive legal regime to be applied to aliénés in the colony.[119] Still the 1918 law assumed an important role. As the only legal regulation around insanity in Indochina, it served as the de facto guideline for mental health care until a more comprehensive legal regime was instituted in 1930. In the meantime, as Jean Adrien Gaston Poulin, the resident superior of Tonkin, stressed in 1921, the principles of the 1918 decree should be applied generally as they have a "broad reach."[120]

Revisiting the 1838 French Asylum Law: The Interwar Years

After World War I, reformers once again sought to develop a legal infrastructure around mental illness in Indochina, one that would go beyond the simple grafting of French law onto preexisting Vietnamese traditions. The French 1838 asylum law, while not officially promulgated in the colony, nevertheless continued to be routinely referenced as the touchstone guiding psychiatric practices in the colony.[121] In a sense colonial officials had to play a game of catch-up—the arrival of the colony's first asylum signaled the need for a comprehensive legal framework to oversee the confinement and release of patients and their treatment, as well as the expansion of services throughout the colony. The focus thus shifted from determining the "true" extent of mental illness as the basis for legal intervention to what kinds of local adaptations the Indochinese context would require. What's more, at this time in France, the 1838 asylum law continued to face intense scrutiny both within and from outside the psychiatric profession. By the turn of the century, progress in psychiatric care and methods of treatment seemed to render the 1838 law all but obsolete. With the broadening of the concept of insanity beyond the idea of the dangerous and incurable individual and the movement toward open-door care and preventive services, critics increasingly questioned the fundamental concept of psychiatric care embodied in the 1838 act—namely, that of treatment conducted by compulsory detention within the setting of an asylum.

The move toward mental hygiene in the metropole also coincided with a major interwar effort to organize colonial policy around the principles of social and economic development, otherwise known as *mise en valeur*, an effort in which public health was envisioned to play a major role. In September of 1925, the minister of the colonies, Albert Lebrun, called for the creation of a commission to advise on the development of psychiatric services across the French empire as "an important aspect of our colonial medical assistance program."[122] Acknowledging the "relatively little advanced knowledge on the subject of colonial psychiatry and the diversity of races in their overseas possession," the commission undertook a comprehensive study of each colony in order to realize the platform first articulated at the 1912 Tunis meeting: the training of colonial psychiatric experts, the introduction of mental health legislation suited for colonial needs, and the establishment of a network of psychiatric institutions.[123]

Colonial administrators in Indochina faced the double task of both improving the 1838 law and adapting it to local conditions. Above all, the law needed to be tailored according to the different racialized legal categories that existed in the colony: Europeans or assimilated and naturalized *indigènes* (for whom the same text as the 1838 law would apply); native colonial subjects; and natives with "protected" status (*indigènes protégés français*).[124] For Governor-General Monguillot, there was also the complicated legal landscape of the colony to consider, a far cry from the "strong centralization and homogenous mentality" of France, where the legislation originated. Indochina's patchwork of oral traditions and customary law and imperial written law "frozen in an archaic formula" alongside French legal precepts together seemed wholly inadequate to address the problem of mental illness.[125] Many, like the director of health in Tonkin, feared that superimposing the 1838 law across all the territories of the Indochinese Union would touch off a whole range of messy legal questions pertaining to property succession, family organization, and competing jurisdictional claims, resulting in "texts that are superimposed and contradictory."[126] Monguillot nevertheless insisted that it should be possible to come up with some sort of flexible legal structure that could account for these internal variations. This preoccupation with local interpretations and applications of the law reflected a central tension faced by the colonial administration over how to effectively govern different kinds of people across a wide territory.

For French administrators tasked with elaborating a legal framework around mental illness in the colony, the challenge to take traditional practices and morals and transform them into a generalizing and overarching framework was formidable. At stake was balancing uniformity with efficiency on limited budgets. Doing so would require establishing a culturally shared understanding of the aliéné as a category of legal personhood deserving of state protection. As the director of the health service in Tonkin put it, the introduction of metropolitan legislation would require more than just "a simple adaptation of vocabulary." He warned that the "spirit of the law risks being misunderstood by the majority of the indigenous population and all the guarantees of administrative and judicial control, instituted in order to safeguard the liberty and protection of interests of the aliénés, are at risk of appearing as irksome and vexing formalities." An important gap in legal norms and practices would have to be bridged. He therefore cautioned that the new law should not be imposed from above but derived from local conditions and "possibilities of action."[127]

Despite these challenges, colonial reformers who participated in writing the legislation—across the civil and judicial administrations as well as the colonial health service—enjoyed more freedom to experiment than their metropolitan counterparts. While other French colonies completely abstained from legislating the question of mental illness or adopted the law of 1838 wholesale or on only certain essential principles, Indochina's government was remarkable in the sense that it drafted new, stand-alone legislation adapted to the particular needs of the colony. The 1930 asylum law adopted many innovations including the expansion of the category of aliéné to include those individuals who suffered from "lighter" or nonviolent forms of mental illness. However, by introducing the aliéné as a new kind of legal category in a vastly different social and political context than that from which it first emerged, the 1930 law presented the colonial administration with new kinds of obligations that would prove to be a major financial challenge and face serious political opposition.

The July 18, 1930, law establishing a psychiatric assistance program in Indochina (referred to hereafter as the 1930 law) was officially promulgated two months later on September 6, 1930.[128] The legislation called for the expansion of the asylum system beyond Biên Hòa to include a second asylum near the colonial capital of Hanoi to service the colony's northern region. Together these two asylums would serve as the basis of a new psychiatric assistance program tasked with the treatment of curable patients, hospitalization of the chronically ill, and the isolation and surveillance of those patients with "antisocial" tendencies or criminal pasts.[129] A number of secondary services run out of civil, military, or private hospitals that radiated into the interior of the colony would supplement the work of these two institutions. They would aid asylum doctors by identifying patients early, putting them out of harm's way, and treating curable cases early without confinement. While open services had existed in France since 1920, pioneered by the psychiatrist Edouard Toulouse and the League for Mental Prophylaxis and Hygiene (Ligue de prophylaxie et d'hygiène mentale), the 1930 provisions in Indochina marked the first time they were formally introduced into French law.[130] The law also called for a strict separation of indigenous and European patients. The parallel system for dealing with the mentally ill, divided along racial lines, would persist within the single space of the asylum. Given the expense of repatriation and small numbers of mentally ill Europeans even eligible for such a journey, the governor-general endorsed the creation of "mixed" asylums in the colony as a way to maximize resources. He insisted that the problem was little more than one of simple architecture. Not all psychiatric reformers—both inside and outside Indochina—were so sanguine about the administration of mixed asylums in colonial settings. They worried in particular over the "delicate" application of the principles of separation to those who defied neat categorization: creoles, *métis*, and natives with French citizenship status, as well as the need, in some contexts, to separate historically antagonistic ethnic groups.[131]

The 1930 law also regulated the procedures for the confinement and release of patients, their care while confined, and the oversight of the asylum to be performed by an independent surveillance commission. The law took particular inspiration from an aborted 1907 project named after Fernand Dubief, a doctor and former minister of commerce in France. The so-called Dubief Law attempted to improve the 1838 law by working to guard against arbitrary confinement.[132] Colonial reformers took up the spirit of the Dubief Law by providing widened scope for the intervention of the judiciary during the process of confinement at the expense of those administrative powers that had been greatly expanded under the 1838 law. When Pierre Dorolle, a French psychiatrist who served in Indochina's health administration in the 1930s, later reflected on the significance of the 1930 law, he praised its commitment to "augment those guarantees provided to the patient and to assure the most humane conditions for the protection of himself and his belongings."[133]

Other features differed from the 1838 asylum law in important ways that signified the innovative qualities of the Indochinese legislation. Most notably, the 1930 law abandoned "isolation" as the sole guiding principle of psychiatric treatment and broadened the legal definition of *aliéné* to include those who suffered from lighter or nonviolent forms of mental illness. Other innovations included the regulation of care of patients at home, psychiatric treatment in ordinary hospitals, and rules regarding the civil capacity and administration of patient property; the provisional character of confinement until a decision was rendered by a tribunal; the possibility of voluntary placement initiated by the patient himself; the regularization of the confinement of epileptics and drug addicts, as well as those criminal patients found irresponsible by reason of insanity.

Just as in the French legislation, families retained the power to pursue the confinement of one of their family members (*placement requis*, or "requested admission"), and the government retained the authority to place in a special establishment any person whose mental state was found to compromise "public decency, tranquility or security" (*placement d'office*, or "mandated admission"). According to the 1930 law in Indochina, however, these internments remained provisional until, at the end of an observation period of six months, a decision of the justice system could prolong the confinement of the patient following expert advice. Furthermore, the new legislation regulated the care of the insane at home and instituted, as another innovation, voluntary placement (without any legal formalities) from the simple verbal demand of the patient himself.

Part of the originality of the 1930 legislation was to provide release even before cure, in the form of "provisional exits" or "trial leaves," which allowed the legislation to "take on a more medical character."[134] Under these trial leaves, patients returned to their families and communities, where medical observation would continue in the form of regular visits by the local doctor, who would administer medicines and advise in favor of or against a permanent reintegration into the community depending on the medical progress of the patient. While officials touted the trial leave as an innovation reflecting a more modern outlook on psychiatric care, in many ways it represented a continuation of precolonial and earlier French colonial practices that relied on family and communal resources to care for the patient as a way to relieve pressure on state budgets. Once the patient was home, the family member or guardian was obligated to address a written declaration to the prosecutor's office accompanied by a medical report dated within the first fifteen days of the patient's release. If home care was found insufficient, the tribunal could mandate that the patient be given to another guardian or placed within a private or public institution.

Despite the law's innovative qualities, challenges still remained in terms of implementation, especially in Tonkin, where there would not be an asylum to receive sick patients for another four years. Dr. A. de Raymond, the director of the health service in Tonkin, explained in October 1930 that contrary to the governor-general's pronouncement, the law in Indochina essentially represented a copy of the 1838 law in France in the sense that it "aggravated and complicated and was barely inspired, as far as the indigènes were concerned, by local necessities." He therefore worried over its application, especially before the opening of the second asylum in Tonkin, and recommended the law's postponement. Raymond, in fact, had expressed his opposition to the expansion of the asylum system from the beginning, warning that it was "too premature."[135]

In the meantime, creative solutions helped fill in the gaps. For instance, Raymond proposed that services for the mentally ill, already in place at the Indigenous Hospital in Hanoi, could be considered a site for observation rather than treatment and confinement, so a simple certification of hospital admission would continue to suffice. This move would obviate legal oversight because patients would be considered free until they were officially deprived of their rights by court order. How to follow the letter of the law when no public or private establishments for the mentally ill existed at the time of the law's promulgation remained a point of serious frustration for those health experts in the north.[136] Until the Vôi asylum and the other secondary centers for assistance opened for business, the resident superior of Tonkin provided assurance that the 1930 legislation would remain a dead letter and that officials should continue to rely on the 1918 law.[137] While in theory the 1930 law offered common prescriptions that could be adapted to the cadre of local laws and royal ordinances that prevailed in different parts of Indochina, in practice the process was not so straightforward. Colonial officials also feared the law might set in motion a wave of more comprehensive changes to the native civil code (*code civil indigénat*). One suggestion for such a project included modeling the protection of the insane after provisions for the protection of minors in the French civil code.[138] Ironically this formulation mirrored the traditional Vietnamese legal code providing that the insane person and minor held the same functional legal status under which "all latitude was left to the parents . . . to act in favor of his personal interests."[139]

Toward a New Era of Asylum Care

By the time of the promulgation of the 1930 law, earlier presumptions that the Vietnamese psyche remained "unscathed" by modernity had long begun to shift. As one asylum director remarked in 1927, "It seems as though all development of civilization is accompanied by a growth in madness which follows in its wake."[140] Colonial officials attributed the increasing visibility of the mentally ill, counted among the thousands of vagrants who flooded into cities like Saigon, to the effects of dislocation and social upheaval under French rule. The heightened visibility of mental illness indexed widespread social and economic change in the colony. This in turn formed the critical backdrop for the emergence of the aliéné as a responsibility of the colonial government. In just a few decades, colonial officials moved from claiming there was very little legal basis or practical exigencies for an asylum in Indochina to achieving one of the most comprehensive mental health care systems in the French empire.

This chapter has discussed this transformation in terms of shifts in the legal definition of insanity. Although at first only dangerous forms of mental illness were considered a requirement for legal intervention, effectively foreclosing early attempts to establish an asylum, this did not mean that in practice people coded as mentally ill by Vietnamese communities and colonial authorities alike did not become a burden to the colonial state. Once hospitals began to increase their capacity to care for these patients, however imperfectly, the availability of services began to generate new demand for their expansion, rendering a problem that was formerly hidden increasingly visible. The opening of the asylum in 1919 therefore gave mental illness a new concreteness that could be captured in official statistics. The concept's transformation into an official category of person, one which required legal protections and access to services, must thus also be understood within a growing health care infrastructure that responded to both local developments *and* international pressures for its expansion. Furthermore, the legal definition of insanity, encoded in the French asylum law of 1838, not only had to be made to reflect more modern understandings of psychiatric knowledge and practices but also had to be translated to a vastly different cultural and institutional context. Indochina's varied legal and administrative regimes, coupled with a lack of funds—which made the inauguration of new services impracticable if not impossible—posed a major practical challenge to colonial reformers.

As mental illness moved from a problem exclusively of social order toward one increasingly focused on social responsibility at the turn of the century, it raised difficult questions about the obligations of the colonial state toward its subjects. Mental health care also had to be carefully weighed alongside other concerns demanding attention and the dedication of considerable resources. After World War I, the target of health care services in Indochina shifted to meet local needs, including public hygiene education campaigns, provisions for clean drinking water and better sanitation in urban centers, as well as the battle against infectious diseases in the form of targeted campaigns against epidemics and the creation of specialized services for lepers, tuberculosis patients, and pregnant women.[141] As late as 1928, the inspector general of sanitary and medical services deemed the promulgation of a comprehensive asylum law premature given the state of the general medical service in the colony, which he found "absolutely insufficient." The project would divert funds from other medical branches whose development pressed much more urgently.[142] Nevertheless, by the 1930s, Indochina's psychiatric assistance program was lauded as surpassing not only the efforts of other colonies but also those of the metropole. Despite these important innovations—as this chapter has foreshadowed and the following chapters will show—there emerged considerable difficulties in putting these policies into practice.

CHAPTER 2

Patients, Staff, and the Everyday Challenges of Asylum Administration

Located on the side of Route 1, about thirty-four kilometers outside Saigon, the Biên Hòa asylum first opened its doors to the public in January of 1919. On approach visitors might have been startled to encounter not a large imposing prison-like façade but a modest white picket gate at the entrance giving way to a wide, tree-lined lane. Once inside, they would have discovered dozens of low-lying buildings, or "pavilions," comprising the entirety of the hospital complex, itself surrounded by a large expanse of rural land with no walls in sight.

A small river cut through the asylum grounds and provided irrigation to land dedicated to the cultivation of rice, rubber, and other crops, as well as the raising of farm animals. Patients may have dotted the landscape, hard at work sowing seeds or harvesting vegetables, painting a tranquil pastoral scene. For visitors to Biên Hòa it was apparently a "surprise . . . to observe that the quarters in which one hears any kind of noise are those of the calm patients on the verge of leaving [for work] for the day."[1] This setup proved key for colonial asylum directors eager to demonstrate to the public that the asylum was not a place of "secrecy, cruelty and injustice" but rather a psychologically sound environment geared toward cure.

Designed as a large agricultural colony, Biên Hòa reflected the vision of its expert planners, who promoted the use of open spaces so as to provide patients with a kind of "semi-liberty" and "comfort in freedom previously

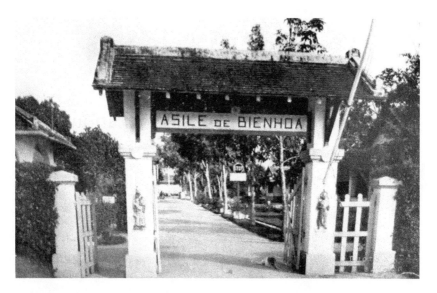

FIGURE 1.   Entrance to Biên Hòa, 1934. ANOM (Base Ulysse).

unknown."[2] Not only did this simulation of the social world reflect a more modern and more humanitarian conception of care than earlier methods of confinement—one that proved useful in improving the poor public image of the asylum—but the appearance of freedom itself was seen as curative.[3] As Biên Hòa's director explained in 1926, the colonial asylum "must form a special milieu, organized exclusively in view of the lunatic, where he will find the care and surveillance necessary without the sensation of being a prisoner, cut off from the world. This setup is almost realized at the asylum of Biên Hòa where patients enjoy liberty in their surroundings which would make them the objects of envy of many asylum patients in the metropole." He continued, "Perhaps in seeing patients well treated, well fed and rejoicing in an expanded freedom more patients will demand hospitalization."[4]

Asylums were seen as harbingers of modernity and progress and therefore figured as important elements in France's civilizing mission. Colonial psychiatrists in Indochina routinely presented themselves as on the cutting edge of their profession, even outperforming their colleagues in France, whose own efforts at asylum reform were mired in political controversy and a maze of antiquated laws. Yet deficiencies in infrastructure and personnel coupled with frequent budget crises hampered the ambitions of Indochinese psychiatry. Plans for the establishment of a second asylum in Tonkin reveal some of the hard-learned lessons at Biên Hòa over the difficulties of surveillance of patients at work and asleep. With the dramatic rise in patient numbers, asylum oversight commissions in the 1930s worried over the severe overcrowding of patient pavilions and a staff that was poorly trained and underpaid. Among the patients themselves, asylum directors encountered resistance. While some protested the terms of their confinement, claiming they were not in fact insane, others found more subtle ways of defying the terms of categorization that governed the organization of asylum space. Colonial asylums were at once spaces of discipline and therapy, open doors and confinement, labor and rehabilitation, boredom and frustration, care and violence. These ambiguities in the functioning of asylums led to episodic crises but also opportunities for flexibility and innovation in psychiatric practices.

Arrival at the Asylum

On January 15, 1919, the Biên Hòa asylum received its first patients, including men and women of both European and Asian descent. This "mixed" model distinguished asylums in Indochina from those in India, where separate asylums were built for Europeans and native populations.[5] It also distinguished asylums from other kinds of colonial institutions in the colony such as schools, prisons, and hospitals that were marked by a dual system segregated along racial lines.[6] Like patients in France, those confined in asylums in colonial Vietnam exhibited a loss of social competence—manifested in extreme or otherwise abnormal behavior—that prompted their families and neighbors, or the authorities, to seek their removal from public life and delivery into the hands of experts. Before they were asylum patients, many had spent months if not years transiting through colonial public health and surveillance networks where they may have suffered from abuse and neglect but also found common cause with fellow travelers afflicted by the stigmas of race and poverty. The exact mechanisms by which patients would enter and leave the asylum—including the important mediating role played by families—will be discussed at greater length in chapter 4. This chapter instead sets out to relate the experience of asylum patients and those tasked with their care and surveillance.

Upon arrival at the asylum, Vietnamese patients were required to give up any personal items, to be returned at the time of their exit, and in return were provided with bed linens, a mosquito net, and a new set of clothes, including a white cotton jacket and pants and a traditional Vietnamese hat. European patients were also provided with new clothes including pajamas, blouse, and pants (cut in a typical European style). In addition, Vietnamese patients underwent a number of hygienic measures. After their heads were shaved, the newly admitted patients bathed and received vaccinations against smallpox and cholera. Doctors often remarked that at the time of their admission a large proportion of the patients arrived in a state of such "physical decrepitude that they could be classified in the category of severe wasting. These unfortunates come to us malnourished having suffered ill treatment at the hands of their entourage."[7] Diagnosed most frequently with skin diseases and pulmonary infections, doctors observed their patients dramatically improve with the sole therapy of sleep and regular food.[8]

Patients then moved to the "admission" building, where either the director of the asylum or the chief medical resident would determine the specific nature of their psychosis. Asylum directors, all French men, were chosen from among the civilian or military doctors in the colonial health service. They had typically served as chief doctors at an asylum or psychiatric clinic in the metropole or, more often, had simply completed a *stage*, or internship, in psychiatry in a French asylum following their medical education in Bordeaux, Paris, or Lyon.[9] Expertise denoted not just specialized training in psychiatry but also knowledge of the local language, considered "absolutely indispensable" when it came to the psychiatric treatment of the indigenous population.[10] Experts who could not communicate directly with their patients would remain incapable of "distinguishing among the thousands of medical nuances" or "thousand nuances of elocution and conversation" that comprised the precious arsenal of the psychiatric expert, as Louis Lorion complained of French doctors practicing in Saigon in 1887.[11] Colonial reformers also continually stressed the need for a "double specialization" in both psychiatric and colonial medicine; advanced training in neuropsychiatry would prove useless if one also remained ignorant of the basic principles of exotic pathology.[12]

All patients fell under the observation of the asylum's director, who would approve recommendations for care and treatment. The director also assured the personal care of European patients. A Vietnamese medical resident stood second in command. Residents, trained at the Hanoi Medical University, were included among the corps of indigenous medical doctors who constituted an essential part of Indochina's medical service. In 1934, the École de Médecine in Hanoi added psychiatry to the curriculum as part of the advanced training of Vietnamese doctors who would come to staff the psychiatric assistance program and eventually assume control once the French left Vietnam in 1954.[13] The medical resident assisted in the medical visits and follow-up examinations of patients, took notes on the course of therapy, and managed the clinical paperwork for each patient.[14] A staff of nurses, guards, and coolies assisted doctors with the daily care and surveillance of patients, the administering of medicines, and the translation of patient demands into French.

After establishing their psychiatric status, the asylum director would direct patients to the appropriate pavilion. Each pavilion at Biên Hòa was named after a famous French psychiatrist, arranged on its own large plot, and surrounded by plants, flower beds, and some trees. Iron rails masked by live hedges separated the pavilions one from the other, with the entire group of asylum buildings also enclosed in the same way.[15] Designed to reduce the risk of patient escapes, these covered rails measured two meters in height.[16] Patient pavilions were segregated by race, by gender, and by the severity of the patient's diagnosis. For Vietnamese men and women, there existed one pavilion each for senile and epileptic patients, two for "calm" patients, and two for the "semi-calm." Designed to hold forty people, each pavilion consisted of two common rooms with a dining hall, bathrooms, and its own watch guard. Patients convicted of criminal charges required a special kind of surveillance and found themselves placed in the "Quartier Morel," named after the famous French theorist of degeneration, Benedict Morel. Twenty individual isolation cells were reserved for the most agitated patients and followed the model of Dr. Clerambault, the medical chief of the special infirmary of the prefecture of police in Paris. (See figure 6)

In 1925, the asylum housed one pavilion for European patients, reserved for men only. Converted from its original purpose as a pharmacy, the pavilion was cramped, consisting of two bedrooms and one isolation chamber, housing ten patients total, a bathroom and water closet, as well as a small garden. European quarters eventually expanded to include ten bedrooms, a dining room, reading and game room, a bathroom and shower for every two bedrooms, and a separate pavilion for female patients. A common physical education room reserved specific hours for use by each gender.

The racial segregation of patients also found concrete expression in the quality of bedding and clothing provided, respective diets, as well as the organization of daily life at the asylum. The regimes for indigenous patients were decidedly modest. They were provided with basic wooden beds and mats for sleeping. At mealtime, they received iron bowls and chopsticks to eat a diet of typical peasant fare, including freshly husked white or red rice of "inferior" quality, fresh or dried fish, pork or beef (or two duck eggs or two Annamite sausages), fish sauce, green vegetables, and tea. Beef was prepared Tuesday, Thursday, and Saturday, while fish was provided Thursday and Sunday. During the rainy season, dried fish substituted for fresh fish or pork. A designated chef, with the help of patient-laborers, prepared all meals and even provided special meals on holidays.[17]

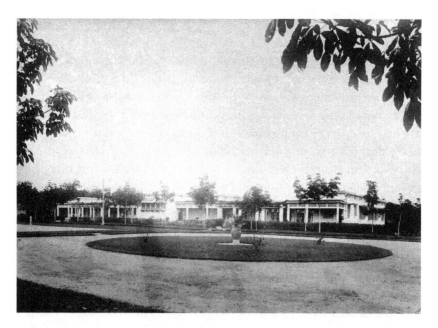

FIGURE 2. European pavilion, Biên Hòa, 1931. Courtesy of user manhhai, Flickr.

European patients, meanwhile, ate meals prepared in the French style. For breakfast, they had black coffee or café au lait, and pastries made with chocolate and butter. For lunch, they enjoyed varied hors d'oeuvres, an entrée of fish or eggs or pasta, meat and vegetables, and a dessert. For their evening meal, they dined on a stew or soup, an entrée, a meat course, a vegetable course, dessert, and bread. In true French fashion, patients were also served "red wine of good quality " and ice cream with their meal.[18] The asylum even installed a refrigerator in order to keep perishables cold. By the late 1920s, beer made with locally grown hops replaced wine as a cost-saving measure. Menus also varied to accommodate the dietary needs of different kinds of patients, from those who arrived at the asylum malnourished to those Muslim patients whose religious beliefs forbade the consumption of pork.[19]

The organization of leisure time also marked a fundamental difference in the experience of asylum life across the patient population. Many indigenous patients labored in the fields or ateliers as a form of work therapy. For these patients, leisure time came in the form of siestas in between work sessions and during holidays. European patients, meanwhile, did not work because of concerns over the intensity of the tropical heat.[20] Scheduled promenades in the large garden adjoining their pavilion, as well as swimming and tennis, provided essential forms of exercise and relaxation as well as indoor games

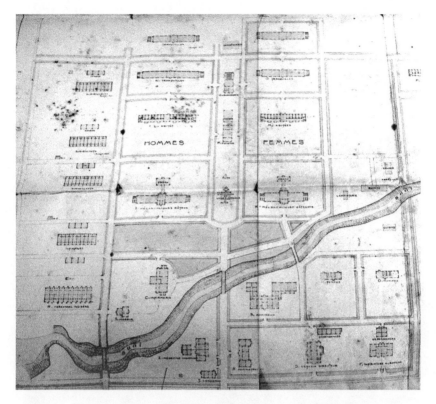

FIGURE 3. Blueprint of the Biên Hòa asylum, Cochinchina, 1927. TTLTQG-1, 73750, Résidence Supérieur au Tonkin, Organisation et fonctionnement d'un Asile d'Aliénés à Bien-Hoa (Cochinchine), Note sur l'organisation générale d'un Asile d'Aliénés par le Dr. Augagneur, Médecin Directeur de l'Asile de Bien Hoa, 1927.

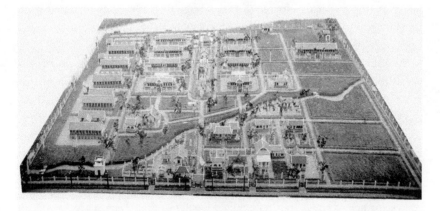

FIGURE 4. Scaled model of Biên Hòa handmade by patients and asylum guards. ANOM, AGEFOM, 554, Assistance Médicale—maguettes d'Asile de Bien Hoa, Exposition Coloniale (Indochine) Paris, 1931–32.

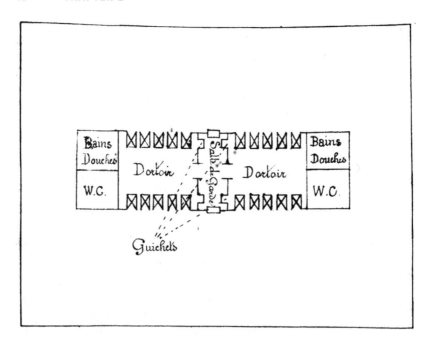

FIGURE 5. Drawing of pavilion for "calm patients," Biên Hòa asylum, 1927. TTLTQG-1, 73750, Résidence Supérieur au Tonkin, Organisation et fonctionnement d'un Asile d'Aliénés à Bien-Hoa (Cochinchine), Note sur l'organisation générale d'un Asile d'Aliénés par le Dr. Augagneur, Médecin Directeur de l'Asile de Bien Hoa, 1927.

for when it rained. Even their room furnishings, which included tables and armchairs, reflected expectations for these patients to engage in reading, writing, and self-reflection.[21] Asylum reports discussed the importance of leisure and entertainment to cheer up patients, European and indigenous alike. In this respect, Indochina's mental health institutions reportedly fell behind those of British India, where football matches, musical instruments, and dance performances helped to distract patients.[22]

Already blurry distinctions between those destined for European and Asian pavilions grew especially complicated with the arrival of *métis*, or mixed-race patients. One patient's story is instructive. The son of a lieutenant in the French army and a Vietnamese mother, Hoang (alternatively referred to in his case file by his French name, Jean G.) was born in Yen Bay province in September 1987. His father left Indochina soon thereafter. Several years later, in 1921, Jean G. moved to Hanoi and without a fixed home, in the grips of mental illness, he became a well-known threat to public order.[23] As a *métis non reconnu*—not recognized legally as French by his father—Jean G. was refused entry to the Lanessan Hospital reserved for the exclusive use of European patients, while physicians at the Indigenous Hospital stressed

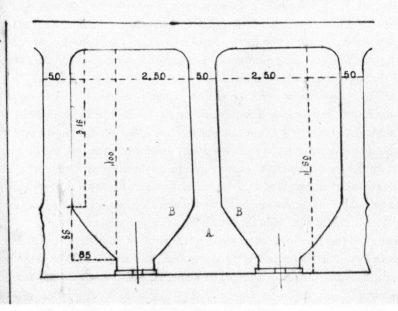

TYPE DE CELLULE

POUR ALIENES

ECHELLE O 02 P.M.

FIGURE 6. Model of the typical cell for patients in the "agitated wing" at Biên Hòa, 1927. TTLTQG-1, 73750, Résidence Supérieur au Tonkin, Organisation et fonctionnement d'un Asile d'Aliénés à Bien-Hoa (Cochinchine), Note sur l'organisation générale d'un Asile d'Aliénés par le Dr. Augagneur, Médecin Directeur de l'Asile de Bien Hoa, 1927.

that they were unprepared to receive a patient of "his type."[24] Although his condition seemed to be improving, the colonial administration in Tonkin found it impossible to keep him in limbo, so it decided to send him south to the Biên Hòa asylum, where he was interned in November of 1922. Confined to the indigenous section of the asylum, the doctor writes in his case file that Jean. G "certainly suffered from this situation." He determined that the "only way to make this situation better was to reclassify him in the category reserved for Europeans" which was accomplished five years later in November of 1927.[25] Another patient's story points to structural deficiencies and the subtle but effective forms of individual agency that prevented the neat racial segregation of patients. A French patient sent to Biên Hòa in 1931 was temporarily placed in the indigenous section because the European quarter was full. He subsequently refused to move to the European pavilion once space became available and so was left to his own devices among the indigènes, much to the chagrin of the asylum staff.

The deficiencies in accommodation for European patients, made worryingly visible in both of these cases, weighed heavily on the asylum administration. Six years after Biên Hòa first opened, in 1925, the asylum's director warned, "This can only be a resting place for those mentally ill awaiting their repatriation. It is impossible to aspire to keep these patients over a period of years without the comfort and space to which they have a right." Worries over the increasing numbers of Europeans and *métis* born in the colony, including those with families already established there, led colonial officials to believe that repatriation was no longer a practicable option. Asylum administrators agreed and continually stressed the "imperious need" for the construction of a new European quarter.[26] To make patients more comfortable in the short term, they proposed the purchase of additional furniture (to make the rooms appear less spare) and the establishment of a library. They also thanked the heads of various local newspapers for donating daily papers to the asylum each morning.[27] However, years later, arrangements for European patients at Biên Hòa remained "insufficient, poorly arranged. . . . The two pavilions that were available in 1927 require two patients to share the same bedroom." Meanwhile there was "no place to put loud or disruptive patients which means that one agitated patient prevents all the others from relaxing."[28]

Asylum directors faced other kinds of practical challenges. Confronted with constant hikes in food prices, clothing, and medication throughout the 1920s, they started to cut corners. A 1925 report references the complaints of patients who accused asylum directors of reducing their daily ration of rice.[29] The clothing worn by patients, of such poor quality that it easily fell apart, prompted the asylum administration to insist on the need for thicker, more expensive cloth, for, "despite all the repairs and a very active surveillance a number of patients tear and do away with their clothing."[30] Otherwise patients were forced to don "patched-up garments that give them the aspect of vagrants, which produces a very bad effect on families who come to pay them a visit. . . . An atelier for repairs works nonstop and despite all that we cannot change patients' clothes as often as is desirable."[31] The power of public perceptions put pressure on asylum administrators, but it also became a useful tool for extracting from the colonial administration those things they needed most.

Unsurprisingly, the question of the asylum's budget continually pitted asylum directors against the administration. Particularly contentious was the organization of asylum finances in such a way that the institution itself had no income. Instead it operated on credit that was then reimbursed from the budget of the colonial public health service, as well as provincial and municipal budgets in proportion to the number of patients treated. According to the 1918 and 1930 asylum laws, a patient's hospitalization was to be reimbursed directly by the patient's family or, more often if the families were indigent, by the budgets of their province of origin. (The amount paid by families relative to that paid by the provinces was vanishingly small. In 1926, for example, the asylum received 2001.50 piasters from the families of paying patients, while reimbursement from the provinces totaled 68,949.50)[32] At the moment of admission, asylum administrators faced the challenge of determining where exactly patients had come from in order to know which provinces to charge—not an easy feat given the numbers picked up on vagrancy charges often far from their family homes and flung across the entire Indochinese Union.

Throughout the 1920s, the actual costs of the daily management of Biên Hòa annually outpaced its projected expenses despite routine requests to the colonial administration for a greater allowance.[33] Over a thirteen-year period, from 1919 to 1932, the amount by which the money spent on hospitalization exceeded the amount reimbursed reached over 40,000 piasters, or an average of just over a 3,000 piaster deficit a year, as one asylum director pointedly observed.[34] Given the high initial operating costs, asylum directors hoped the budget would achieve an "equilibrium" point once the asylum population passed four hundred patients, which occurred in 1927.[35] Yet regional increases in the costs of food, agricultural tools, and general upkeep continued to spiral beyond control even as the number of personnel was kept as low as possible.[36]

In order to ease the institutions' already-strained finances, in 1928 asylum administrators successfully advocated for an increase in the daily tariffs of hospitalization for both European and indigenous patients.[37] They envisioned the expansion of the asylum's "paying service" into three class divisions for European patients and one for indigenous patients. These new classes of patients would not only encourage families to send patients in the belief that they would receive better treatment but also serve as an important source of revenue. Creating a "paying service" would, however, require an increase in the number of personnel and lodgings to conform to the wider variety of regimes associated with each new category of patients. A 1934 decree later expanded the categories of paying European patients from three to four.[38] It also specified that the two pavilions at Biên Hòa, named after the French psychiatrists Emmanuel Régis and Gilbert Ballet (previously occupied by Europeans who were moved to their new wing), would receive two new categories of indigenous patients in which members of the Vietnamese and Chinese bourgeoisie could find "all their desired comforts" for a cost of between 1.00 and 1.50 piasters per day.[39] Indigent patients, meanwhile, were to be kept in "common rooms" away from the paying patients. Ten years later, the fees for paying patients would continue to creep upwards but nevertheless fail to keep pace with the "real cost" of treatment, as the resident superior of Tonkin cautioned in a May 1938 note. Because of the often lengthy confinements of patients, it would be impossible to charge a high daily rate as general hospitals did, yet asylums were still forced to pay the same salaries for their employees and market prices for goods.[40] Asylum directors yet again created a new paying category for indigenous patients set at 0.50 piasters per day. They hoped this move would help displace the burden from provincial budgets onto those of families for whom the costs of internment had previously been out of reach.[41] Still, the amount received from families never represented more than a fraction of the operating budget of the institution. Other solutions to make asylums more productive and efficient were also pursued aggressively, the subject of the following chapter.

Diagnostic Practices and Treatment Regimes

Annual asylum reports provided meticulous data to the colonial administration on patient backgrounds, length of stay, diagnosis, and rate of cure. These data provided the basis for new scientific knowledge about mental illness in the colony that was published in both local and metropolitan medical journals. It also testified to the need for continued state investment in colonial mental health care, even if the efforts to secure more resources were never more than partially successful. Read alongside individual patient case files, these reports provide an important picture of shifts in the demographics and psychiatric profile of the colonial asylum population throughout the interwar period.

By the end of its first year of operation, Biên Hòa had treated 138 patients. Over the following ten years, asylum directors would witness a dramatic rise in patient numbers. In 1924, five years after Biên Hòa opened its doors, the asylum treated 325 patients. By 1928, the asylum treated 473 patients for a total of 157,086 days of hospitalization for the year.[42] The number of hospitalization days is perhaps a more accurate measure than absolute patient

Années	Nombre des hos- pitalisés	Nombre des journées d'hos- pitalisation.
1919	138	5.639
1920	159	10.040
1921	190	62.871
1922	241	79.242
1923	264	88.538
1924	326	107.909
1925	360	126.157
1926	379	131.282
1927	428	144.284
1928	473	167.086
1929	468	173.484
1930	532	177.690
1931	590	202.775
1932	622	216.851
1933	660	234.039
1934	636	235.538

FIGURE 7.   Table of patient numbers and days of hospitalization at the Biên Hòa asylum (1919–34). TTLTQG-1, IGHSP, 51–07, Rapport annuel de 1934 sur le fonctionnement du Service de l'Assistance Médicale de Biên Hòa, Sai Gon, Bac Lieu, 1934.

numbers of the true burden on the asylum staff, given the tremendous fluidity of the patient population.

The large majority (82%) of those who left the asylum in 1927, for instance, had been residents for less than two years.[43] This was not a fluke but rather indicative of a general pattern that would continue into the 1930s. In 1934, for example, out of a total 801 patients, 141 entered Biên Hòa, while 101 were released. Thirty-five percent were released after less than ten months in the asylum and 92 percent after two years.[44] Patient turnover reflected less the efficacy of psychiatric treatment than the various pressures facing asylum directors to remove patients from their care.

The asylum administration kept data not only on those who arrived but also on those who left and under what conditions. In 1928, sixty-two patients were reportedly cured, while forty-nine died and one escaped. It should be

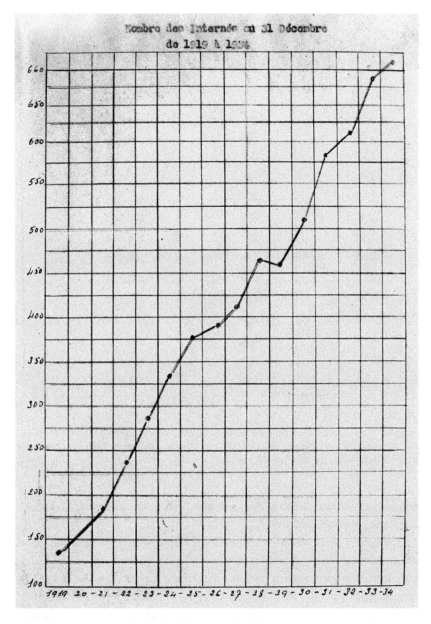

FIGURE 8. Chart of annual patient admittances at the Biên Hòa asylum (1919–34). TTLTQG-1, IGHSP, 51–07, Rapport annuel de 1934 sur le fonctionnement du Service de l'Assistance Médicale de Biên Hòa, Sai Gon, Bac Lieu, 1934.

pointed out that "cure" often meant that the patient's symptoms had subsided enough that he or she could return to normal life, not that the patient was clinically free of the underlying disease. Certain psychoses could be dramatically improved, but there was always a risk of a relapse, even in the long-term future. One psychiatrist in 1934 even admitted that it was "probable" that among his patients many would make multiple visits to the asylum.[45] For the period between 1919 and 1934, the number of cures almost always exceeded the number of deaths at the asylum, except for a slight rise in patient deaths in 1924 and a dramatic rise again in 1931 and 1932. Perhaps the asylum received more sickly patients as a result of the economic crisis in the region during this period. According to annual asylum reports, most died of pulmonary tuberculosis, wasting or malnourishment, or meningitis and kidney disease, conditions that had most likely plagued these patients since well before they found themselves at the asylum. Suicide, it should be pointed out, was an extremely rare occurrence among patients.[46]

Annual data on the racial background of asylum patients, listed as a "predisposing cause" of psychiatric illness, offers a valuable metric of the diversity of 1920s Indochina. By 1928, of the 1,009 patients who ever entered the asylum's doors, the majority (827) were of Vietnamese origin from the region immediately surrounding Biên Hòa in Cochinchina and neighboring Annam. Patients were also sent from Tonkin (22), Cambodia (56), and Laos (2). There were 56 patients of Chinese origin, as well as 5 Hindus and 2 Malays, most of whom had found their way to Indochina as passengers or navigators on steamships, or engaged in commerce that was booming in the major port cities. Most were sent back to their place of origin upon falling ill. For those foreigners without families, the cost of their confinement was typically covered by local congregations. As for the European population, asylum reports counted 16 French patients who entered between 1919 and 1928, in addition to 13 métis who were accordingly classified as Franco-Cambodgien, Franco-Annamite, Franco-Tonkinois, and Bourbon-Annamite.[47] Either unemployed or working as farmers, coolies, and day laborers, most Vietnamese patients were poor, or as the report's author bluntly put it, "that is to say those natives whose lives are the most miserable, who suffer from a deficient diet, whose conditions of material existence are mediocre."[48] Doctors often spoke of good hygiene and improved quality of life as prophylactics against the development of psychoses.[49]

The maximum frequency of mental illness occurred between the ages of twenty-six and thirty, followed by thirty-one- to thirty-five-year-olds, and twenty-one- to twenty-five-year-olds. Common beliefs regarding the "precociousness" of Asian populations meant the twenty-six to thirty age bracket was considered the "normal period of activity of middle age." Other factors included considerations of climate, with most admissions observed during the hot and dry season. Being unmarried also seemed to predispose individuals to psychopathic illness.[50]

Between 1924 and 1931, the main categories of psychiatric classification expanded from three to five, and subcategories also grew increasingly specific over time. The first category of *psychopaths infirmités* was initially defined according to the degree of impairment and included those suffering from dementia and "degeneration."[51] While degeneration as a diagnostic category had fallen out of use in the metropole by the interwar period, it continued to be frequently employed in Indochina. By 1931, these categories had splintered into more precise clinical designations based on etiology and presentation of symptoms. The second, and most common, category belonged to general psychopathic disease, which included various forms of paranoia, depression, mania, mental confusion, and schizophrenia (*démence précoce*).[52] It is perhaps no surprise that these were the most prevalent disorders; they tended to be associated in annual statistics with those violent behaviors that precipitated police involvement. At the Vôi asylum in 1936, a third of the total asylum population was diagnosed with démence précoce. Psychiatrists observed no significant differences between their European and Vietnamese patients: the condition mostly appeared before the age of thirty, and the symptoms and prognosis differed very little. Forms of paranoia were rare and tended to express themselves in grandiose or "mystical" ideas that carried a certain cultural valence in the colonial context but expressed nothing "inherent to the race."[53]

The last category included a mixed bag of unrelated disorders that eventually coalesced into three categories: nervous disorders such as epilepsy, psychopathic illness caused by intoxication (associated with alcohol and opium addiction), and psychopathic illness caused by infections including "general paralysis."[54] Closely linked to syphilis, this last diagnosis was the most common diagnosis among French patients in the 1920s. It also reinforced calls for better prevention of venereal disease in the community.[55]

The rates of mental illness were also strongly gendered. Almost twice as many men as women entered Biên Hòa (595 men versus 388 women) between 1919 and 1928. The same proportion held true on a larger geographic scale.[56] Even as the number of hospitalizations continued to grow at Biên Hòa, the relative proportion of men and women remained remarkably constant (429 men to 231 women in 1936, and 528 men to 298 women in 1938).[57] This is all the more striking given the feminization of the asylum population during the interwar period in France, where women came to outnumber men by upwards of 30 percent. Aude Fauvel attributes this transformation to changes in the medical discourse on madness, specifically the treatment of female criminality, as well as the emergence of the first crop of female psychiatrists in France.[58] We do not see similar processes unfolding in colonial Vietnam. Furthermore, given that doctors often explicitly couched the goals of psychiatric treatment in terms of improving economic productivity and policing efforts, it is not altogether surprising that young men garnered the most attention from colonial experts.

Doctors also observed differences between men and women in terms of the kinds of triggers for psychotic episodes. Patient case files reveal the fascinating observation that psychotic episodes among men were connected to the dispossession of their land.[59] Doctors attributed higher rates of mental illness among men to the fact that they performed more intensive work and therefore had higher rates of alcohol consumption, which predisposed and intensified the expression of psychiatric illness. Nearly a third of patients at Biên Hòa (303 out of 1,009 patients) were classified as alcohol abusers. Alcoholism concerned colonial doctors because of its easy accessibility to the lower classes, whereas opium addiction remained mainly among the Chinese population.[60] Reduced prices as well as to the efforts of "bootleggers" and clandestine operations that proved impossible to regulate, especially the introduction of potentially toxic substances, were to blame.[61] Asylum directors recommended raising taxes on alcohol as a deterrent to drinking among the lower classes, an unpopular proposal given alcohol's budgetary importance to the tax revenue of the colonial administration.[62]

For women, doctors considered complications related to childbirth—whether in terms of pregnancy, abortion, or menopause—or the loss of a child or family member as important triggers for mental instability. Vietnamese medical thought also associated childbirth with temporary forms of insanity; these points of conceptual overlap may have facilitated the entrance and exit of this specific class of female patients from asylum care. Among the 388 women who entered Biên Hòa between 1919 and 1928, psychiatrists counted 16 cases of psychosis brought on by post-childbirth infections. They almost all resulted in a "speedy recovery."[63] Other typical female disorders took on a more serious and permanent character. One particular case of a forty-year-old female patient provides a useful illustration. Can was sentenced to five years of hard labor for the attempted poisoning death of her husband and neighbors by mixing arsenic with their food.[64] In the course of an expert medical exam to determine whether she could be held responsible for her actions, Can claimed that she had been possessed by genies or spirits that led her to commit the crime. She was subsequently diagnosed with "menstrual psychosis," a mental disorder characterized by a cycle of periods of calm followed by acute crisis episodes brought on by the arrival of the menstrual period. Her case file reports, "Here we find a typical clinical expression of violent delirium, that is more or less disordered accompanied by mild confusion" caused by a slow and progressive "genital auto-intoxication of the organism." The medical exam found that Can was of a "primitive nature," which made her especially vulnerable to delirious dreams and mystical influences that ultimately caused her to commit a violent and impulsive act. Her doctor therefore concluded that Can had lost all consciousness of the gravity of her crime and was therefore innocent, meriting confinement at the Biên Hòa asylum for continued treatment.[65]

Deviance from gender norms—and especially instances of openly challenging them—was also taken as evidence of insanity. In 1935, Nga, a twenty-three-year-old female patient, was brought to the Indigenous Hospital in Hanoi after causing a public disturbance.[66] She was described as having the "appearance of an eccentric," with a boy's haircut and sporting masculine clothes. Doctors observed that when left to her own devices, she would sing, imitating a masculine voice, aping all the attitudes of boys. She would also twist and wriggle, talk without stopping, and at times cry out without saying why. She would recount stories about her three sons, students at the local school, whom she would gaze at through the window as they studied. It was almost as if she wanted to be in their place but, as a woman, found herself excluded from pursuing further education. Nga's case file reported that she would clearly make up stories during her psychiatric examination, which would make her laugh as though she was "conscious of her lies." Together these symptoms painted the portrait of a compromised mental state that, in the eyes of her psychiatrist, made her dangerous to others and necessitated her confinement.

As for treatment, doctors administered a variety of drugs including sedatives and calming agents such as opium, chloral, and bromides.[67] They reported special success with the use of *somnifère*, a kind of sleeping agent administered by intravenous injections in the case of violent agitation. Its use resulted in the "absolute suppression" of mechanical forms of restraint such as the straitjacket that was used only as a last resort. The drug allowed asylum staff to equally avoid the "onerous use" of padded rooms, prohibitive in Cochinchina because of the "numerous parasites that would destroy even the best surfacing in a matter of hours."[68] Doctors also practiced certain forms of hydrotherapy, or the use of the physical properties of water such as temperature and pressure to calm nerves and stimulate blood circulation.[69] The construction of a large pool (20 meters by 50 meters, at a depth of 1 to 1.6 meters) with a sandy bottom allowed patients to clean themselves and play after they were finished working out of doors.[70] Meanwhile, those agitated patients not employed in asylum labor schemes would be enveloped in a damp sheet as a kind of calming device, an easy method that required

no additional installation and could be entrusted to the surveillance personnel, who proved themselves "perfectly comfortable with performing this
technique."[71]

Psychiatrists in Indochina also began to experiment with more intensive
forms of therapy, including treatment by shocks, which was becoming
increasingly popular in Europe and North America.[72] By the early 1930s,
somatic therapies represented the cutting edge of psychiatric treatment. The
idea behind shock therapy was to use a physical stimulus in order to provoke
a rise in body temperature and thereby jolt the brain—and the mind—out
of an illness state.[73] At Biên Hòa, colonial psychiatrists injected patients with
Dmelcos (also known as chancroid vaccine) and even milk![74] They tried out
paludotherapy—the use of the malarial vaccine for the treatment of ter-
tiary syphilis—but only with "extreme prudence." Despite or in some cases
because of the higher prevalence of malaria in Southeast Asia, colonial doctors feared that indigenous patients would be exposed to different kind of
risks than those patient populations of France and Europe. (The technique
had been abandoned altogether in Japan.) Doctors also injected cardiazol to
induce seizures as a treatment method for schizophrenia, a technique learned
from Dutch psychiatrists in Batavia. The interruption in the sourcing of cardiazol during the early years of World War II, coupled with the treatment's
dramatic side effects including cardiac arrest and irreversible coma, led colonial psychiatrists to experiment with electroshock therapy in its place. By
January of 1942, doctors at Biên Hòa had commenced electroshock treatment on fifty-five subjects of different races, ages, and genders. Thirty-eight
patients received the full treatment of ten or twelve sessions, totaling 390
induced seizures. Doctors reported some "very nice results" in the pages of
the Hanoi-based *Revue médicale française d'Extrême Orient* later that year—
achieving success previously not considered possible—and recommended its
more general use.[75] The enthusiasm for ECT in Indochina, similar to what
Richard Keller observed in French Algeria, "expose[d] a general pattern of
metropolitan caution and intense experimentation on the periphery."[76]

Learning from Biên Hòa

The growth in the demand for psychiatric care throughout the 1920s
exposed the defects in the original planning of Biên Hòa, but it also gave
new urgency to move forward with plans for a second asylum. The distance separating patients from their families, especially those arriving from
the north of the colony, was cited year after year as an inconvenience for
those family members who wished to visit the asylum as well as a major

disincentive to those who would do their best to hide patients rather than bring them in for care.[77] Stressing this point may have also proved strategic for Biên Hòa's asylum staff, who would benefit from the establishment of a sister institution that could absorb the rising numbers and costs of patients. The gaze therefore turned northward to Tonkin, where plans for a second asylum had been discussed since the turn of the century.[78] When in 1927 the proposal was taken up with renewed energy, the director of the health service in Tonkin requested Dr. André Augagneur, the director of the Biên Hòa asylum, to serve an advisory role.[79] Augagneur, a former clinical instructor at the Faculty of Medecine in Lyon, France, had attained the title of Commanding Doctor of the Colonial Troops. He served as the director of the Biên Hòa asylum between 1925 and 1933. In his capacity as adviser, Augagneur supplied the Tonkin administration with maps and blueprints, as well as advice on planning and organization. His guidance stemmed from difficult lessons learned during his tenure at Biên Hòa, revealing many of the early challenges of asylum management in the colony. In this way, Biên Hòa would serve as both model and cautionary tale for this next experiment in asylum care.

The first question facing the Tonkin administration concerned the physical placement of the institution, for which there were many requirements. The site must have easy access to water yet still be well protected from floods. It must also be flat, especially the area for patient pavilions, in order to facilitate surveillance. Proximity to an urban center (but not too close) would provide easy access to food supplies, hospitals, and laboratories and would ease recruitment of both European doctors and an indigenous medical and surveillance staff.[80] The dedicated plot must be large enough to accommodate space for the individual buildings and rice fields, which could be easily annexed to the asylum. This would have the "double advantage" of providing occupations to calm patients interned at the asylum. In terms of anticipating the future extension of the asylum, it made more sense to purchase a larger property straightaway than to buy adjacent territory later, at a high price. This was a hard-learned lesson for the Biên Hòa asylum, which found itself in constant need of expansion due to rapidly rising numbers of patient admissions and severity of overcrowding not anticipated by the original planners.[81] Expanding early would also have the immediate advantage of creating a "zone of protection" immediately surrounding the asylum, which would help prevent the smuggling of alcohol to patients and asylum staff, as well as minimize the distractions of noisy neighbors.[82] Finally, individual buildings should be separated by a distance of no less than thirty meters in order to improve surveillance.[83] Biên Hòa's asylum director and his family apparently found it impossible sleep on certain nights because of the cries of female patients, whose pavilion stood at a distance of only ten meters away.[84]

In Tonkin, colonial administrators fielded several proposals for sites for the establishment of the asylum, including a proposal to transform the Quảng Yên Hospital into an asylum for the mentally ill, blind, elderly, and incapacitated.[85] The director of health for Tonkin, Dr. de Raymond, suggested placing the asylum in close proximity to the Qua Cam leper village in Bắc Ninh province. The principal architect for the project agreed with

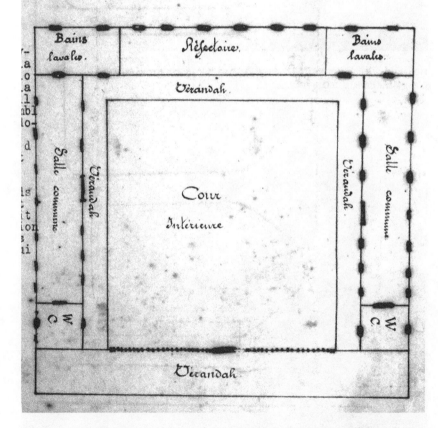

FIGURE 9. Plans for a U-shape pavilion, to be installed at the Vôi asylum in Tonkin, 1927. TTLTQG-1, 73750, Résidence Supérieur au Tonkin, Organisation et fonctionnement d'un Asile d'Aliénés à Bien-Hoa (Cochinchine), Note sur l'organisation générale d'un Asile d'Aliénés par le Dr. Augagneur, Médecin Directeur de l'Asile de Bien Hoa, 1927.

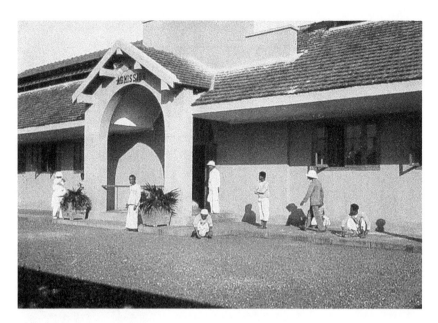

FIGURE 10. Admission building at the Vôi asylum, Tonkin. ANOM, "Assistance psychiatrique, Bac Giang (Asile de Voi)," ICO, 8 Fi-498.

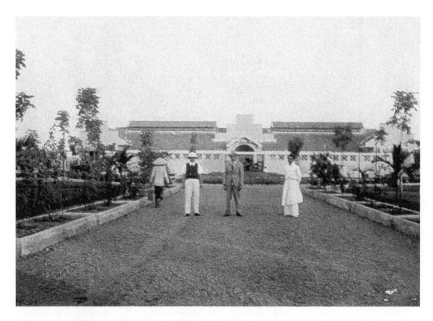

FIGURE 11. Inside courtyard of the Vôi asylum, Tonkin. ANOM, "Assistance psychiatrique, Bac Giang (Asile de Voi)," ICO, 8 Fi-498.

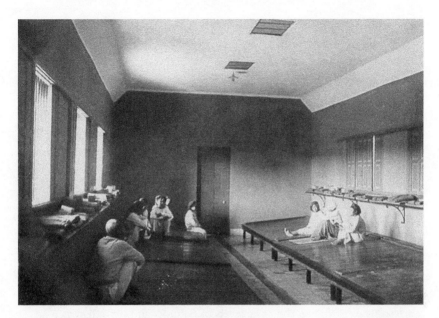

FIGURE 12.   Inside of a pavilion for "calm" Vietnamese patients at the Vôi asylum, Tonkin. ANOM, "Assistance psychiatrique, Bac Giang (Asile de Voi)," ICO, 8 Fi-498.

Raymond, especially given the possibility of annexing land for rice paddies on the opposite side of the road in direct view of the diverse pavilions that would comprise the establishment.[86] The neighboring leper village formed the only inconvenience. He suggested constructing a fence around its perimeter in order to avoid all contact between the lepers and the tranquil patients working in the neighboring fields.[87] The fact that this site was singled out in the first place reflects how these different projects for the care of the chronically ill and socially marginalized were linked in the colonial imagination. In the end, the colonial administration chose a site in Bắc Giang province in what proved to be a serious miscalculation. Construction started in 1928 with an anticipated finish date of 1930. Frequent delays, caused most notably by the discovery of a severe infestation of malaria-carrying mosquitoes in the local area, pushed the opening of the asylum back to 1934.[88]

While the project may have appeared "ill-fated" from the beginning, to borrow Raymond's words, the plans for Vôi carried forward.[89] In addition to choosing the site, the buildings where patients lived and received treatment would need to undergo a significant redesign. The admission building at Biên Hòa, for instance, was described as a "veritable heresy from a medical point of view," distinguished by "many tortuous corridors creating the ideal conditions by which patients could not be guarded and placed in obscurity."[90]

The peculiar setup of patient pavilions also made it very difficult to observe what happened inside. A watch room in the center of the pavilion separated two dormitories on either side, flanked by bathrooms and showers at the far edge of the building, out of sight of the guards in the very middle, and therefore the most common route for patient escapes. While during the daytime it was difficult for guards to keep track of those coming in and out of the dormitory, at night it was even more challenging. With only one window on either side of the central watch room looking onto the adjacent dormitories, and with the mosquito nets mounted above the beds blocking their view, the guards were not able to see past the first bed to the interior of the room.[91] Most pavilions also did not have proper ceilings, in spite of asylum regulations, resulting in a number of successful escape attempts whereby the patient climbed to the rafters and easily displaced the tiles to be set free. The heat in the pavilions reportedly became quite intense from the sun heating the tiles, which were placed in such a way that no breeze could enter to provide relief. The fact that patients were often found "jammed in" to these spaces only exacerbated the basic levels of comfort and surveillance.[92]

The problem of how best to "decongest" these buildings spoke to closely linked concerns over security and hygiene, as well as to the determination of the colonial administration to cut costs from the very beginning. Asylum buildings required constant repairs and upkeep: they were covered with defective tiles that became easily damaged during the rainy season, the hearth of the kitchen was fashioned out of ordinary brick instead of more heat-resistant material, and the maintenance of the septic system mounted a "heavy charge and an unenviable task for the workers, which could have been avoided if the construction of the water tower had been done less economically and doubled in size." The installation of a new system, compared with that of a few years earlier, would double the cost of the original system, not to mention the costs of continued upkeep.[93]

These mistakes served as a cautionary tale for the planners of the Vôi asylum. For the patient pavilions, Augagneur recommended abandoning the Biên Hòa model altogether. Instead he suggested that the Vôi asylum planners adopt a U-shaped model, which mandated the installation of multiple windows and a narrow verandah that circled the perimeter and allowed the watch guard to see in an instant the entirety of the pavilion. Such a design would prove "infinitely more practical" by allowing for a more comprehensive surveillance. The pavilion would include a dining hall that would double as an atelier to keep patients occupied with different kinds of work such as basket making and embroidery. During the dry season, those patients who were not employed in outside labor were able to rest comfortably in a new interior courtyard where one wall had been replaced with mostly iron bars, allowing the patients to look out. It also had the appreciable advantage of allowing those calm patients to rest "outdoors" at night during the summers.[94]

In order to ensure a continuous surveillance, Augagneur emphasized the importance of electric lamps protected by metal or unbreakable glass. Power outages were frequent at Biên Hòa, especially during the rainy season, when interruptions lasted minutes if not hours. In 1928 for example, 172 interruptions were counted, resulting in 244 blackout hours. While service marginally improved over the following years, as of 1933, there were still 95 outages a year (or 137 hours without service).[95] One of these outages led to a critical lapse in surveillance, resulting in a patient suicide.[96] Without access to a steady electric current, the asylum staff was often forced to use the asylum's power reserves to illuminate lamps on the property so that the pavilions could stay lit and patients would remain supervised. Electricity was also expensive, costing 6,000 francs per month on average. In order to conserve energy, the asylum staff increasingly sought to "modify the distribution so as to only allow those lamps strictly essential for the guards to stay illuminated" and rotate throughout the asylum space. Doing so, they hoped, would reduce consumption of electricity by nearly a quarter. In 1926 asylum administrators had already began to express the hope for the negotiation of a better contract once the current one expired (in 1937) that would result in better rates and less frequent interruptions.

Concerns about pavilions for European patients centered less on surveillance and more on ensuring comfort. In turning his attention to lodgings for European patients, Augagneur stipulated that they should remain entirely separate from those for indigenous patients. European pavilions should consist of two sections, one male, one female, with each section including ten bedrooms (with a bath and water closet for every two rooms), its own dining room, a room for reading and games, and between the two sections a dedicated kitchen. A common room for physical education with hours reserved for men and women should also be provided as well as a large garden for walking.

Staff Worries

In 1931, three doctors, including one French asylum director and two Vietnamese medical residents, cared for 580 patients at the Biên Hòa asylum. While their service was lauded for assuring the daily function of the asylum in an "irreproachable fashion and with zeal and devotion worthy of praise," the job had nevertheless become "more and more burdensome, [with doctors] working for four years without interruption."[97] In his annual report to the colonial administration, the asylum director drew on details of a British asylum in Rangoon to illustrate by contrast the paucity of caretakers in Indochina's asylums.[98] The demands of a fast-growing patient population proved challenging not only to the asylum's medical experts but also to the large Vietnamese staff charged with the day-to-day functioning of the asylum. Their duties were complex and onerous: to ensure a well-regulated institution that provided protection and security for patients; to balance firmness with compassion, moral qualities with technical expertise; and to exert oversight of others while also subjected to disciplinary action by their superiors. Tasked with providing care and oversight of others below, asylum staff also endured recriminations from above. The oversight of the surveillance staff itself, rather than solely that of the patients, emerged as a crucial question of asylum management.[99]

At issue was not just how to grow the staff but also how to prevent excessive staff turnover.[100] Low pay and relative isolation were blamed for the successive and rapid passage of doctors, rendering the asylum, "a little favored post where one wants to spend as little time as possible." The asylum suffered when "at the precise moment he acquires a good practice of psychiatry, the doctor leaves his post."[101] Vietnamese doctors apparently also considered the position a disgrace, given the distance of Biên Hòa from the city center, and did everything in their power to transfer. At the moment they had received the requisite training in psychiatry to be useful and had grown acquainted with their patients, they were gone. Recruitment efforts at Biên Hòa were further hampered by competition from other higher-paying jobs.[102] This held equally true for both medical experts and the surveillance staff, whose recruitment was characterized as "very mediocre, the good ones having been taken by plantations who offer much more interesting salaries than those we could offer."[103] As one asylum director put it, "20 specialized wardens are worth more to patient surveillance than 25 *ignorants* who do not accept the work to which they are obliged."[104]

Staff issues jeopardized not only the quality of care of patients but also possibilities for their surveillance. The night service—charged with policing asylum grounds between the hours of six at night and six in the morning—particularly suffered.[105] Because of deficiencies in staff numbers, at the end of their overnight tour many night guards worked the day shift. Deprived of sufficient rest, guards were permitted to bring material for sleeping such as mats, pillows, and covers to their overnight post, a measure that only "tempt[ed] the weak" and resulted in some "unfortunate errors over the years."[106] As the 1927 report from Biên Hòa noted, "It has taken two years of efforts to arrive at the point where the night watch does not fall asleep."[107] While the number of guards at Biên Hòa rose steadily throughout the 1920s, reaching a maximum number of seventy-eight in 1930 (to serve 532 patients), by 1933 the number of guards had been reduced to sixty-seven, although the total number of patients had risen to 658.[108]

Asylum directors were often frustrated in their attempts to recruit and maintain a competent nursing staff. A 1931 report noted that, with rare exceptions, the nursing staff proved generally to give the "minimum efforts with the maximum pretensions." Serving "with regret in a post they consider without interest, they are only ephemeral guests at the asylum; one might say they resemble those who are making a holiday in a country that bores them." Apparently they considered their role as "one limited to providing a vague kind of oversight, making their work fall to those in the personnel of surveillance." Meanwhile their technical education and understanding of French remained very limited and, in some cases, "it is to be demanded if during their internship [stage] they are given the least notion of order and asepsis."[109] In general, asylum directors preferred recruiting nurses after they had completed an internship in a hospital or clinic and received their professional certification after passing exams, if not for their advanced knowledge at least for acquiring a more realistic set of expectations. Whereas a student who had completed a stage before entering the profession knew more or less what to expect, those admitted to school with a simple certificate arrived largely ignorant of the demands and inconveniences of the profession. As the same 1931 report underscored in reference to their poorly performing nurse staff, "Even if some are satisfied, a good portion will not continue their studies with great zeal, or do so only grudgingly, without knowing why. Assigned to a provincial health service after their exit from school, they arrive with exaggerated pretensions imbued with the superiority that they believe to have because of their diploma. They work like amateurs without enthusiasm."[110]

Confronted with an inadequately trained and poorly motivated nursing staff, asylum directors began to look for solutions elsewhere. At various points they proposed promoting male and female guards, or *surveillant(e)s*, to the hybrid position of *infirmier-surveillant* based on seniority and performance. They hoped such measures—an honorific gesture at first, later accompanied by an increase of salary—would introduce a new level of economy and result in a more permanent cohort who possessed the requisite knowledge for working in the special conditions of an asylum.[111] The idea was not exactly groundbreaking. While in theory the asylum staff divided into distinct medical and surveillance units, in practice their functions overlapped substantially. Guards were responsible for the general upkeep and orderliness of patient quarters as well as the provision of meals, the supervision of patient labor, and the surveillance of asylum grounds at night. Every morning they would register observations about the patients in a notebook, including complaints and demands from the patients themselves, which the asylum director then reviewed. Those patients signaled by the guards as needing medical attention were then brought to the infirmary.

In 1924 the colonial government put into force an official decree to improve and standardize the recruitment of a special indigenous corps of asylum guards. The decree's language reflected what were considered the special demands of asylum work.[112] Declared unlike any other branch of the colonial administration, the occupation of asylum guard was described as particularly delicate. At once in the service of patients, the guards were also tasked with enforcing their obedience. For this reason, it was important to recruit personnel of high moral quality. "To win the confidence of the patient in order to then direct him, to order him in such a way as to think that the direction and order are in his interest, is an often difficult task that requires much patience and devotion."[113] Given the influence they held over the patients, guards played a critical role in the treatment and rehabilitation process. They were required to be conscientious, attentive, and capable of discerning the particular needs of patients while also treating them with gentleness, patience, tact, and firmness. Their task proved undoubtedly "arduous . . . delicate and extremely tiring as the least weakness, the least negligence, might result in a serious accident. This is why the number of guard stuff must be increased and their situation improved."[114]

According to the 1924 decree, an asylum guard must be a French colonial subject, follow a "good life" and exhibit morals that could be verified by a clean criminal record, and demonstrate his or her physical capacity to restrain others. Preference was given to former military personnel. Hired guards would first assume a temporary post, after which they were expected to finish a one-year stage and, upon its completion, join the local health service with a permanent position. Those who proved inept or badly behaved would face a range of penalties including restriction to asylum grounds for a period of one to ten days, the noting of an official warning in their dossier with the possible delay of promotion by one year, or a demotion or dismissal.[115] While on duty, their uniform consisted of khaki pants and a jacket with badges embroidered "AB" (shorthand for Asile de Biên Hòa) in yellow cotton. The chief wardens wore stripes in silver in a reversed V pattern to indicate their seniority, while ordinary guards wore stripes in yellow cotton also in the form of a reversed V. The female guards wore a blouse in white khaki with a single band of yellow linen across the chest; female chief wardens wore two bands.

Despite the introduction of the decree, and with the exception of a "few very good agents," the average guards in the service of the Biên Hòa asylum remained mediocre at best, and the kind of care they provided was alternately described as "coarse" and "repulsive." Apparently, in the words of one dispirited asylum director, "certain employees considered their occupation as closer to that of a guard in the penitentiary service."[116] As asylum directors deliberately recruited their surveillance staff from among former prison guards, this is hardly surprising. Soon the asylum administration began to strongly crack down on staff violations and to pursue severe sentences for any brutalities inflicted on patients.[117] While the indigenous personnel "must be submitted to a necessary purification" in order to obtain an effective surveillance, the problem could not be fixed by removing bad eggs alone. It was also undoubtedly a problem of education. Biên Hòa's 1926 annual report cites the work of the famous American physician and medical reformer Oliver Wendell Homes, who described the chronic patient as a "vampire sucking the blood of able-bodied people. While this opinion is a bit exaggerated it can, however, be applied in part to the mentally ill. To make a guard understand that the aliéné whom he harasses, without leaving him a moment of respite is a patient, that is the most difficult thing above all, especially in this relatively primitive country where the spirit of devotion and solidarity only appears to be in its faint beginnings."[118]

By 1927, asylum directors began to organize frequent conferences in order "to make the staff understand that the patient is not a convict and that he is a patient and it is therefore important to be patient, gentle and devoted."[119] An ideal asylum guard should possess the following qualities:

1—Absolute respect for the discipline of the establishment, a strict discipline being indispensable for the good functioning of the asylum;

2—To be "well-balanced" in order to be capable of occupying a special milieu made up of diverse kinds of patients, those who are unclean whom it is necessary to bathe incessantly, others who are violent, turbulent, vindictive, malcontent or insidious;

3—Able to exercise a constant surveillance during long periods of time, a surveillance that is often very thankless as a result of long periods of inaction;

4—Rigorous cleanliness on account of frequent contact with patients suffering from contagious disease, syphilis and tuberculosis;

5—Absolute discretion as much toward the patients as those strangers to the service;

6—To maintain authority, not to impose oneself brutally on the patients but to have an air of letting him follow by guiding;

7—To be courageous; the situations which demand this quality are most often unexpected and also very frequent.[120]

These principles rejected violence and mechanical restraint in favor of displays of kindness, gentleness, and watchfulness.[121] Expected to serve as models of behavior for patients, guards and the question of their recruitment forced asylum directors to articulate exactly what a good model should look like and in so doing revealed deep ambivalences about the racial hierarchy within the asylum. While at first guards who could read and write French were preferred, asylum administrators ultimately found them to be "in general pretentious and not very hardworking." It would now be better to recruit guards who could read and write *quốc ngữ* (the romanized Vietnamese script) only and who also possessed useful skills such as mason, carpenter, basket maker, weaver or farmer. In short, those occupations geared toward physical as opposed to intellectual labor.[122] Furthermore, the delicacies of guaranteeing surveillance in a "mixed asylum," especially in those cases when the use of physical force proved necessary, posed a special kind of challenge. Vietnamese guards charged with the oversight of European patients found themselves placed "in an awkward position because they did not have any authority over the European patient, even if he was mentally ill; on the other hand, the weak constitution of the indigenous guard does not allow him, most of the time, to take control of the agitated European who possesses a certain physical force." In order to remedy the awkwardness of this situation, the head of Indochina's health service proposed the creation of a new position for a European male attendant, "whose force and constitution, combined with the prestige of his race, can naturally impose on this category of patients."[123]

With the elimination of "certain undesirables," little by little the service at Biên Hòa began to improve. Salary increases also helped staff recruitment given the relatively high cost of living outside Saigon.[124] Female guards who performed the same work, took the same risks, and faced the same worries as men, not to mention the fact that female patients were apparently "often much more disagreeable than the stronger sex," saw their salaries improve to match those of their male counterparts in 1925.[125] Soon thereafter, the service of the women guards was considered "much better assured" than that that of the male guards.[126] Asylum administrators also proposed new

bonuses for guards as necessary incentives for advancement within the institution.[127]

Despite some success in establishing a "friendly collaboration" between
the surveillance staff and patients, there was still much to be done to improve
the moral character of the asylum's Vietnamese employees.[128] The lack of
attention to detail, born of a casualness and frivolity and "childlike silliness,"
posed considerable impediments to a more efficient service.[129] Even so, as
one asylum report stressed, "From the purely psychological point of view it
is remarkable to witness how easy it is to influence and train the indigenous
personnel. The spirit of a 'sheep herder' must not be lost from view." The
creation of a new position for an officer who would be charged with maintaining a vigilant discipline among the guards offered one potential fix.[130]

The staff's affection for gambling proved especially worrisome. In 1926
asylum administrators went to the extent of surrounding the lodgings for
the guards with wire fencing (exactly as they did with patients) in order to
separate each building, making participation in popular nightly card games
more difficult.[131] While the asylum administrators may have eventually succeeded in suppressing gambling inside the asylum, they found themselves
largely unable to prevent their staff from playing outside its walls. Solicited
by the "unrepentant" and notorious managers of local bars and inns, those
guards who spent their nights gambling also tended to indulge in "profound
napping" during the day. There was also the disconcerting presence of debt
collectors who waited at the asylum's door on paydays.[132]

Asylum administrators also proposed improvements to the quality of life
at the asylum so that the staff would not seek distractions elsewhere. This
was not an easy task as "one is obliged to stimulate them constantly."[133] General instruction courses for staff in written and spoken French were offered,
as well as a series of special night courses for the professional development of
guards and medical personnel alike.[134] Administrators organized film screen-
ings and constructed a library and two tennis courts, funded by the collection of dues from the personnel themselves. A nursery and school allowed
for the supervision of the children of female guards for much of the workday
(about thirty children attended the school in 1928).[135]

In this way we see the deliberate attempt to fashion the asylum as a world
unto itself, a world that replicated many of the same features of colonial society but in miniature. The physical separation of pavilions for indigenous and
European patients and the creation of parallel psychiatric regimes—one premised on work and surveillance, the other on comfort and convalescence—
reflected colonial racial ideology. And yet, much as in the world outside its
walls, these hierarchies within the space of asylum were constantly being

undone by tight budgets and unruly employees, misbehaving subjects and crumbling infrastructure. Pressures on psychiatric institutions pushed down from above but also bubbled up from below.

System under Pressure

By 1933, Biên Hòa housed 660 patients, well over twice the 300 patients for which it was originally designed. Awaiting the much delayed opening of the Vôi asylum in Tonkin, as well as badly needed improvements to Biên Hòa itself, asylum directors warned the colonial government they would soon have no choice but to refuse patients whose confinement was demanded by their families. Such a predicament would lead only to dire—perhaps even fatal—consequences.[136] As it stood, they had trouble maintaining order and effecting a rational treatment of patients depending on their mental and physical state. The surveillance commission charged with Biên Hòa's oversight routinely emphasized this point in its annual reports to the colonial administration. Composed of a diverse array of French and Vietnamese elites—including among others a judge, doctor, engineer, lawyer, entrepreneur, and philosophy professor—the commission made regular visits to the asylum, where its members witnessed firsthand the breakdown in psychiatric classification.[137] Asylum regulations mandated a "partitioning and absolute separation" between patients according to different racial, gender, and diagnostic categories, including the "calm, agitated, epileptic, senile and recovering, as well as those antisocial types under criminal investigation."[138] Despite official pronouncements, the director of the health service in Cochinchina complained about the lack of space at the asylum, which meant that patients were "literally crammed together and [slept] on mats on the floor in an unhealthy promiscuity."[139]

The "uneasy" surveillance that resulted from overcrowding clearly unnerved Biên Hòa's surveillance commission, which complained about the presence of an excessive number of patients in the common room, leading to "bloody confrontations. . . . In trying to separate these 'brother enemies,' the personnel, to whom falls the responsibility of reestablishing good order, are exposed to the danger of being struck and hurt."[140] A rise in the number of agitated male and female patients, who, given the absence of a sufficient number of dedicated pavilions, mixed freely with the rest of the patient population, exacerbated an already fragile situation. The risk to patients was made worse by mixing with the criminal element of the patient population (those acquitted by reason of insanity and sent to psychiatric care instead of the prison). Contrary to the regulations set forth by the 1930 law, the asylum's thirteen female criminal patients continued to be lodged in various pavilions with ordinary patients. By 1934, the sole pavilion dedicated to male criminal patients reached almost double the original intended capacity, topping out at 79.[141] Patient overcrowding led to concerns over security but also worries over the increased risks for the spread of disease. The infirmary, for example, desperately required improvements, including the addition of an isolation pavilion for contagious patients. Apparently many tuberculosis patients lounged about in the common rooms, putting others at risk.

Patient Protest

> They tell me that I am crazy. It is false. I never did anything extravagant.
> I did not strike anyone. They insulted me and were violent with me and
> I retaliated. They were unjust in my regard and I protested against the
> arbitrariness [of their treatment]. They concluded that I lost my mind.
> (Patient case file, Huân, 1938)[142]

Asylum directors felt the pressure from surveillance commissions, but they also faced resistance from patients. Voices of patient protest, gleaned from the pages of case files, offer a narrative of resistance against unjust confinement that challenges official accounts of due process, scientific expertise, and the protection of public security. Not only do these voices give us privileged insight into a patient's experience, both within and outside the walls of the asylum, but they often expose the underlying gaps in knowledge and weaknesses in surveillance that plagued the asylum administration. Huân, a thirty-eight- year-old farmer, strongly opposed the terms of his confinement and even tried to escape, using a piece of broken glass to upend the tiles under his cell door. While eventually recaptured, he counted as one of ten patients who attempted escape from Vôi in 1938 alone.[143] For his doctors, Huân's unsuccessful bid for freedom only served to confirm his mentally ill status despite his protests to the contrary.

Patient protests, while interpreted as a symptom of mental illness, also served as an index of insecurity, both for the patient confined against his will and for the doctor whose authority he openly opposed. Take the example of Lâm, a thirty-nine-year-old courthouse clerk in Hanoi. In June 1932, he began to write alarmed letters to the colonial administration, offering information on illicit schemes by European bureaucrats and their Vietnamese accomplices to embezzle government money. He claimed he was now the target of a vast conspiracy to silence him, authored by his family and his wife's family, a campaign coordinated across "all five regions of the Indochinese

Union" by a "society the most secret, the most powerful, the most rich, the most savage and the most dangerous for public security for Annam and for the Franco-Vietnamese collaboration."[144] On March 6, 1933, against his will, Lâm entered Lanessan military hospital in Hanoi for observation. Two weeks later, Dr. Naudin, the resident psychiatric expert who oversaw Lanessan's neuropsychiatric clinic, offered the following diagnosis: "delirious ideas of hypochondriasm and persecution, *psycho-motrices* and *psycho-sensorielles* hallucinations, a leaning toward language and above all pathological writings, a progressive systematization of delirium and the beginning of a penchant for defensive reactions."[145]

When we read Lâm's own handwritten letters, however, an alternative patient perspective of this clinical encounter comes into view. Lâm instead relates how on the day of his arrival at the hospital, Goirau, the doctor in charge of treatment, "after examining me, said that 'My health is good' and told me after a long consultation that 'He is sure that [I have] no mental illness.'" When relating these interactions, Lâm carefully specifies the race and rank of his doctors; he also describes the others present in the room who bore witness to these encounters. Lâm further reports that during his time at the hospital, which constituted the better part of four months, Dr. Naudin, whom he refers to as a "specialist of the brain," visited him only twice in quick succession. After both visits, Naudin simply said to wait a few days while waiting for the results of the medical exam but otherwise did not indicate "anything abnormal in my speech." Quite the opposite, in Lâm's telling, Naudin described his deameanor as "absolutely calm, courteous and respectful," marked by a "tranquil conscience, good sense and reasonable logic." At the end of March, after being told he could finally leave for good, Lâm describes his utter surprise when, suddenly, "several European nurses closed me into a cell in the insane wing, despite my explanations and reasoning."[146]

In the first fifteen days of his confinement, from March 27 to April 10, Lâm refused to eat or drink. After a week, soldiers and nurses came into his cell to force him into a straitjacket. He decried the arbitrary and "cruelly unjust" terms of his detention and, upon viewing the order for his provisional confinement at the hospital, accused Naudin of having falsified his medical certificate and thereby "compromised the prestige of the medical corps." Lâm proceeded to offer all sorts of proof of his sanity: testimonies provided by various doctors, nurses, and guards (both European and Vietnamese) regarding his intelligence and "irreproachable conduct." He emphasized his role as a loyal bureacrat who had "always given satisifaction to my bosses." Lâm also claimed his own letters as evidence of his sanity; indeed, it is possible, given the meticulous level of detail with which they were written, that he had this very argument in mind from the beginning. "The state of my brain which permitted me to make this request and demonstrate in a mathematical way the false nature of the medical certificate in question largely proves not only that I am not suffering from mental alienation a thousand times over but also that I have . . . not even light mental troubles or the least imbalance [*désequlibremment*] of the brain." His doctors claimed the opposite—that in their content and in their volume, the letters provided clear proof of his insanity. The letter writing itself was declared "pathological," as noted in his medical certificate.[147]

Moreover, the inconsistency of expert opinions exposed the fragile scientific basis for his confinement. On March 31, for instance, Lâm writes, "Guirau told me 'You aren't crazy' but three months later, he told me that I am crazy." During this period, Guirau allegedly called Lam into his office to serve as an interpreter and declared, "You will teach me Vietnamese." The implication of this anecdote is clear—why would the doctor make such a request of a mentally ill person? Lam also learned that the results of his medical exams, including a lumbar puncture, were "excellent" and "prove[d] that I don't have a brain disease." Lâm even charged that during his entire stay at the hospital, he received no medical care. These facts all added up to insurmountable proof that the information provided on the medical certificate was, in his words, "absolutely false."[148]

Lâm charged that he presented no security threat but rather it was his doctors, in collusion with his family, who presented the real danger; in locking him up, they tried to push him to the edge to commit suicide. However, it is clear from his family's reaction that there is yet another story at play. His wife, Phuc, requested his release in late June, and his brother made the same request a week later. Phuc claimed that Lâm fell sick as a result of mental exhaustion caused by his job with the colonial courts; in her words, he worked "too conscientiously." She did not dispute his illness but nevetheless emphasized that Lâm did not betray any signs of violence during his confinement and argued that only the joy and care a family could provide would greatly hasten his cure.[149] As a result of these petitions, the family succesfully delayed Lâm's transfer to the asylum until the administration of a new mental exam. The original diagnosis was eventually confirmed, and he was sent away.

While the 1930 law may have helped to formalize the procedures surrounding the confinement of patients, it also multiplied the pressure points where doctors, patients, judicial officials, and family members could stake their own claims about expertise, morality, and the function of law. Lâm interpreted his experience as one of a victim of a vast conspiracy, while his doctors claimed he suffered from "persecutory delusions" that could turn violent. It is possible, likely even, that neither tells the entire story and that the "truth" of this encounter is better realized in the presentation of multiple, fractured, sometimes overlapping and, at other times, conflicting viewpoints. Lâm's sense of persecution and his "penchant for defensive encounters," as noted in his medical certificate, perhaps speak to deeper anxieties about the colonial encounter being filtered through these two-way exchanges between a Vietnamese patient and a French doctor. Indeed, a sense of precarity lingers throughout much of this file, a feeling that remains unresolved long after Lâm's transfer to Biên Hòa in August of 1933. Months later, he persisted in writing letters of protest to the colonial administration.

Patients like Lâm most acutely suffered from the precarity produced by their social marginalization. Yet nurses, guards, and doctors—both Vietnamese and French—who confronted violently mentally ill patients were also made vulnerable by the conditions of their workplace marked by insufficient space and inadequate resources. Much of what drove the daily experience of psychiatric confinement must therefore be understood less through the prism of rational treatment than through the calculus of risk management.

Continuing challenges

The opening of the Vôi asylum in 1934 did immediately relieve some pressure on Biên Hòa after two sets of patients were dispatched north in July that same year and again in February 1935.[150] Even so, administrators cautioned that it did not become any less necessary to create specialized psychiatric services in hospitals across all parts of the colony.[151] Biên Hòa remained overpopulated, especially among the population of "indigent natives" whose families were unable contribute to their upkeep, thereby exacerbating the institution's financial difficulties. Biên Hòa's administrators insisted on the necessity of constructing another asylum in Cambodia. By 1934, the asylum housed seventy-three Cambodian patients, including sixty-three men and ten women. Furthermore, as one asylum director put it, "for Cambodian patients, to find themselves in a milieu that is more conformed to their moral and cultural traditions, where they will not feel exiled like at Biên Hòa, will right away act as a favorable influence on their morale and facilitate their psychiatric rehabilitation." In the meantime, Biên Hòa hired Cambodian guards as a way to provide a unique kind of comfort to their Cambodian patients as well as to train them for future employment at the new asylum in Cambodia, which eventually opened in January of 1940.[152]

Vôi meanwhile continued to grow well beyond its theoretical capacity of 300 patients. By 1937, asylum directors counted 424 patients in their care.[153] A report issued by Vôi's oversight commission subsequently discovered many of the same problems that had plagued Biên Hòa over the years:

> The buildings that exist now and those that are in the process of being constructed will together turn out to be clearly insufficient after the completion of the works. The patients are piled up like prisoners in common rooms in contempt of any kind of psychiatric classification: the epileptics are neighbors with the senile, the impulsives with the depressed. This situation, due to the lack of space, is very detrimental to their well-being. Despite the construction of new pavilions, it remains impossible to classify the patients by their mental categories. . . . Rooms will be needed where each patient will have his own bed, doctors to supplement the present staff, able to take on the specialized services, a laboratory and annexed pharmacy.[154]

Even the shift in official nomenclature from "asylum" to the more modern classification of "psychiatric hospital" in 1937 could not mask the grave problems that continued to plague asylums in colonial Vietnam.[155] Cramped quarters, the deterioration of physical buildings, constrained budgets, and the poor caliber of the asylum's staff all required a certain amount of flexibility and improvisation on the part of asylum directors. That financial imperatives routinely trumped the dangers of overcrowding and category mixing was not a unique feature of colonial asylums. In his study of the colonial prison system in Indochina, which suffered from many of the same structural problems, Peter Zinoman understands the failure to invest in colonial prisons as evidence of the "relative weakness of the disciplinary impulse within the colonial project as a whole."[156] Here I suggest an alternative reading: frustrations over the lack of funding at their disposal forced colonial psychiatrists to innovate and seek opportunities to elaborate their field's disciplinary impulse outside the physical walls of the institution. Under tough circumstances, asylum administrators tried to make do by blurring the functions of guards and nurses, expanding the different pay grades of patients, and improving the design of patient pavilions. By the 1930s, they also came to rely on open psychiatric services in major hospitals and family care in the community, as well as agricultural colonies attached to asylum grounds, as a way to ease overcrowding and generate important sources of revenue. In their attempts to bring their institutions into line, however, asylum directors drew mental hospitals into increasingly unpredictable and unwieldy networks of care and economy.

CHAPTER 3

Labor as Therapy

Agricultural Colonies, Study Trips, and the Psychiatric Reeducation of the Insane

Hampered by budgetary constraints and an unruly staff, psychiatrists in colonial Vietnam nevertheless insisted that the function of the asylum should be more than one of just a *garderie*, or child's nursery, where patients were kept indefinitely with no hope of cure. Instead they argued that there was a role for experts in treating chronic patients as well as those suffering from more acute forms of mental illness. Therapeutic solutions were sought in the development of pharmaceuticals, but they were also located in older strategies that relied on the calming power of outdoor labor. This chapter examines how rural spaces, mental health, and productive work were reimagined in the everyday life of the colonial asylum. Drawing on a rich psychiatric discourse in the metropole about the virtues of patient employment and lessons learned from their study trips to Java, first in 1904–5 and again in 1916–17 and 1937, French experts in Indochina designed the colony's asylums as large agricultural colonies where patients could work the land on the path to healing and eventual liberation. In spite of its early origins, the *colonie agricole* seemed to offer colonial psychiatrists a modern conception of psychiatric care that promised not only "cerebral hygiene" and discipline through physical labor but also, in simulating the appearance of freedom and normal life, a kind of moral reeducation.

By integrating the economy of asylum care within the wider regional economy, agricultural colonies could also yield significant financial and administrative benefits to the asylums themselves. The agricultural colony can therefore be considered not only a site for discipline but also a model of capitalist production driven by the demands of a largely agrarian plantation economy that promoted the exploitation of labor. Annual asylum reports reveal the ways in which psychiatrists in Indochina framed the therapeutic and economic imperatives for labor and how they came to articulate a vision of psychiatric rehabilitation that blurred the distinctions between patients and laborers, between spaces of confinement and release. In simulating real life outside the walls of the asylum, the agricultural colony was designed to create a kind of continuity between the discipline of institutional order and social life in the community. In so doing, it provided patients with a path to rehabilitation and colonial psychiatrists with the challenge of articulating a vision of what the aims and forms of this kind of rehabilitation should look like.

This chapter therefore takes us one step further away from the heart of the institution by examining those liminal spaces of patient labor that orbited the asylum's grounds. It also follows French psychiatrists as they traveled along their own transimperial orbits within Southeast Asia in ways that vitally shaped their patients' experiences of asylum care. Early study trips went far toward establishing Southeast Asia in the minds of indigenous and colonial experts alike as a coherent entity, a shared object of knowledge that could be investigated, managed, and exploited using similar methods. For French and Dutch physicians caring for the insane, these insights informed critical assumptions about the possibility of transferring therapeutic labor regimes across empires and the development of a specifically regional knowledge of psychiatry.

Lessons from Abroad

In 1898, Dr. Edouard Jeanselme, a professor of medicine in Paris and expert in tropical diseases, took an extensive research trip to the Far East, traveling to Indochina, Yunnan, Thailand, Java, Burma, and Singapore. Appointed by the French ministers of education and the colonies to study the means of reducing the incidence of leprosy in the French colonies, he soon broadened his mission to include investigations of other diseases, including beriberi, syphilis, and mental illness. During his travels, Jeanselme made special note of Java's mental asylum at Buitenzorg (today's Bogor), where the Dutch colonial administration had established an asylum surrounded by a large agricultural colony in 1882. Writing in the *Presse Médicale* on his return, Jeanselme marveled that despite the absence of any restraint or coercion,

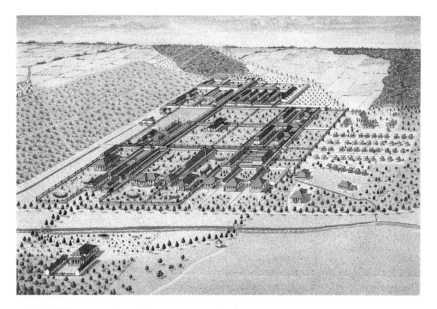

FIGURE 13.   Overview of the insane asylum near Buitenzorg. Lithograph from around 1890. KITLV/ Royal Netherlands Institute of Southeast Asian and Caribbean Studies, Leiden. Image 50N8. Leiden University Library.

there had been "no suicide, murder, or even escape, meanwhile the asylum is not enclosed by walls."[1] Buitenzorg represented the first systematic application of this kind of care for the insane in Southeast Asia in which the principles of moral treatment, and especially the use of labor as therapy, featured most prominently.

For Jeanselme, this research trip underscored the rudimentary state of mental health care in the French empire as compared with that of other colonial powers whose programs were, he warned, "growing more and more refined every day."[2] At the time, the Dutch boasted the highest number of available places in psychiatric institutions per capita in all of South Asia and Southeast Asia.[3] For French physicians in charge of psychiatric institutions in Indochina who saw in neighboring Java fundamental ethnological and geographical similarities, Dutch successes signified the prospect of incorporating many of the same practices within their colony's first asylum, Biên Hòa.

Jeanselme's voyage to the East Indies was one of several study trips French experts undertook (and would continue to undertake) to the Dutch colony. Between 1891 and 1904 no fewer than twenty-five French study missions visited colonial Indonesia. These fact-finding journeys surveyed everything from the management of the métis population and the specifics of grafting rubber trees to the linguistic and legal training of Dutch bureaucrats and the creation of botanical gardens. In fact, this story is part of a much older tradition of French interest in the Malayan world that long predates official French colonization in the region. From 1878 to 1886, for example, a group of scholars founded the *Annales de l'Extrême-Orient*, which was dedicated to the Indonesian archipelago and Malaysia, as well as India and Indochina. The French restoration of Angkor Wat relied on techniques developed by the Dutch to preserve their own colonial ruins in Central Java, in particular the Borobudur and the Prambanan temples.[4]

French officials clearly felt they had something to learn. Even as they criticized the Dutch for failing to espouse any sort of colonial ideology tantamount to a civilizing mission, French accounts nevertheless generally presented a rose-colored picture of the Dutch as benign and effective bureaucrats. In his 1900 work entitled *Java and Its Inhabitants* (*Java et ses habitants*), Joseph Chailley-Bert, then director of the French Colonial Union, emphasized the utility of looking to France's rivals for models that could be adapted to suit French needs. He wrote in the preface, "Why pretend to invent when the invention already exists? Much better to look around us; I add: even to look behind us."[5] France's own colonial past, as well as the accomplishments of rival empires, could prove useful. Chailley-Bert's project of what he termed a "comparative colonialism" underscores the importance of the development of new forms of transnational and transcolonial expertise that were seen as vital in administering the empire.[6]

When French physicians sought to expand institutional care for the insane in Indochina, they did not look to other parts of their own empire. Instead, they traveled to the Dutch East Indies to study what they saw as an effective model of modern psychiatric care.[7] What attracted Jeanselme and others was the effective use of labor as the primary form of treatment for indigenous patients—successful in reducing agitation, restlessness, and outbursts of violence among patients, in promoting beneficial agricultural productivity among them, and, additionally in the eyes of thrifty colonial administrators, in reducing expenses and generating income for institutions. With the expansion of plantation economies in the region, institutions that transformed troublesome "natives" into productive colonial subjects appeared unusually promising to both Dutch and French colonial administrations. The story of how French experts came to be interested in Dutch practices does not fit within the narrative typically told by historians of colonial science and medicine, which tends to emphasize the relationship of metropolis to colony as the most important axis of inquiry. By contrast, this chapter draws those forms of interimperial scientific exchange that have received little albeit growing attention in the historiography, especially among scholars of colonial Africa and the Caribbean.[8]

Throughout the late nineteenth and early twentieth centuries, the agricultural colony model proliferated throughout Southeast Asia as penal colonies for political prisoners, reformatories for juvenile delinquents, and sites for the occupational training of poor white settlers and for the rehabilitation of the mentally ill.[9] The Dutch experiment at Buitenzorg was part of an international flourishing of agricultural colonies and other forms of "open door" psychiatric care that spread throughout France, England, Belgium and Germany, as well as to the United States, Canada, Argentina, Japan, and Norway in the late nineteenth and early twentieth centuries.[10] The establishment of these *colonies agricoles*, or small farms attached to psychiatric hospitals, first emerged in Europe as a response to broader calls for psychiatric reform dating from the mid-nineteenth century. With mounting concerns over asylum overcrowding and accusations of patient negligence, psychiatrists began to experiment with alternative forms of patient care that relied on new uses of space and the environment; instead of chaining or isolation cells, psychiatric reformers argued that putting people to work in the fields, in the open air, would be more humane and therapeutically effective. Fresh air, sunlight, and exercise gave labor a moral dimension, one that coincided well with the new emphasis on treating the psychological and emotional causes of mental illness, otherwise known as "moral treatment."

At the heart of discussions about the uses of labor as therapy was actually a much older idea rooted in antiurban discourses and a vogue for experimental farms dating from the early 19th century. The first colonies agricoles were introduced in France as rural outlets for a revolutionary urban underclass and as penal colonies for orphans and juvenile delinquents, including the famous colony of Mettray. Early discussions about the colonies were marked by a condemnation of urban, industrial society and a countervailing valorization of the countryside as a site for the restoration of authority, order, and social discipline in the wake of the 1848 revolutions throughout Europe. Reformers embraced these agrarian utopias but for reasons that went beyond an appreciation of their aesthetic or romantic qualities. As the French historian Ceri Crossley writes, "Rurality was not so much emblematic of an earlier, simpler world as constitutive of a passive citizenry. This was not the countryside as escapism: agricultural work—with religion in support—was understood as a process of socialization."[11] As a model of socialization, the agricultural colony was premised on a set of distinctions between urban and rural life that guided psychiatric reformers in their efforts to rehabilitate abnormal populations. In contrast to the disorienting effects of city life, the agricultural colony would instead provide patients with a "life out of doors" and a daily routine structured around principles of regular exercise and discipline. A reorganization of the external social world would produce a reordering of the interior private one.[12]

Nineteenth-century reformers believed that rather than confinement itself, it was the act of working that would transform the criminal, destitute, and mentally ill into industrious, disciplined, and fully integrated members of society.[13] The introduction of labor in asylums in early nineteenth-century France also promised its own kind of moral transcendence, allowing the mentally ill to regain not only their sanity but also, in so doing, the ability to be free. In the opening to an 1873 study of agricultural colonies, the French psychiatrist Firmin Lagardelle quotes the work of the renowned nineteenth-century French alienist Jean-Baptiste-Maximien Parchappe, writing, "Work is an invaluable blessing, and liberty, a need which cannot afford to be misunderstood. . . . The word is holy and that which above all is the most desirable, but liberty in all its forms and all its degrees presupposes a state of reason."[14] This emancipatory rhetoric illustrates the ideological weight given to labor, even as it was promoted as an invaluable economic resource for sustaining these new institutions. The political implications of this line of thinking in a colonial context, however, remained politely ignored.

Before the 1930s, patient labor was one of the only treatment methods available to colonial psychiatrists, apart from a handful of drugs and prolonged bath therapies, which were widely practiced and praised. Nevertheless, in tracing the genealogy of the international consensus with respect to work therapy, Indochina's psychiatrists worked hard to present themselves as modernizers who not only had inherited the expertise of their French forebears but stood at the vanguard of progressive psychiatric care. Asylum directors repeatedly evoked the Dutch experience in the East Indies as evidence that this model of patient care could work in Indochina, but they also drew extensively from international studies, conferences, and publications that heralded labor therapy as *the* universal standard of psychiatric treatment. Remarking that when it came to patient labor there was a "unanimity that is rare among doctors especially concerning therapeutic methods," André Augagneur, the Biên Hòa asylum's longest-running director from 1925 to 1933, quoted widely from the early nineteenth-century works of the celebrated French alienists Pinel and Ferrus to the latest studies emerging out of Belgium, Germany, Italy, the United States and Canada. Citing a 1926 international conference in Geneva where patient labor received top billing, Augagneur concluded in his report, "Today it is recognized by all psychiatrists that work is the best therapeutic agent for psychosis, some even going so far to say that it is the only therapy that the director of an asylum should use."[15] In spite of this insistence on the consensus of the psychiatric community about the merits of the agricultural colony, the organization of patient labor continued to be vigorously disputed among French psychiatrists in the metropole. Throughout the nineteenth century, debates over therapeutic labor served as a forum for broader contests over ideas about the curability of mental illness, the need for different treatments of chronic and acutely ill patients, how best to balance economic imperatives and medical goals of institutional care, and how to achieve the most effective surveillance of patients.

Putting Patients to Work

The ease with which labor therapy was adopted and transferred across the globe, despite important differences in medical contexts and cultural expressions of mental distress, demonstrates the extent to which psychiatric experts saw labor as a kind of panacea for an ever-widening spectrum of mental disorders.[16] For colonial psychiatrists in Indochina, the fact that the majority of their patients were already farmers generated a sense of optimism about the special therapeutic value of agricultural labor.[17] It was seen as an important factor of cerebral hygiene on account of its physical, outdoor qualities and for the impact of repeated movements on the motor skills of the brain. The act of gardening, in particular, was thought to yield valuable results, demanding constant and meticulous attention. If patients were left idle, as one psychiatrist warned, their physical degradation would only accelerate their psychiatric degradation. By contrast, labor would "channel" the unutilized energy of the insane for more productive ends.[18] One asylum report from 1931 thus framed patient labor as "indispensable for the organism, a method of physical education which is to be valued above all others. The distraction it creates works against ideas that are obsessive, melancholic, or depressive. It withdraws the patient from a delirious world and restores him to a sane reality."[19]

Annual asylum reports describe the application of patient labor in a rational and organized manner, just like any other therapeutic technique. For instance, asylum directors assigned patients to any one of several labor activities based on their "professional and physical aptitudes, as well as their type of psychosis."[20] In making their assignments, asylum directors adhered to a typology of work choice, developed in the metropole, in which patients, depending on their diagnosis, were thought to derive a certain kind of benefit from certain kinds of work.[21] Labor in this way was transformed into a kind of therapeutic agent that asylum directors prescribed and whose effects they were able to observe and measure. The language used by one asylum director in 1933 displays a medicalization of work choice that stands in sharp contrast to former methods of treatment, "From a medical point of view, work constitutes a powerful distraction and an excellent method of treatment that is easily implemented. Methodically organized, *bien dosé* [well dosed], and judiciously applied to able-bodied patients, it avoids the sad spectacle of those who are idle, crammed into rooms, or wandering in the corridors."[22] In theory, this categorization of work choice represented a natural addition to asylum life organized around the principles of division and separation. For patients already classified into different pavilions based on their race, gender, and form of psychosis, work assignments would easily follow. In practice, sending out patients to work during the day proved a welcome solution to the serious overcrowding of patient pavilions that had begun to seriously plague the institution by the late 1920s.

While agricultural therapy was originally conceived in the metropole for patients suffering from chronic conditions, psychiatrists in Indochina came to advocate for its application to a broader asylum population. For them, the "modern asylum" should provide care "not only to dangerous and chronic patients with no hope of cure but it must also assure a therapy based on rational measures in the best conditions possible for those whose psychiatric troubles are both transitory and curable."[23] As a result, therapeutic labor was prescribed for tranquil or chronic patients as well as those who suffered from greater states of agitation and acute psychiatric episodes. Labor was thought to transform passive and apathetic patients into active beings while also calming those who were more disruptive. It was even observed that, contrary to what might have been assumed, those patients who were the most agitated also made the best workers.[24] For "excited maniacs" it was important to start work as early as possible in order to space out their periods of agitation. Manual work for the "confused" meanwhile was seen to reduce the period of their isolation. For others, the effect was less immediately therapeutic than practical. Senile and epileptic patients, for instance, were tasked with the specific chores of cleaning, sweeping alleys, gathering dried leaves, and transporting water. As one psychiatrist wrote,

> This is clearly not a labor force of choice, with much activity, but this work presents an advantage in letting them leave the pavilions, where they otherwise rest unoccupied, because this inaction is always a source of arguments which easily degenerate into fights, especially in the women's quarters. In using them for work of no importance, we are able to guard them outside all day and only let them return to the pavilions for meals and at night. A day in liberty, in the great outdoors, is a serious supplement to any other therapy.[25]

While asylum directors drew on evidence from study trips and international conferences to support patient labor, these findings went only as far
as supporting the uses of labor for the indigenous populations on account
of the perceived special vulnerabilities of Europeans to the local climate.
(This is especially interesting given the fact that many of these studies drew
their conclusions based on experiences with white European patient populations!) The intensity of the heat and sunlight, for instance, was thought to
predispose European colonial settlers, especially men, to a condition known
as "neurasthenia," a kind of mental disorder characteristic of the tropics,
marked by physical degeneration and a weakening of the "moral sense."[26]
Psychiatrists worried that the inactivity of European patients on account
of the climate was exceedingly harmful to their recovery, "Witnessing how
much idleness is detrimental to our European patients, rest of the body is not
a very favorable condition for the rest of the spirit."[27] For some psychiatrists,
such observations confirmed claims that neurasthenia could be considered
not just a pathology of climate but an affectation of people who simply had
nothing to do. As a result, asylum directors complained about the European
patients who, segregated in their own pavilions, "currently do nothing and
pass the days smoking, resting sprawled out; it is necessary to create for
them some sort of occupation."[28] Instead physical education took the form
of outdoor leisure activities in the practice of sports like tennis, swimming,
and other outdoor activities.[29]

Patient employment also provided a kind of moral reeducation that, psychiatrists hoped, by approximating the habits of ordinary life would better
prepare patients for life outside the asylum. For asylum directors, outdoor
work proved useful in preventing the patient from becoming "absorbed in
false ideas" and experiencing mental degeneration but also in warding off
those "habits of laziness which, in the case of cure, would be deplorable for
him and for society."[30] This notion of inactivity formed a major preoccupation in which concerns over psychiatric treatment bled into broader anxieties about the social organization of indigenous life and the development of
a productive local labor force. A 1931 study on mental illness in Indochina
reported that men between the ages of twenty-six and thirty, in the prime
of their working years, experienced the highest rates of mental illness in
the colony. It drew attention to the high rates of opium, and especially alcohol, consumption among young men, observing that, "The existence of
the Native is in general rather disorganized. While his days are dedicated to
some ordinary kind of work, he dreams only of resting for the coming night.
To use a vulgar expression, one could say that in general the Indigene 'lives
life in the fast lane [*vie de patachon*].'" The report continues,

It is the night when life is the most intense: Annamite or Chinese the-ater, gambling, interminable conversations, such is the existence of city dwellers. Peasants pay visits to friends who live more or less far away, play, or take advantage of cool weather to do certain kinds of work or to hunt or fish. As a general rule, the Indigène sleeps little with the exception of the hot hours during the day and one is struck by the number of people that one meets at night going single file on paths, covering distances that are too long in order to visit friends or to see some sort of spectacle.[31]

The agricultural colony, which promoted the inculcation of rigid bodily discipline and values of hard work, was intended to serve as a powerful model for behavior by way of contrast. In sharp contrast to the decadence and intensity of this social world, the rhythm of asylum life in Indochina was strictly organized, at least as presented in official reports. Patients woke at 6:00 in the morning; they received their breakfast and would proceed with cleaning the pavilion, watering, folding mats and mosquito nets; and then head to work until 10:30 a.m. They would then return to the pavilion, where they would lunch and take a siesta until 2:00 in the afternoon. They would then work again until 4:45 p.m., when they would return to the pavilion for supper and sleep. It was stressed that patient labor, at a maximum, would last only six to seven hours a day. This rigid daily routine was described as producing a kind of metamorphosis in patients previously considered dan-gerous or incurable, "From a psychological point of view, the patient who, on entering does not recognize anyone, cannot eat alone, is incapable of walking, can now leave the pavilion, eat alone, learn again how to talk and even to read . . . is a major improvement. We try to reeducate this kind of patient without much hope for the rest."[32]

Even for those with no hope of cure, psychiatrists believed that approxi-mating the habits of ordinary life would serve a kind of harmonizing func-tion. Part of the ambiguity around the use of therapeutic labor derived from the fact that a cure was not the only or even necessarily the primary goal—indeed, for some chronic patients a full recovery was considered impossible. Rather, psychiatrists believed that the sense of accomplishment and confi-dence a patient derived from finishing a task, no matter how minor, repre-sented a "precious moral benefit" that fought against the more harmful and destructive symptoms of mental illness. In 1936 one psychiatrist remarked, "The more they work, the better the morale of the inhabitants."[33] A similar position was taken in regard to the care for lepers for whom treatment—never mind cure—was out of reach before the 1940s and for whom physical segregation was a life sentence. The idea to replace traditional leprosaria with agricultural colonies gained some traction within the colonial health service by the end of the 1920s. Doctors saw that by providing patients with some of the freedom and routines associated with normal social life, the colonie agricole was lending a certain humanization to the confinement of lepers.[34]

Earlier beliefs about the uses of labor to occupy and distract thus became reframed in the 1930s as no longer the most important outcomes of therapy. Instead asylum care increasingly concerned itself with attempting to "readapt the patient. This reeducation must interest the patient and awaken his initiative. For this goal we must do what we can to guide him, and reward him when he is finished."[35] Agricultural labor, as well as work in ateliers or workshops, therefore helped not only to promote a kind of psychiatric rebalance but also to arm patients with those professional skills that would allow them to secure work after their release.[36] Psychiatrists recognized that patients who left the asylum often needed special guidance during the first period of transition back to normal life. They therefore recommended the creation of a special form of social assistance specifically designed to help patients once they left the asylum.[37] One proposal even suggested the creation of a kind of "village of transition" adjacent to the asylum where a number of patients could live in simulated families and learn how to live independently on the path to full emancipation.[38]

Embedded in the discourse on reeducation was a colonial vision of what normal social life should look like. The internal organization of the asylum—from the segregation of pavilions along racial criteria to the strict schedule of daily labor, even the meals provided to different classes of patients—reflected a particular vision of colonial order aimed at patients on their journey from confinement to release.[39] This order not only reflected assumptions about the racial hierarchy of colonial life but also came to be inflected with class-based notions about the distribution of labor. Europeans did not labor, but neither did the members of the Vietnamese bourgeoisie who came to occupy the old European wing when a "paying service" for indigenous populations was inaugurated at Biên Hòa in 1934.[40] The ways in which the agricultural colony obscured the distinction between life inside and outside the asylum held the key to the therapeutic promise, and rehabilitative potential, of this model of care. At the same time, its capacity to blur boundaries between spaces of freedom and spaces of surveillance, between patients and laborers, introduced fundamental ambiguities into the meaning of freedom and treatment in the everyday practices of the colonial asylum.

Economics of Patient Labor

In 1936, two years after the Vôi asylum opened outside Hanoi, colonial officials proposed that the asylum generate its own revenue, given the "abundant
labor force put at its disposition," here referring to the captive patient population.[41] Patient labor had proven successful in keeping the Biên Hòa asylum
(mostly) solvent, and the economic importance of this particular form of
therapy was not lost on its northern partners. As the comment above makes
clear, the agricultural colony was always more than just a model of care. It
was also a model of capitalist production that responded to the dynamics of
a colonial economy that promoted the deepening exploitation of labor. The
agricultural colonies established in association with mental hospitals can be
viewed as part of a continuum of colonial labor practices aimed at transforming the indigenous population into a disciplined and loyal workforce. In
French Indochina, as in the Dutch East Indies, the financial survival of the
asylum hinged on the economic productivity of its patient-laborers.

Asylum finances also depended on swings in the wider regional economy.
By the 1920s, Indochina's economy was booming, driven primarily by the
commercial rice trade and rubber production in the south, as well as other
big market crops like coffee, sugarcane, and peppercorn, in addition to min-
eral mining. From the early 1900s, rubber plantations had expanded quickly
throughout Cochinchina, Cambodia, and southern Annam as industrial
demand for latex grew apace, introducing a new engine for colonial development into the region but also the swift transformation of local economies and
ecologies. The granting of large concessions resulted in the concentration of
land in the hands of wealthy Vietnamese landowners and French investment
firms, displacing thousands of people from their ancestral lands. Between
1908 and 1940, the amount of land devoted to rubber production increased
from 200 hectares to 126,000 hectares in 1940. By the late 1920s, French
Indochina became the third-largest rubber exporter after British Malaya and
the Dutch East Indies.[42] Between 1925 and 1929, the rubber boom produced
a jump in cultivated acreage from 18,000 hectares to 78,620. The industry
employed a total of seventy thousand "coolies," contractual workers from
Tonkin and Annam, and free workers (those employed as casual laborers)
recruited locally.[43] The rapid growth of the plantation labor system led to
massive labor migrations from the Red River delta in Tonkin to the Mekong
delta in the south. The southern population increased from 2.2 million in
1895 to 2.8 million in 1900 and 5.6 million in 1943.[44] That laborers abandoned
the relative security of their home villages to find wage-paid employment on
rubber plantations can be attributed to the socioeconomic transformation

of agrarian relations in the northern countryside, particularly the growing polarization of land ownership as the result of colonial economic policies.[45]

The social effects of the plantation system can be traced, in part, to the extra burden placed on the local health system around Biên Hòa. By 1928, local medical officials remarked on how the massive influx of migrant workers, attracted from all corners of Indochina by the growing demand for plantation labor, was straining resources and access to regional hospitals, including the Biên Hòa asylum.[46] Asylum administrators now received requests for confinement not only from police and, occasionally, from families and communities but also increasingly from European owners of big commercial rubber estates. Madame de la Souchère, the owner of a nearby rubber plantation spanning Long Thành and Xuân Lộc provinces, wrote the colonial authorities in 1927 in order to request the transfer of one of her coolies (Van N. or "Number 22.597") to Biên Hòa. She claimed that because his contract did not stipulate mental illness as a protected condition, she could not be held responsible for supporting the costs of the coolie's confinement. Moreover, he had worked only 114 days; he still owed her 1,059 days plus the costs of recruitment.[47] The asylum administration was left with no choice but to bill the patient's home province to cover the expenses. In order to keep up with the surge in the patient population, as well as the rising costs of food staples, clothes, and medications, Dr. Augagneur requested that the colonial government increase the daily rate of hospitalization from 2 to 3 piasters for European patients and from 0.50 to 0.60 piasters to cover the care of the indigent.[48] As we saw in the previous chapter, multiplying the number of categories of paying patients was continually employed as a revenue-raising measure in 1928, in 1934, and again in 1938.[49]

The arrival of the Great Depression in Indochina in 1930, fueled by the precipitous decline in rubber and rice prices on world markets and excessive speculation, deepened the asylum's budget woes. With the loss of tax revenue, the colony's general budget fell from 108 million piasters in 1931 to 60.9 million in 1934; local budgets fell from 69.6 million to 43.6 million piasters.[50] The mandate that Indochina's colonial economy be entirely self-supporting fell by the wayside as the metropolitan government, together with the Bank of Indochina, intervened to stabilize the economy. Public expenditures were cut by 42 percent. Indochina's budget dedicated to health and sanitation dipped precipitously after 1931, a drop further amplified by the devaluation of Indochina's currency, the piaster.

These cuts in funding exacerbated the long-term frustrations of asylum directors over the lack of sufficient funding put at their disposal. From the mid-1920s, asylum directors had sought greater autonomy to control the

institution's finances, first by insisting the institution possess its own trea-
sury.[51] Then they decided to take matters into their own hands, transforming
the scale of agricultural labor from simple self-sufficiency into a genuinely
expansive revenue-generating operation that targeted urban markets. Following asylum directors in France who had come to favor more intensive
forms of cultivation, ensuring year-round harvests, colonial psychiatrists
also called for the diversification and escalation of crop production beyond
rice, including the cultivation of tobacco, cassava root, and potatoes, which
required little care and attention. Preliminary attempts to expand the annual
harvest yielded promising results. Seeds imported from France—including
varieties of lettuce, cabbage, carrots, celery, and watercress, as well as green
beans from Dalat—were tested in order to guarantee a "sure output." Of
critical importance was the installation of a dam on the stream that traversed
the asylum grounds and ensured the abundance of clear, pure water even
during the dry season. The shift to cultivating fresh vegetables required a
more intense and careful effort on the part of "patient-workers" (as they
were often called) in terms of preparing the land, planting seeds, watering
plants twice a day, weeding out harmful herbs, and setting out protective foils
and garden stakes.[52]

Expectations for profits were high. Asylum directors proposed the sale of
vegetables on a subscription basis to colonial settlers and bureaucrats, as well
as to shopkeepers in Saigon, in order to establish an "easy flow of all quan-
tities of vegetables."[53] The sale of fresh vegetables at the Saigon markets,
estimated at 600 piasters per year, would join with the proceeds from the sale
of rice and tobacco, rubber and pork, projected to total an additional 3,100
piasters. Not only would patients receive more fresh vegetables above the
normal ration, but the expansion would also create a critical revenue stream
for the asylum that could be used to purchase machines for the ateliers,
improve agricultural tools, increase the indemnity given to patients upon
release, and assure supplementary funds for special holidays. As one French
psychiatrist remarked, "Happily the labor force of the asylum works well.
Without it, the upkeep and repairs would represent an important loss."[54]

The organization of patient labor also proved remarkably efficient. In
order to remedy the persistent problem of patients sleeping on the floor, in
1932 it was decided that patient-laborers would construct a number of new
beds out of wood. Teams were formed under the direction of the guards
and a carpenter, and the work was divided into specialized tasks, with some
teams sawing the boards to size and others charged with sanding the wood
for a smooth and even finish. The planks were then passed to assembly
teams, who would adjust the size of the feet and the frame. In a matter of

days, they had managed to build two hundred beds. If purchased locally, the price of the beds (including transport costs) would have come to 5 piasters each. Using their own labor force, asylum directors were happy to learn that they had procured sturdier beds for half the cost.[55]

As in Europe, asylum administrators in the Dutch East Indies and French Indochina continually promoted the therapeutic value of labor even as the scale and intensity of patient labor deepened in the struggle for economic profit. By 1934, nearly a third of all patients at Biên Hòa were kept busy performing tasks associated with every aspect of the daily running of the asylum: from the harvesting of rice and vegetables for meals to the construction and painting of new pavilions, laundry and the sewing of patient clothing, making baskets, husking rice, manufacturing bricks and the production of latex from rubber trees grown on the asylum's grounds.[56] This expansion in scale and efficiency of patient labor recalls Daniel Hémery and Pierre Brocheux's likening of 1930s Indochina to an "agro-industrial factory," marked by the Taylorization of labor, the rationalization of space, and the use of increasingly advanced technologies for extraction.[57] To give a sense of the massive scale of the work, the annual rice harvest at Biên Hòa grew from 1,800 kilograms in 1924 to almost 7,000 a decade later. Crops expanded to include twelve thousand tobacco plants, nearly one thousand rubber trees,

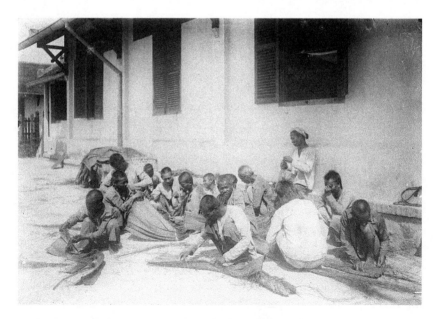

FIGURE 14.   Patients weaving mats at Biên Hòa. Courtesy of user manhhai, Flickr.

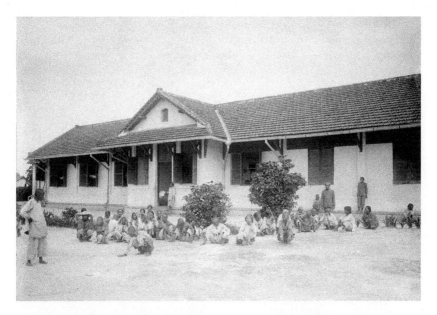

FIGURE 15. Patients in the courtyard of Biên Hòa. Courtesy of user manhhai, Flickr.

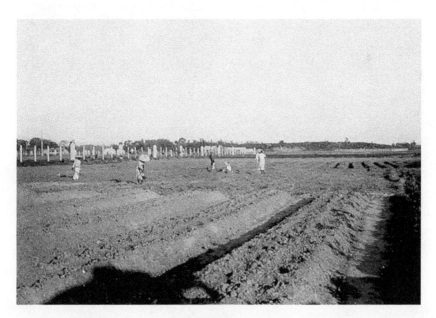

FIGURE 16. Patients tending to a vegetable garden at the Vôi asylum, Tonkin. ANOM, "Assistance psychiatrique, Bac Giang (Asile de Voi)," ICO, 8 Fi-498.

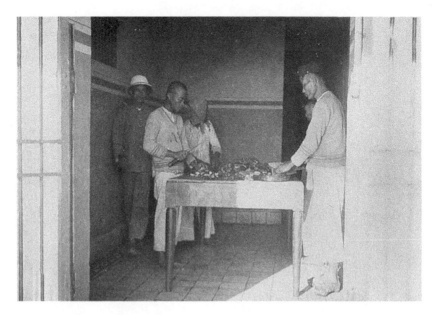

FIGURE 17. Patients helping with the preparation of meals at the Vôi asylum, Tonkin. ANOM, "Assistance psychiatrique, Bac Giang (Asile de Voi)," ICO, 8 Fi-498.

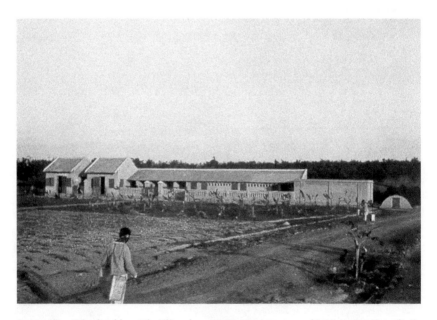

FIGURE 18. Animal stables at the Vôi asylum. ANOM, "Assistance psychiatrique, Bac Giang (Asile de Voi)," ICO, 8 Fi-498.

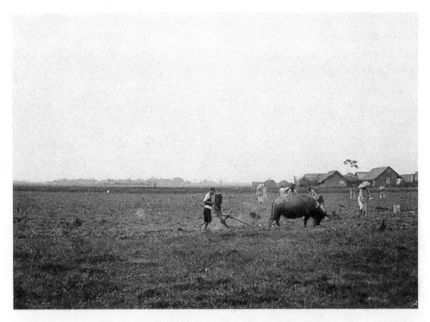

FIGURE 19.   Patients at Vôi preparing the fields for rice cultivation. ANOM, "Assistance psychiatrique, Bac Giang (Asile de Voi)," ICO, 8 Fi-498.

fifty lemon trees, as well as evergreens and coffee plants, covering two acres of forest. By 1929, the administration of the asylum was described as "flourishing," and in 1931, while continuing to suffer from financial setbacks, it produced in enough quantity in order to "greatly lighten its budget."[58]

The embrace of labor as therapy thus reveals the alignment between the institutional discourse of rehabilitation and the economic imperative to cut costs by increasing production, as well as the general economic imperative of the 1920s to increase the *mise en valeur* of the colonies by extracting profits from the cheap and plentiful supply of indigenous labor. Asylum labor also exposed the uneasy tension between coercion and therapy, a constant preoccupation of asylum directors, who routinely insisted that labor was, first and foremost, prescribed for its therapeutic value and that under no circumstances were patients ever forced against their will to work.[59]

Coercion or Encouragement? Tackling the Ethics of Patient Labor

Between 1919 and 1934, the Biên Hòa asylum treated a total of almost 1,600 patients. Of those who had left the asylum, 80 percent were classified as cured, or roughly a third of the total asylum population ever admitted. In their annual reports to the colonial government, asylum directors attributed their therapeutic successes in overwhelming measure to the colonies agricoles and requested funds for continued land acquisition in order to expand employment opportunities for patients.[60] Yet the different goals of therapeutic labor often slid uneasily together in annual asylum reports. To take one example from 1933, "The work of lunatics is one of our dominant preoccupations. This form of treatment is not only a method of distraction but also a valuable resource for the establishment. It constitutes an important part of the functioning of the asylum. To provide an occupation to the largest number of patients in order to improve and perfect the conditions of work, that is our goal."[61]

While acknowledging the financial benefits of the practice, asylum directors also routinely insisted that the organization of patient labor was for medical purposes first and foremost and that in no circumstances were patients coerced into working. Throughout the 1920s and 1930s, psychiatrists stressed that only those "able-bodied and voluntary lunatics" who requested to participate were eligible for work outdoors. They even framed work as something that was actively pursued by the patients themselves, who had come to appreciate its medical value. One psychiatrist, for example, noted that when therapeutic labor produced an improvement, no matter how slight, the patient would "demand to know the kind of work with which he was to be entrusted."[62] Despite the greater freedoms permitted patients, who worked often at long distances from the asylum grounds and only under limited surveillance, only three patients escaped in 1926. In the eyes of asylum directors, this fact testified to the acceptability and success of therapeutic labor.[63] Nevertheless, betraying some lingering anxiety, they stressed the importance of closely watching over patients as they labored and ensuring tools were safely stowed away at night.[64]

Much of the energy devoted to insisting on the voluntariness of patient labor exposed an underlying sensitivity shared by asylum administrators to accusations of mistreatment. They surely knew of the pressures facing psychiatrists in France, who confronted charges of patient labor as inherently exploitative. Sometimes these charges came from the patients themselves. In 1910, reports of a bloody revolt at the agricultural colony of Chézal Benôit in central France described a group of patients who, misled by the appellation of a *colonie*, were apparently "disillusioned" to find themselves barricaded in and sent to the fields to labor rather than resting comfortably in the homes of the local peasantry.[65] In Vietnam, the anticipation of such critiques produced some anxiety in the pages of annual asylum reports. For example, at

Biên Hòa in the 1920s, some patients were employed with the banal task of removing rice husks. This incredibly labor-intensive chore also had the lamentable effect of forcing patients to work in what was described as a "very dusty atmosphere." As compared with those patients exposed to the clean air of the open fields, a fundamental tenet of work therapy, those husking rice were found to be in a "regrettable" situation. In 1927, as a result, the director of Biên Hòa invested in the installation of a more useful (and efficient) Groundhand machine for processing the rice that had been harvested on asylum grounds.[66]

This sensitivity to charges of exploitation is striking in a colonial context where labor abuse was commonplace, particularly in settings of confinement. The use of prisoners as a source of plentiful, cheap labor began in Indochina as early as 1862. Prisoners were put to work digging irrigation ditches and building roads. The colonial state also farmed them out to private contractors as a revenue-generating measure. Poulo Condore, the notorious prison colony, represented the extreme end of forced labor in Indochina: physically taxing work, long hours, poor diet, and high mortality rates from diseases such as malaria and dysentery. Such punishing working and living conditions provoked prisoner rebellions and public outrage and did much to undermine claims about the rehabilitative goals of punishment.[67] Corvée, the requisitioning of labor for large-scale public works, also drew the ire of the colonized population and resulted in periodic protests as early as 1908 and helped fuel the rise of left-wing activism in the colony from the late 1920s. The practice was eventually outlawed by the French government in 1937 following the arrival of the Popular Front to power and mounting international pressure to sign the International Labor Organization's forced labor convention of 1930. The careful promotion of patient labor thus unfolded in the context of local protests as well as growing international consensus around the prohibition of "unfree labor."[68]

Asylum directors may have stressed the entirely voluntary nature of asylum labor, but their insistence belied the actual use of a range of persuasive and coercive measures to encourage patients to work. In 1921 a decree mandated that those interned at the asylum would receive a pécule, or bonus, of two cents a day in compensation for their labor. Patients would receive one-half each Sunday in order to purchase cakes, sugar, cigarettes, and other goods subject to official approval. The other half would be noted in individual registers and returned to the patient following his or her release from the asylum. Three cents would also be reserved from weekly wages in order to cover the costs of food.[69] In 1934 at the Biên Hòa asylum, 230 patients performed 62,392 days of work and were compensated an annual total of 1,247.84 piasters.[70]

The practice of the pécule derived from a metropolitan law in France that formally regulated labor in asylums. The 1839 law, later revamped in 1857, developed in response to concerns about the protection of patients from exploitation, especially around the introduction of *la grande culture*. The regulation specified work as a "method of treatment and distraction" but also "limited, if necessary, the length of work" and assured "general working conditions and related sanitary precautions." Patients could not be employed for labor that required the exclusive use of muscular force, and the workday could never exceed eight hours in the winter and nine hours in the summer. The pécule was intended as a kind of "remuneration for workers, not only for the execution of good work but also for the recognition of the effort made by such and such a patient, even if the outcome is minimal." Patients were therefore not compensated for actual work output, like normal workers, but for the additional energy that they put into the work as patients of the asylum.[71]

In colonial Vietnam, as a source of "precious encouragement," the pécule clearly succeeded. "As soon as they are able, improved patients submit to work therapy. No difficulty here; on the contrary, work is solicited because it is compensated."[72] Asylum directors would also encourage patients to work in teams by giving those with the best results supplementary rations of tobacco, fruits, and cakes. Asylum administrators did not shy away from using a range of techniques to encourage patients to work. In a 1926 report the director of Biên Hòa noted, "Labor is, moreover optional, any patient who does not want to work is left at the pavilion. While they are laboring if the patient stops himself and does not work anymore the guards have been ordered to not force him to work. They should find out if he is tired, in which case he is brought back to the pavilion, if not they are to wait to see if he would like to take up his task again. Ordinarily this pause does not last for long, the patient being encouraged by the other companions of his team."[73]

How to balance the directives for labor, framed at once as an important benefit to the individual and to the institution, with the ostensibly voluntary nature of patient employment presented a challenge to colonial psychiatrists. In many ways, the art of convincing rather than forcing the patient to work emerged as the most suitable strategy. The asylum personnel were charged with this important yet "delicate" task of navigating the different impulses of patient care around both a firm discipline and compassion. As one asylum director explained, "To win the confidence of the patient in order to then direct him, to order him in such a way as to think that the direction and order are in his interest, is an often difficult task that requires much patience and devotion."[74] However, the fact that the guards themselves often participated in the manual labor of the asylum alongside their charges and benefited from its revenues complicated their use of authority to encourage patients to work. Asylums also often hired back a number of patients as coolies who were deemed "cured" and ready for release but did not have families to return home to. Such an arrangement allowed these patients to continue to be an object of surveillance, yet in their new role as coolies they were also entrusted with the supervision of labor and the exercise of the surveillance of other patients at night.[75] The fluidity of these hierarchies within the asylum's walls worked to disrupt ideas about what it meant to be a patient and what it meant to be an employee, as well as the notion of labor itself as a therapeutic strategy reserved for the sick.

While some patients required encouragement to work, psychiatrists wondered at those patients who "work with an activity and conscientiousness truly astonishing in a country where work at a slow pace is the norm" and often remarked on their "punctuality, tranquillity and silence."[76] In one instance, the labor of ten patients was thought to have resulted in an output superior to that of the work of twenty coolies.[77] A 1925 report admitted, "It would seem paradoxical to claim that we find less difficulties with the patients than we would with another labor force" for "certain patients work with a real care and enjoyment."[78] The ability to work also emerged as a major prerequisite for release and constituted critical evidence of improvement of the patient's condition. Those who were viewed as uncooperative were much less likely to be considered cured and ready for a return to normal social life. Indeed, the inability or unwillingness to work was often cited as a reason to reject requests for release initiated by family members or by the patients themselves.[79] Here the more coercive aspects of an institutional logic guided by labor as therapy emerge the most clearly.

Back to the Dutch East Indies

Faced with dire overcrowding, psychiatrists in Indochina once again looked to the Dutch East Indies for solutions, signaling a second wave of French interest in Dutch practices. In August of 1937, Pierre Dorolle, a colonial psychiatrist and future deputy general of the World Health Organization, took a study trip to Java. He traveled as the secretary of the Indochina delegation to the Intergovernmental Conference of Far-Eastern Countries on Rural Hygiene held in Bandung, a meeting that historians now view as a milestone in the development of international initiatives for rural public health.[80] Organized by the League of Nations Health Organization, this regional conference capped what historians Theodore Brown and Elizabeth Fee describe as a "surge of interwar interest in rural hygiene [that] in several ways fore-shadowed the WHO's famous Alma Ata Conference."[81] In particular, the 1937 conference addressed concerns over what to do about the vast major-ity of Asia's population that lived in poverty in the countryside, far from modern hospitals and with limited access to modern medicine. The confer-ence stressed the importance of prevention—including public health educa-tion and the establishment of small clinics focused on maternal and child health—instead of expensive, technology-intensive curative approaches that remained outside the reach of most indigenous peoples. It also emphasized the need to pay attention to the languages, cultures, and traditions of local populations, as well as broader issues surrounding economic development and land reform.

During the first half of the twentieth century, international concerns about health in Southeast Asia intensified, creating many opportunities for travel and the exchange of ideas and practices. The Far Eastern Association of Tropical Medicine (FEATM) provided an important early organizational framework for medical experts in Southeast Asia to meet and exchange ideas and for medical knowledge to travel in the region. Interest in tropical dis-eases followed a number of breakthroughs in tropical medicine around the turn of the century, including the discovery of the role of insect vectors in the transmission of malaria and yellow fever and the isolation of the cholera bacillus.[82] From its first meeting in Manila in 1908, FEATM regularly brought scientists and physicians together to discuss progress in the understanding and control of regional diseases like beriberi, malaria, smallpox, and yellow fever.[83] At the same time, the International Health Board of the Rockefeller Foundation organized a number of demonstration projects focused on pub-lic health education in several parts of Southeast Asia.[84] The International Health Board also supported the International League of Nations Health Organization. As Sunil Amrith has argued, it was through the variety of these international health initiatives in Southeast Asia, culminating with the Bandung conference, that local practices and expertise were transformed into a new international discourse on health.[85]

Before the start of the conference Dorolle made a satellite visit to Len-teng Agung, halfway between Batavia and Buitenzorg, to visit a new kind of stand-alone agricultural colony, which had been established in 1933 on 325 acres of land, under the direction of the P. M. van Wulfften Palthe, professor of neurology and psychiatry at the Batavia Medical School. Two hundred calm, chronic psychiatric patients had been successfully transferred from the asylum at Buitenzorg to Lenteng Agung, where they worked in the fields under minimal supervision. Following the famous Belgian model at Gheel, seventy patients were later placed in the homes of villagers who housed and fed patients in exchange for their labor.[86] Not only did this hybrid model of care encourage patients to readapt to normal Javanese village life, but it also helped to relieve the financial burden of caring for the insane. Moreover, in what was a real innovation, the project was entirely organized as a private, philanthropic initiative rather than by the colonial administration or the Dutch East Indies Public Health Service (it was partly financed out of lottery profits).

After visiting Lenteng Agung and attending the Bandung conference, Dorolle became convinced that van Wulfften Palthe's "colony asylum" model (or *asile colonie*) could work in Indochina, for several reasons that he recorded in his report to the French colonial administration upon his return home. He noted fundamental similarities, particularly with the countryside of Tonkin, citing the dispersed population, bare hills mixed with those covered with grass, and the dedication of low-lying lands to the cultivation of rice. Beyond topography, the striking ethnological similarities between the Tonkinois and local Indonesian populations and their local economies (which shared comparable salaries for indigenous medical staff) gave Dorolle hope. In one particularly ardent passage he wrote,

> Nothing resembles more, in effect, a southern Indochinese village than a Sundanese village. Nothing resembles more the countryside of Lenteng Agung than the hills of Phu-Tho, of Vinh-Yên, of Bac-Giang, and certain regions of Bien- Hòa and Thu-dâu-Môt. The diet of patients is, with only minimal difference, the same in Java as here. . . . That which has succeeded perfectly in Java, with remarkable results from an economic point of view, will succeed equally in Indochina.[87]

Prior study trips had gone far toward establishing similarities across populations and geographies of both colonies. Dorolle's exercise in comparison can be interpreted as being part of a long intellectual tradition that connected the two colonial territories as parts of a single region.[88] Some of the challenges the Dutch had faced in implementing this model of care, specifically how best to expropriate land from village ownership and irrigate land of poor quality, could serve as important lessons for the French. For Dorolle, the Dutch experience underscored the importance of selecting land in collaboration and agreement with both agricultural experts and indigenous authorities—earning community trust would be key. Dorolle observed that the local Sundanese population, "afraid like any other people in a similar situation around the world," at first protested against the establishment of this "colony of lunatics" without the protection of a wall or any

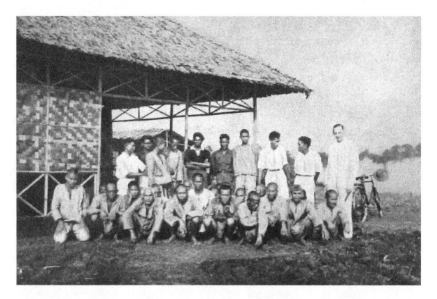

FIGURE 20.   Newly arrived patients at the asile colonie of Lengteng-Agoeng in 1934. ANOM, Guernut 22, "Note sur la colonie agricole d'aliénés de Lengteng-Agoeng [Java] par le Dr. P.M.Dorolle," October 1937.

kind of fence. The villagers barricaded their houses at night, fearing some "horrible strike from their neighbors." Yet, Dorolle recounts, "Very rapidly, however, in part due to the entanglement of the land belonging to the *colonie* and that belonging to the villagers, the peasants recognized that the *colons* were not dangerous and worked peacefully in the fields. They began to converse and got to know each other, and in a matter of months the villagers perfectly accepted the idea of welcoming one of these patients into their homes."[89]

Dorolle cautioned that sites should be selected in areas of low population density and close enough to the asylum to facilitate urgent care but far enough away so that transferred patients would "have the impression that they had truly left the asylum for a new existence."[90] Yet for Dorolle, having villages nearby was indispensable to pursuing family placements, which he viewed as the "second step" of the program after the initial transfer to the colonie. On his return home, he summarized his findings in a report that included a series of photographs of mental patients from the colony working in the fields and eating meals at communal tables. Relying on the Dutch experience, Dorolle argued that in Indochina the removal of the chronically ill from asylums and the creation of these separate colonies would reduce by six to eight times the cost of patient oversight, and up to ten to fifteen times the overall cost of care.[91] The report said little about charting patients' therapeutic progress or comparative rates of different psychiatric disorders; instead it was the potential for cost savings and the practicalities of daily management of the asile colonie that attracted Dorolle's attention.

His enthusiastic report met with a decidedly mixed reception. Many French officials balked at the idea of boarding out patients, given the prejudices of the local population and the difficulties of medical surveillance and control. Yet the Dutch experience demonstrated that halfway measures in a semidetached colony were practicable in a colonial context, even if they dispensed with certain elements and replaced them with others. Rather than placing former patients in the homes of peasant families, the commission in charge of reforming Indochina's asylum system approved the creation in 1938 of a village of recovering patients designed to simulate family country life, under active and continuous medical surveillance.[92] In a letter to Indochina's governor-general, Edouard-André Delsalle, the resident superior of Tonkin, wrote, "There is room to conceive of the envisioned agricultural colony, not as an actual village that is more or less autonomous but rather as a special kind of agglomeration organized according to rural and familial ideas, but where the action of the family would be replaced by that of the doctor and asylum personnel." With the director of the asylum serving as a benevolent benefactor, three or four patients would live together in individual homes, simulating a Western European nuclear family structure. With seeds and tools furnished by the local agricultural cooperative, they would work during the day under appropriate supervision and sell their harvests to help ease the asylum's operational costs. The experiment was envisaged as a kind of "center of reeducation through work" in which the therapeutic logic of labor would extend beyond the asylum's walls and into the community. Villagers would have the chance to exercise the skills they had learned while working at the asylum, all while under supervision as if they were still hospitalized.[93]

Yet this paternalist vision had its critics, who believed that it sanctioned a fatal kind of dependence upon the state. They were especially critical of the monthly allowance that all patients would receive to supplement their incomes. According to one of the plan's many skeptics, this would not only waste resources but also "put into their heads" that the administration had decided to pay them a salary until the end of their days and thereby "liberate" them from a future of having to perform any type of difficult work.[94] The issue of surveillance also became an object of grave concern. Two guardians would be required for every fifty settlers. Furthermore, those patients described as "most neighboring normal" were to serve as a kind of "reinforcement system for surveillance" and be held responsible for maintaining village cleanliness and discipline. To mark their authority vis-à-vis the other inhabitants, they would receive honorary titles (such as *lý trưởng*) matching those in ordinary Vietnamese villages and live in small, independent lodgings. They would receive a higher allowance and, with prior authorization, would be allowed to live with a partner and start a family. Yet such visions of family life had their limits, and regulating the sexual lives of the villagers was the single biggest concern voiced by critics of the plan. The director of the health service in Tonkin, for instance, warned that inhabitants "either through '*la vie en ménage*' or through accidental sexual relationships with the habitants of neighboring villages" must be prevented from "breeding descendants who are more or less defected and crazy." For this reason, asylum personnel would have to subject the villages to a particularly severe surveillance.[95]

For its chief supporters, the village concept, in proposing a domestic family model of care to promote cure and reintegration, formed the next logical step in patient recovery. For Dr. Roger Grinsard, the director of the Vôi asylum outside Hanoi, the project represented a "social work of reeducation allowing the recuperation of a social life by individuals currently confined. This creation, new in the Far East, has a humanitarian goal on which it would be pointless to insist."[96] Still, some critics rejected the idea outright as a complete waste of resources. A crucial point was that the Dutch model relied on the generosity of private benefactors, of a sort that never gained traction in Indochina. Given the project's costs, with no foreseeable financial benefit to the colonial administration, many urged that the burden should instead be placed on families by urging them to take back patients as soon as possible.[97] And while the governor-general approved the creation of the villages in 1939, only a year later the commission in charge evidently had a change of heart, arguing that it was "inappropriate, from a social point of view."[98]

While the asile colonie ultimately failed to take hold in Vietnam, the debates among physicians and psychiatrists over five decades reveal what they thought to be commonalities across imperial spaces, particularly in terms of shared challenges as well as the kinds of adaptations Indochinese society would require. In particular, the decision to model the village and its organization on a Western family model underscores a key difference between French and Dutch styles of colonial administration. Whereas the Dutch adopted a pragmatic solution to the problem of asylum overcrowding as part of broader efforts to "indigenize" the health service, French officials in Indochina pursued a modified version that corresponded to a different kind of colonial vision in which they aimed to remake native subjects in their own image. Their attempt to reproduce the social relations within the asylum outside the formal space of the institution offers an intriguing account of how they thought normal social life should look in the French colony. The fact that this family model of care was eventually found to be unworkable—given concerns over surveillance, cultural prejudice, cost, and sexual promiscuity—marks the limits of scientific exchange across empires.

In comparing the two colonial settings, however, Dorolle and others not only contributed to a specifically regional knowledge of psychiatry but also entered into a long-standing expert engagement with Southeast Asia as a space that superseded the boundaries of empire. The movement of psychiatric knowledge and practice across empires yielded not only practical, concrete effects in terms of the management of asylum patients—in ways that ultimately set Indochina apart from the rest of the French empire—but also helped to shore up Western understandings of what we understand today to be "Southeast Asia." Such a perspective offers a way of thinking about French colonial Vietnam as part of an emerging transnational network of experts that was not only colonial and not only French. Instead, imagined as part of Southeast Asia, Vietnam's public health landscape was shaped by regional exchanges of information that increasingly took place within the framework provided by international health organizations.

Spaces of Therapy, Spaces of Labor

Located on the margins of asylum grounds, the agricultural colony signified the last step in patient recovery and reentry into colonial society. By drawing our attention to those liminal spaces between confinement and release, the history of the agricultural colony reveals the fluidity of mental illness as an object of medical knowledge—a state that could be cured or at least improved through rational treatment—and highlights broader French debates over what kind of subjects the colonial state sought to mold. Recasting discussions around the development of a healthy and productive colonial workforce, psychiatrists in Indochina claimed that the act of labor itself was an indispensable therapeutic mechanism for ridding individuals of mental illness. They argued that putting asylum patients to work would not only result in important health benefits but also equip patients with the moral principles, self-discipline, and technical skills that would prove essential upon their liberation. Yet the discourse of patient freedom and work therapy clashed with the everyday imperatives of surveillance and economic profit that governed the administration of the colonial asylum. In some instances, asylum directors viewed these apparent contradictions as a practical challenge of asylum management, and in others, a real tension of practice that required more careful attention.

For historians of psychiatry, these coercive aspects of patient labor serve as powerful reminders of the abuses of the asylum system.[99] Yet the dynamics of patient labor itself—the kind of work patients did and how it was organized, what they planted, and whether they were compensated—tends to be overlooked in the historical literature.[100] In this chapter, I have argued that we cannot separate the history of patient labor from the history of labor relations in the region. Colonial asylums were embedded in local and regional economies that structured the kind of work that patients engaged in, its integration into daily institutional regimes of care and surveillance, and the reliance on this labor to ensure the financial solvency of the institutions. With the partial exception of Madagascar, Indochina was the only French colony (and the only other colonial territory in Asia) to follow Dutch leads by adopting patient labor as the central organizing principle of care for the insane. The fact that the colonie agricole achieved pride of place in Indochina's psychiatric assistance program, to an extent not witnessed in other parts of the French empire, points to the distinctiveness of the Southeast Asian context. In part this can be attributed to Dutch leadership, which shaped French expectations about the potential success of this treatment in their own colony. It must also be grounded, however, in the development and intensification of the plantation economy in the region, which explains the enthusiasm among colonial asylum directors for this particular form of patient therapy.

CHAPTER 4

Going In and Getting Out of the Colonial Asylum

Families and the Politics of Caregiving

In 1931, Dr. Augagneur quoted the words of Gaëtan Gatian de Clerambault in the introduction to the asylum's annual report: "There are no arbitrary confinements, there are only arbitrary releases."[1] Clerambault, a French psychiatrist who had worked in the 1920s as the head of the Infirmerie du Dépôt in Paris, was defending his profession against accusations of capriciousness and neglect that forced in some instances the early release of patients. Like the directors of Parisian asylums in the late nineteenth and early twentieth centuries, those of psychiatric institutions in colonial Vietnam throughout the interwar years also faced problems of serious overcrowding and public pressures to both confine and release the insane. Suffering from insufficient space and resources, asylum care in Indochina came to be marked out of necessity by high rates of patient turnover. Even at the height of psychiatric activity in Indochina in the 1930s, annual asylum reports clearly reveal that the majority of the insane spent their lives not confined in psychiatric institutions but circulating in and out of asylums, jails, hospitals, poorhouses, and family homes.

This chapter traces the patient's journey to the asylum and, in some cases, back to family homes. It argues that the ways in which people moved in and out of psychiatric care in Indochina were not arbitrary but were instead shaped by complex negotiations between psychiatrists, colonial authorities, and the public, especially families. Confronted with the reality of few experts living in the colony, French bureaucrats and doctors developed mechanisms regulating the confinement and release of the mentally ill that provided for, and indeed depended on, the critical participation of families and communities for information, surveillance, and care. Examining the processes of going in and getting out of the colonial asylum reveals the ways in which laypeople participated in the negotiation and exchange of ideas around what it meant to be "abnormal" as well as disputes over what it meant to be "sufficiently improved," in the words of one French psychiatrist, as to return to society. Debates revolved around the mental health of the patients but also the capacity of the families to assume their care upon release and the asylum itself as the most appropriate site for treatment and rehabilitation. I argue that paying attention to exchanges that transcended the asylum's walls allows us to witness debates over the legitimate aims and forms of colonial psychiatric practices, the historical relationship between families and the colonial state, and evolving ideas about what it meant to be a normal productive member of society in French colonial Vietnam.

Colonial psychiatrists often commented on the role of families—as either ignorant or obstructionist—but as nevertheless critical to their ability to confine patients. They were struck by the hundreds of visits paid by families to loved ones at the asylum, and they complained when families were not available to care for patients once they returned home. The attachment of patients to their families (or demonstrated lack thereof) also informed clinical judgments about the mental health of the individual. The inability to name close family members or, more significantly, express any concern about what had happened to their family would provide doctors with justifications for prolonged confinement.[2] Vietnamese psychiatrists later in the century also recognized the power of families to transform efforts to diagnose and treat. As one Saigon-based psychiatrist writing in the 1970s put it, "[The] family is not an accessory to treatment but the crux of the matter."[3]

I should emphasize here that my use of the term "family" does not imply a self-evident or stable category but rather a network of shifting relations among immediate family members and extended kin.[4] An individual's route to clinical diagnosis and confinement in an asylum was not always precipitated by a "crisis" episode or mental breakdown; or, more precisely, the possibility of any single crisis initiating confinement was often tied to more fundamental crises associated with changes in family fortunes and disruptions to communal life that accelerated under French colonization. Just as the history of mental health in Vietnam does not start with the arrival of the French colonizers, psychiatric care did not begin with the entrance of patients into formal medical institutions. Instead, seeking out the assistance of experts, whether local or foreign, was part of a much longer-term process mediated by families that is not reducible to the prerogatives of state institutions. Indeed, French psychiatrists continued to compete with indigenous healers well into the 1930s even as the colonial state increasingly worked to restrict the practice of traditional medicine and to promote widespread and exclusive recourse to Western medical care. Here I argue that colonial-era asylums must be seen as part of a long-term strategy of household care as much as they constituted spaces of abandonment.[5]

This chapter looks specifically at the relationship between families and the asylum in order to trace the development of a kind of colonial "micropolitics of care" using patient files, community surveys, and asylum reports. While colonial asylums housed indigenous and European individuals of both genders, I focus my attention on Vietnamese patients, particularly men, who formed the overwhelming majority of the asylum population.[6] The first section, "Going In," discusses the role of families and communities in shaping the process of confinement and how their role changed with the shifting norms of institutionalization. The next section, "Getting Out," examines letters written by family members requesting release of patients and how these requests were assessed based on determinations of both patient health and the caretaking ability of the family. Embedded in these assessments, offered by doctors *and* families, were competing notions of what it meant to be normal enough to live in society and the nature and function of surveillance outside the walls of the institution. By paying attention to the daily dynamics of institutional practice, the asylum emerges less as a blunt instrument for the social control and medicalization of colonial society than as a valuable historical site for reframing narratives of colonial repression and resistance.

Going In

In 1927, a fifty-seven-year-old farmer named Cac was found guilty and condemned to fifteen years of hard labor for setting a fire that killed a nine-year-old child. Following a psychiatric exam that found Cac irresponsible by reason of insanity, he was sent back home to live with his family. In response to a request from the colonial provincial resident about the possibility of his internment at the Biên Hòa asylum as a "preventive measure," the local director of health called for a new administrative inquiry that would look into Cac's "attitude, his acts and his sociability" since he had reintegrated into his village, as well as a medical certificate describing signs of dementia that could justify his internment. The author of the inquiry, conducted in the village of Gia Hòa in Sơn Tây province, where Cac resided, reported back, saying, "The mandarin let me know that since his return to the village, Cac has lived a peaceful life, without experiencing any new crises, and is not doing anything abnormal."[7] The doctor's mental exam also found no signs of psychiatric disturbances but warned that the crises could reappear in the future. On the basis of these eyewitness *and* expert reports, the local director of health expressed serious doubts about renewing Cac's confinement. Internment in an asylum, he argued, "could be justified only by actual mental troubles, or by default, by a *fonds démentiel* that allows one to conclude the risk of a relapse that could endanger the security of persons or the public order."[8]

This episode highlights how lay accounts were as important as expert opinions in shaping the decision to confine the mentally ill in Indochina. In particular, the power to confine patients depended on the assistance of families and communities who could provide doctors with critical information about long-term behavioral patterns and the specific circumstances surrounding a recent crisis. In the 1930s, when French psychiatrists working in Indochina began to speak about the virtues of preventive care and the need to create a clientele for psychiatric services, the role of the family became reshaped. The idea of a fonds démentiel—literally a demented foundation or background—signaled not only a shift in the norms of institutionalization but a growing concern among doctors to identify early warning signs so as to avoid confinement entirely, a process in which the family was envisioned to play a major role. The concern here is therefore to situate the process of confinement within a social landscape marked by a diversity of actors that contributed to shifting colonial ideas about what it meant to be abnormal, and to demonstrate the extent to which expert practices relied on the intervention of the public.

Mandated Placement

Before the first asylum was opened in Cochinchina in 1919, the colonial state relied almost entirely on families and communities for information and surveillance of the mentally ill, with only the most extreme cases sent to special pavilions in hospitals or repatriated to France.[9] In 1887, the administrator of Thủ Dầu Một province wrote to the director of the interior service, complaining of the lack of expertise and the continued absence in Cochinchina of any decree prescribing the legal process of confinement, "Since the beginning of the year three lunatics have already been sent to Chợ Quán Hospital. . . . It is impossible for me, given the absence of a doctor, to testify as to the mental state of the patients that I send to Chợ Quán; I am obligated to bring back the testimony of their families, their neighbors and the authorities of their village."[10] Investigations were often prompted by the concerns of community members, as in 1912, for whom "this individual is a continual source of anxiety, [and] his neighbors are in effect obligated to exercise on him a continual surveillance in the fear that he will set fire to the village and would be very happy to see him locked away."[11] Given the scarcity of experts, the observations of notables, in addition to those provided by the police, attained their own kind of authority, prompting one police commissioner to declare, "It appears to be superfluous to submit [the patient] to a medicolegal exam."[12]

This practice of *enquêtes*, or administrative inquiries, continued throughout the asylum era as procedures for internment became increasingly formalized. As in France, there were two principal ways people could find their way into the asylum. A *placement ordonné*, or "mandated placement," was requested by the administrative authorities, while the other, a *placement requis*, was initiated by the patient's family, relatives, or friends. Each required a medical certificate confirming an insanity diagnosis and issued only on a temporary basis. At the end of six months, confinement could become permanent depending on the medical progress of the patient. Psychiatric expertise became routinized as part of the internment process, working to expand the legitimate terms of confinement. The 1930 law, for example, extended the grounds for confinement under a placement ordonné from disturbing public security, tranquillity, or decency to include more medically grounded justifications for those who risked their "own security or possibility of cure."[13]

Local investigations to determine what happened to provoke internment represented a key first step in initiating a *placement ordonné*. After an incident, the police commissioner would call for a "small inquiry in the quarter. . . . If an inoffensive mad person, recommend stay with the family. If not sure, send to hospital for an exam."[14] In this way, nonexperts continued to play a powerful role in framing diagnosis and establishing the basis for confinement. In some instances, anticipating possible objections by families and other colonial officials required doctors to adopt an essentially defensive posture when pursuing internment. As the governor-general urged in 1928, in order to avoid "any later complaints," it is "indispensable to establish for each patient whose internment is initiated by public authority an order of placement expounding the motivating circumstances which make it necessary."[15]

These "motivating circumstances" were established by community surveys that inquired after the mental state of the soon-to-be, or just recently, admitted patients. Distributed by asylum directors to local notables as a

routine part of the confinement process, survey questions in the 1930s followed a newly standardized format:

1. Do you find (person) abnormal? If so, since when?
2. Has he or she committed any eccentricities? In the affirmative, what
   kinds?
3. Is he or she capable of working?
4. What is their conduct toward the other habitants in the village and
   the members of their family?[16]

The answers to these surveys provide a rare glimpse into how families
and neighbors, in being asked to offer their own impressions of the mentally
ill in their community, contributed to the development of colonial psychiatric knowledge. In a 1934 letter accompanying a survey of local inhabitants,
one asylum director asked, "Have you heard people say in the quarter that
Phúc is abnormal? Interrogate neighbors on this subject." And "Have you
yourself ever noticed any eccentricities by this individual and if so, which
kinds?" In response, Tin, the chief of Phúc's quarter in Hanoi, noted his
neighbors insisted on his good conduct and claimed that he never violated
the law. However, Tin shared his own impressions of strange behavior, an
allure anormale, that contradicted observations by Phúc's neighbors, suggest-
ing they might have tried to protect him from the asylum: "[He] breaks into
the houses of his neighbors without motive; left school; wanders all day in
the streets; when there is a procession or a vaccination doctor in the quarter, he pretends to be very knowledgeable even though he has no idea. And
finally, from time to time, he plays tricks on his parents as one does with
small children."[17] This idea of an allure anormale underscores the kinds of
eccentric but innocuous behaviors that the community had coded as deviant
but had clearly learned to accommodate.

For those individuals who routinely antagonized their community, the
results from the inquiries left no room for interpretation. Acts of violence,
theft, or arson represented the most common reasons for families and communities to seek confinement for the offending patient. A 1926 report from
the chief of security in Bạc Liêu province found that according to the local
population, André G. was considered "cracked"; he was without profession,
injured anyone who refused him charity, and would ride in a rickshaw for
hours and for payment, hit the coolie. A métis abandoned by his French
father, André had become such an object of terror in his community that
one doctor insisted on his confinement in an asylum rather than imprisonment because "weakened or disabled in the head, André is resistant to

sanctions as is shown by the numerous times he has been their object."[18] In some cases clear conflicts emerged between the patient and community, shedding light on the strategies each would pursue in their representations to colonial authorities. In response to the notables of one village whose report declared that Hoc had been "always crazy" for at least the past three years, the doctor noted the inconsistency with the patient's own statement who countered "that besides those periods which he had signaled, he stayed absolutely normal."[19]

Families were also in a position to offer specific information that psychiatrists used in making their diagnoses. Interrogating the family and neighbors of the patient both before and during a crisis was important because as one French psychiatrist pointed out, "It's the element that we are missing."[20] For example, the father of one patient named Hang described a turning point when his son began to suffer from strange episodes. He provided quite a detailed account of what French doctors later deemed epileptic fits that "began only three years ago, suddenly when Hang had a bizarre crisis, sat on the ground, swaying his body, his legs trembling and in the end declared himself a God." Neighbors and communal authorities later confirmed that Hang had indeed been "caught by madness." They reported that these crises appeared on a recurring basis, every month or two, during which Hang, possessed by spirits, would run wildly down the street and unfailingly attack the passersby.[21]

Doctors clearly took these lay observations about symptoms and behaviors seriously and incorporated them into their own diagnosis. While Hang's psychiatrist later noted that Hang displayed no symptoms during a twelve-day period of observation, he nevertheless underscored the regularity of the fits reported by the communal authorities and diagnosed Hang as a "para-epileptic" with a probable cerebral infection. Cases like Hang's also reveal the points of consensus that emerged between families and doctors over the presence of mental disability that required responsible oversight. Hang's father, for instance, reported that he would notice the onset of symptoms warning of an impending crisis and would be entrusted by his neighbors with Hang's surveillance until the period of danger had passed. He also periodically cut his son's long unruly hair as a way to "refresh his head." What Hang's doctor took as evidence of a shared notion that illness was rooted in the brain— the act of cutting hair—probably carried a different valence for Hang's family. Knotted hair (kết tóc) is closely associated in Vietnamese culture with insanity (bị điên) marked by an inexplicable and sudden change in character, a form of punishment caused by vengeful spirits.[22]

Moreover, in contrast to Western conceptions, it is the belly (bụng) rather than the head where thinking and reflection take place.[23] While beliefs in the causes and remedies of mental disturbances may have varied, the notion that public displays of antisocial behavior flagged an individual in trouble nevertheless provided common ground for making claims about insanity. Doctors' observations of Hang's father's efforts to remove knotted hair also indicates how cultural misreadings produced further justifications for confinement.

Not surprisingly, given the proximity of social relations, much of the violence committed by mentally ill individuals targeted other family members. Mental crises could be triggered by interpersonal crises—such as the loss of a child or spouse—or they could manifest in forms of intimate violence that ripped households apart. At twenty-eight years old, Nam was brought to the insanity wing of Huế Hospital by her husband and father after murdering her mother-in-law. After days of receiving careful assurances, she offered the following declaration of events to her doctor, providing rare access into the firsthand experiences of a patient's breakdown:

> That day, I was busy feeding my kids, my husband being absent. Then, taken by vertigo, I sank to the ground. All of a sudden, transformed by a spur of energy, I stood up and ran to the door. I then hastily arrived at the house of my mother-in-law, my neighbor. *I was like in a state of drunkenness.* I don't remember anything of what happened next for when I awakened, I found myself in my own home, surrounded by official agents who had come to arrest me. They told me that I had struck my mother-in-law with a machete and that the victim had died from her injuries. Me, I had no memory of any of that. I assure you that I never did anything to feel guilty about. I killed her in a moment of complete stupefaction [*abrutissement*].[24]

While the doctor may have described her testimony as "timid," Nam's wording leaves no question about her absolute denial of responsibility. The evidence provided by her family helped to provide broader context for the tragic event. Much like Hang's father, Nam's father confirmed a history of epileptic fits, starting at the age of thirteen, during which she would lose all consciousness, then eventually come to but forget what had happened. Though as an adult she now lived in a different household, her husband confirmed these crises had subsided but the aftereffects lingered and would reappear every few weeks or months: vertigo, nightmares, the habit of spacing out for seconds if not minutes. The doctor discovered she had a sister, also an epileptic, who had died at the age of nineteen, and one of her three children, a daughter, similarly suffered from epileptic fits. A long history of epilepsy within the family, including both direct ancestors and indirect relatives, helped doctors affirm the need for her to be placed at the Vôi asylum.

Kin networks not only mediated the process of confinement but also offered straightforward explanatory models for mental illness.

Colonial psychiatrists clearly became frustrated, however, when they believed families willfully fed them ambiguous or misleading information,

> We've only been able to receive rather vague information on the acts and movements of our subject, watched over by the members of his family since the moment he was returned the last time until the day he was found guilty of the crimes that he is now accused of. How did he comport himself throughout this one-year time lapse, exactly what did he do? It's difficult to know, as we estimate that it would be childish to absolutely believe the words of people who lie by nature and who, better yet, have a reason to hide more or less the truth. It might be better to believe entirely what the accused has to say himself.[25]

Despite doubts as to the quality of information they received, the clear frustration expressed here nevertheless underscores the extent to which psychiatrists depended on those who knew the patient best. It also reveals how some families and neighbors did all they could to obstruct the efforts of colonial authorities from sending patients back to the asylum. In one extreme case, on the evening of the sixth or seventh of February in 1909, a patient was kidnapped by his own family in order to prevent his confinement in a psychiatric ward at Chợ Quán hospital. By the ninth, despite leads from local notables, he had yet to be found.[26]

Requested Placement

By the 1920s, the seeming reluctance of families to present the mentally ill for care became a major concern for French colonial psychiatrists, who worried that they were receiving patients only after they were beyond hope. French experts attributed the hesitation of families to popular stigma against mental illness and imprecise notions that the "mad" were less gravely ill than they were in reality. Scores of colonial texts from the period remark on the superstitious and "credulous" nature of the Vietnamese people, who were said to trace the origins of mental illness to divine retribution for a prior sin.[27] As one provincial chief explained, "According to native beliefs, the cause of madness is entirely spiritual, such as the poorly chosen site for ancestral burial grounds, the unfortunate orientation of the family tombs, the breach of diverse rites or forms of worship, all causes that indispose the spirits and lead them to pursue the guilty individual."[28] Other "misdeeds" included passing under the shade of a large tree, bathing in a creek in the midday sun to the chagrin of water deities, and the wrong selection of dates for marriage or the construction of the family home.

According to these texts, in Sino-Annamite mythology, large numbers of gods, genies, and spirits were anthropomorphized and endowed with human-like qualities, including a weakness for pious attentions, flattery, and vengeance. They would seek divine reprisals on earthly sinners in all sorts of ways but most often through sickness. Mental illness, which could assume a variety of forms, was therefore considered the work of "evils that emanated from the spiritual world whose invisible agents strike those human beings without distinction of social class or rank, from the king to the commoner, the rich to the vagabond, the savant to the illiterate." But these gods, due to their "merciful and magnanimous" nature, would not seek the death of the sinners but merely demand they repent and express contrition for their mistakes. In order to determine the origins of this mysterious evil (known as the *ma quỷ*) and obtain the pardon of the outraged spirit, the family was compelled to seek out the help of a soothsayer or sorcerer to administer a cure.[29]

Mental illness implied not only a condemnation of the individual but also an indictment of the honor of the whole family, who was charged with the duty of caregiving.[30] As the manifestation of the past sins of ancestors, it also held important implications for the social future of the family. The discovery of a family history of mental illness, for instance, could jeopardize marriage contracts. While some French accounts describe the careful attention given to patients at home, others depict more brutal responses offered in powerful contrast to the rational and humanitarian character of modern French methods: one French doctor reported that in order to exorcise the genies who had "ravished" the soul of the person as punishment for some misdeed or sacrilegious act, the Vietnamese engaged in a range of brutal practices including flogging, violent dances, and forced baths. Even after multiple failed attempts at cure, the "unfortunate" remained the family or village's responsibility.[31]

For French doctors, how local understandings of the etiology and cure for mental illness came to be grounded in the honor of the family helped to explain both the widespread social stigma associated with mental illness and the reluctance of families to give up the patient. "For these reasons," as one 1903 report underscored, "families probably will not voluntarily consent to entrusting the insane to the administration in order to place them in a special asylum. They refuse to believe that our doctors can cure them."[32] Reinforcing these views was the unfavorable image of asylums propagated in the local newspapers that likened the asylum to a prison and the personnel to prison guards who were "preoccupied only with guarding as many patients as possible."[33] According to one doctor, concerns over exposure to the other mentally ill in the asylum prompted many Vietnamese to declare, "to be enclosed here and not become completely mad!"[34] And, as another stated simply, "prima facie the thought of a long confinement scares families."[35] As a result, the public tended to envisage the asylum only as a place of last resort: "All of these prejudices, these inaccurate critiques have created a frame of mind of which the principal result is that confinement is envisioned only as a final measure. A number of patients have waited until the last moment when it is too late and . . . often irreparable."[36] Anxieties about the coercive power of colonial prisons, well documented in the Indochinese press, may have also shaped Vietnamese perceptions about the risk of sending family members to the asylum.[37] Doctors often complained that the patients they did see included mainly the poor who sought free lodging and food, cure being "the smallest of their worries"; dilettantes driven out of curiosity and the opportunity to "intermingle"; and those who were simply "forced" by their families or employers. Secretaries and village notables, meanwhile, seemed to appreciate the benefits of modern medicine only when it offered a vacation from work. The director of the health service in Annam grumbled, "Consultations are frequented only by the most miserable of the population . . . the majority of whom don't know why they come."[38]

Concerns that the majority of the mentally ill remained out of reach, especially those in isolated rural regions, continued to plague colonial psychiatrists throughout the 1930s. Yet some began to express hope that the local population had grown more accustomed to the necessity of psychiatric care.[39] For these optimists, the increasing relative numbers of placement requis signaled an apparently "profound modification in the indigenous mentality toward the insane."[40] In 1928, the director of the Biên Hòa asylum reported that after making two tours of remote villages, the asylum personnel had easily been able to convince families to allow their loved ones to be confined at the asylum.[41] Six years later, a 1934 report noted that in the province of Bắc Giang, out of sixteen internments that year, fourteen originated with the families and only two were ordonnés. In all other provinces, the proportion was reversed. The proximity of the asylum and a firmer understanding of its purpose were thought to be significant factors in encouraging families to present their family members for care. One psychiatrist hoped that as knowledge and awareness increased, more families would demand placement rather than conserve the insane in their villages in such "lamentable conditions."[42]

Dr. Pierre Dorolle, a psychiatric expert and tropical medicine specialist working for the colonial health service in Cochinchina, was especially surprised that "the indigenous population has understood more rapidly than we would have believed the goal, the point, of the Asylum and they are more and more frequently receiving visits from family who come to demand the formalities necessary for internment, bringing patients in for an opinion and, after cure, maintaining relations with medical personnel in order to continue the required treatments. Also, patients who were given their liberty have solicited their own readmission."[43] For French doctors, the contact with families was invaluable as a "source of precious information." Their participation revealed that

> Annamite families, even of modest classes, are neither more nor less limited in their inability to understand than European families—I say even, much less. With a little patience, it's always possible to obtain useful information, and it's exceptional that families fail to surrender to our reasons when we explain the necessity of an internment or a prolongation of hospitalization. Little by little, they constitute a veritable clientele of service: those with intermittent crises are brought to us periodically by their families at the first sign of a relapse.[44]

Open Services

With the creation of a clientele of psychiatric services, French psychiatrists in Indochina hoped to shift the focus of treatment from long-term asylum care to early prevention and an "open door" model that relied on the family and the incorporation of new uses of space and the environment in treatment regimes. This more flexible and dynamic approach to mental illness projected the cosmopolitan attitude of colonial psychiatrists who sought to participate in the growing international movement around mental hygiene and, in some instances, to position themselves as even more progressive than their metropolitan counterparts.[45] In France, for instance, the League of Mental Hygiene, founded in 1920, campaigned for major reforms to the asylum system based on a more flexible conception of mental illness as an avoidable and curable disease. Under the direction of Edouard Toulouse, the League advocated for comprehensive services focused on prevention and rapid treatment as well as an expanded role for families in psychiatry and for psychiatry in society.[46] Whereas psychiatry's early founders in France considered families a source of mental distress and their continued presence an obstacle to recovery, the turn of the century brought a reconsideration of the role of the family as now an important ally of the psychiatric expert.[47]

As an essential complement to the asylum system, Indochina's first outpatient clinic for indigenous patients was established at Chợ Quán hospital in Saigon in 1928, followed by the expansion of similar services in major hospitals throughout the 1930s, including René Robin hospital at Bach Mai, located in Hanoi, as well as a Service des Aliénés located at hospitals in Huế (Annam) and Phnom Penh (Cambodia). Lanessan Hospital, a military hospital in Hanoi, opened its own neuropsychiatric clinic for both European and Indochinese soldiers in 1930.[48] Whereas the asylum would receive chronic cases that took years to resolve, these open services would assure triage and treatment *en cure libre* for milder cases as well as those who demanded more immediate attention. Respect for the principle of individual liberty was of utmost importance to ensure the service's success—that one could not maintain the patient against his will or against that of his family and that once a demand for release was formulated, he must be released if his mental state permitted. This "absence of all coercive character, the simplicity of admissions and exits have had a lot of success for the service . . . by encouraging families to entrust their patients before antisocial reactions which mandate their internment."[49] Not only would the service rely on families to facilitate the early detection of mental illness and prevent more serious forms from developing but it would also reduce costs associated with confinement and assure for those less serious cases (*petits malades*) a more rapid "social recuperation."[50] It would also play an important preventive role in the protection of public safety. Those patients whose state was determined by the resident doctor to compromise public security *or* his own cure would immediately become the objects of a regular procedure of confinement in an asylum. Open services would also help to habituate families to the idea of a lengthy confinement if necessary.

The colony's first open services at Chợ Quán Hospital grew out of what had previously been a kind of holding ground for individuals, picked off the streets and suspected of mental illness, awaiting transfer to the asylum. By 1934 the psychiatric service was described as "strewn" all over the hospital and consisted of a small room without amenities (neither showers nor toilets nor garden) for calm patients; at the other end of the hospital a former pavilion for prostitutes and prisoners was converted into space for calm female patients. In the middle of the hospital stood two groups of cells for agitated patients, including one old building that resembled a prison, which housed only the extremely agitated, and a modern building with a small barred-in, shady courtyard planted with grass and flowers, where patients would spend their days. In neither of these buildings was it possible to separate men from women. Next, found in the interior garden of the hospital, stood an isolated pavilion that served as the examination room and office for the service as well as two bedrooms for paying patients. A separate section was later created for the examination and treatment of criminals and juvenile delinquents. Described as a "psychiatric annex" to the prison, this kind of service, while enthusiastically supported by criminologists and psychiatrists alike, had yet to arrive in France.[51] In Cochinchina, by contrast, both accused and convicted criminals suspected of mental illness were hospitalized in the prisoners' wing at Chợ Quán while also placed under clinical surveillance by the specialist personnel in the adjacent psychiatric service. This development was touted by colonial doctors and administrators alike as a true innovation.

Between 1928 and 1934 the clinic doubled its patient load while decreasing the average length of treatment to just fifty days. The service also reduced by more than half the number of confinements in the asylum by hospitalizing those who could be cured more quickly. The numbers of patients leaving the service for reasons other than internment—such as cure, improvement, or repatriation—also jumped from 2 in 1928 to 110 in 1934.[52] These improvements were attributed to the specialization of the services personnel, which permitted a "more rational treatment of acute psychopaths." While the service was intended for the early and rapid treatment of mild mental disorders, out of the 287 patients treated in 1934, the majority (123) suffered from manic-depressive psychosis with 86 particularly expressing the manic form. As further evidence of gains in patient care, there was a fall in the relative number of deaths of patients despite the rapid growth in the number of admits (in 1928 for instance, there were 18 deaths for 110 admits while in 1934 there were 12 deaths for 256 admits). During the course of 1936, close to 400 patients reportedly received treatment and by 1939, 689 patients.[53] Of those 544 patients who left the clinic in 1939, 151 were deemed fully cured, 145 improved enough to return home to their families. Fourteen were repatriated to another health institution in their province of origin, 23 escaped and 57 died. That relatively few (121 in total) were transferred to an asylum is striking and demonstrates the extent to which the open service proved successful in treating and diverting patients.[54]

As clients of psychiatric services, families were asked to more actively participate in psychiatric care. For French psychiatrists, this required the Vietnamese to share basic understandings about mental illness as something that could be prevented and cured under the proper surveillance of experts. Indeed, the organization of an open service aimed at deliberately shifting the perspective of those families who continued to "hide their lunatics, drag them from pagoda to pagoda, from sorcerer to sorcerer, before bringing them to us in such a lamentable state that all our methods are ineffective and there's nothing more to do from a therapeutic point of view."[55]

While some family members remained reluctant to present patients for care, others adopted a more insistent role, even challenging those experts who refused their requests for confinement. For example, one man attempted to place his nephew, Phien, in psychiatric custody by bringing him to the Service for Municipal Hygiene in Hanoi in February 1942. After the examination, under the pretext of Phien's not being a "raving lunatic," the doctor concluded that his hospitalization would be too expensive for the administration (18 piasters per month) and consequently denied the uncle's request. Despite the legal regulations around confinement, in practice, psychiatrists continued to favor those who proved an imminent or dangerous threat. In protest, the uncle wrote to the governor of Tonkin, complaining, "A quarter of an hour contact with one suffering from mental illness would not allow the determination of his true morbid state. Rather it's necessary, in my humble opinion, that a serious observation be made at the Service of Psychiatry so that they can provide with all knowledge an authorized report on the state of the patient, that would allow the administration to subsequently decide to keep him in treatment or give him his liberty."[56] In general, however, doctors considered the service's open reputation as crucial to securing their relationships with families, viewed as an important part of the service's success.[57]

What the French took as an evolving agreement over the existence of mental illness does not imply that the French and Vietnamese also held similar beliefs about the etiology of the disease or the appropriate cure—far from it. While Jonathan Sadowsky in his work on colonial Nigeria understands this overlap in the social recognition of mental illness as demonstrative of the universal validity of psychiatric disorders, he also underscores the ways in which agreement nevertheless continued to be framed in Western terms and served as a powerful means to control socially deviant populations.[58] My focus here concerns more how this overlap created a common space for negotiation over care. While the categories of normal and abnormal continued to be framed in Western terms, I want to bring attention to the fact that the content of these categories critically relied on the kinds of information Vietnamese were willing or thought relevant to tell French doctors.

The rise in the numbers of patients treated at Chợ Quán Hospital therefore raises important questions about the impetus driving the growth of psychiatric services in Indochina. Were families truly becoming more accustomed to psychiatry, as the French suggested, or were there other social forces at work, such as the financial crush of the depression of the early 1930s, which prompted families to confine the insane? Did the expanding availability of open services generate their own demand, or did the growing demand reflect a more profound transformation in the perceptions of the local population? As Patricia Prestwich argues in the case of late nineteenth-century France, the fact that families increasingly presented patients for care does not necessarily mean that they had come to accept the dogma of psychiatric authority. Rather, as Prestwich writes, "It suggests that families had integrated the asylum into their own well-established systems of treatment for the mentally disturbed or chronically ill, systems that made skillful use of various formal and informal resources available in the family, neighborhood and the larger community. When these resources failed, they turned to the asylum, but not necessarily as a permanent or long term alternative."[59]

The same level of caution should be applied to interpretations of the upswing of voluntary admissions in the Vietnamese context. Throughout the interwar years, Vietnamese families increasingly resorted to institution-based mental health care when traditional healers did not work, or in the event of the failure of asylum care, recommenced the search for alternative therapies. Indeed, the decline in family admissions to the Vôi asylum in Tonkin, from a third of all new admissions in 1935 to less than 10 percent three years later, may be tied, at least in part, to the expanded availability of alternatives to asylum care, including open services.[60] However, one element that is distinctive here—as compared with France—is the dual uptake of Western biomedical and local healing practices, which reflects the complex and dynamic patterns of therapeutic pluralism of colonial Vietnamese society.[61] In the context of mental health care, therapeutic preferences shifted with the availability of new forms of treatment in ways that served to broaden rather than replace precolonial strategies for the management of mental illness.

As psychiatric activities diversified and expanded from the treatment of acute mental illness to the identification of underlying abnormalities, a greater reliance than ever was placed on the participation of families and communities. Families continued, however, to pragmatically pursue their own strategies in ways that both facilitated and constrained the ability of colonial psychiatrists to identify and care for the mentally ill. Rather than abandon their relatives to the care of French experts, families continued to write to doctors, visit patients in open services and asylums, and demand their release or transfer to institutions closer to home.

Getting Out

Families played an important role in determining patterns of discharge in colonial Vietnam. Confronted with the pressure to treat more acute cases, psychiatrists depended on family resources to support temporary or permanent releases for those patients deemed "sufficiently improved." Once the family agreed to assume responsibility for his or her care, the patient would be repatriated to his or her home village. Under the 1930 law, this practice became regulated as a definitive discharge (*sortie définitive*) when the patient was declared cured and released from the asylum or, more often, as a temporary discharge (*sortie provisoire*) when the patient was subject to a six-month probation outside the asylum. Indeed the sortie provisoire quickly became the dominant mode of exit from the asylum; at the Vôi asylum, for instance, four years after its opening, over 80 percent of patients who left were approved for release on a provisional basis only.[62] Under the sortie provisoire, patients would be sent home and placed under a "sanitary" or "medical surveillance" of either weekly or monthly visits by the local doctor, who administered medicine, kept track of the patient's progress, and eventually recommended a sortie definitive or reintegration back into the asylum.[63] This system of provisional exits resembles the use of "administrative surveillance" in the colony, which restricted where ex-prisoners could live, work, and travel upon release and mandated they present themselves weekly to the local *sûreté* office.[64] Whereas the practice of administrative surveillance attempted to sever former prisoners from their family and friend networks, the sortie provisoire instead explicitly relied on family networks to provide care and vigilant oversight.

Dr. Pierre Dorolle emphasized in 1937 that this period of supervised release should be viewed not as a break with the asylum but rather as an extension of it: "The *congé d'essai* [trial leave] therefore does not suspend completely the effects of internment from the point of view of restrictions on individual liberty."[65] The 1930 legislation, by permitting premature exits from the asylum "even before cure," worked to protect the interests of those chronic patients who would not otherwise benefit from a long confinement. He therefore lauded the innovative quality of the temporary or provisional charge as lending the psychiatric assistance in Indochina "a more distinctly medical character." The legislation also allowed the patients, their spouses, friends, or family members to put in their own request for release and, if denied, to petition the decision to a tribunal for a second expert opinion. Examining the letters by family members requesting release and the responses they received reveals how the sortie provisoire became a flashpoint for extensive negotiations between families, communities, doctors, and colonial authorities. These included competing definitions and assessments of the patient's ability to live in society—of which medical diagnosis formed only one of many considerations—as well as the ability of their families to take care of them. Whereas confinement allows us to look at how the abnormality of patients became established through a range of both lay and expert opinions and strategies, the process of discharge raises a different set of questions about what it meant to be normal enough to live in society and the nature and function of surveillance outside the walls of the institution.

Letter Writing

French doctors often claimed in their reports that the Vietnamese were humiliated by the presence of mentally ill family members. The archive of patient case files, however, reveals large numbers of family members, men and women, who petitioned for the return of their loved ones back home. As David Wright argues, letters by families in psychiatric archives, while little explored, nevertheless provide rich source material for uncovering those subtle negotiations inherent in the discharge process. These letters typically appear in Vietnamese with a French translation attached to the original copy. Most letters were almost certainly written not by the family members themselves but by a professional they had hired, pointing to the additional forms of mediation that shaped the negotiation of patient release across multiple registers of culture and power.[66]

Letters tended to follow a particular format in which families pledged responsibility for the future actions of the patient, enumerated their caregiving qualifications, and stressed their affective ties to the patient. Family members reassured doctors about the kind of care the patients would receive at home—most important, protection of the patients and others from danger. In 1887, a parent wrote, "I engage to watch over my son very closely and to avoid any mishap if he once again falls mentally ill. I will engage moreover to keep him at my House at Phước Lý where I live and not let him come to Saigon."[67] One father assured doctors that under his "personal surveillance," he would not let his son near any firearms and would allow him to be cared for by the doctor at the medical assistance service in Ninh Bình, where he worked.[68]

In their pleas for release, letter writers would stress their qualifications as responsible caregivers, including claims of their loyalty and devotion to the administration. Many would invoke the support of local notables with ties to the colonial administration to bolster their case, "I come here today to request to allow me to withdraw my son from this health establishment. The notables have certified that I am a good father and capable of properly feeding him."[69] Access to local elite networks represented an important boon, especially to indigent families, as they advanced with their petitions.[70]

Others took more extreme measures. In Cholon in 1927, three brothers of a woman treated at Biên Hòa wrote in their request for her release, "We have reserved for her a small house in the form of an asylum on our property, well aerated, with a garden, in the country, and we give you our formal assurance that the public will not be worried or disturbed."[71] It was even argued that home possessed some important advantages over the asylum for "the country air and family joy will contribute largely to hastening the cure."[72] These attractions of home relied on declaring the strength of affective ties while also warning of the risk of emotional harm to both patient and family as the result of a prolonged separation. Personal pleas to colonial administrators reached the point where the petitioners above claimed, "[Because of] our brotherly . . . love, we will fall into the same state as the person of interest, which is to say suffer from the same mental troubles because of the separation," and the health of the patient will never improve.[73]

In the event of a refusal of request for release, families would continue to negotiate with asylum directors around certain aspects of patient care. Should her husband not be discharged from the asylum, one woman (after multiple requests for release over many years) asked that he be moved into the "paying wing" where he would be provided with better care.[74] In another instance, before the Vôi asylum was opened to the public in 1934, a family, "panic stricken," asked the governor of Tonkin to prevent the transfer of a patient to Biên Hòa in the south. They requested "the favor of leaving us, in Hanoi or in the province of Tonkin, our unhappy Mân, where he will rest locked up until his death, we only demand the near presence of his family—so that we can have news and bring him whatever is necessary, and on his death, to arrange the necessary ceremonies that are demanded by our Buddhist religion." Although he was eventually sent to Biên Hòa, a visit by his wife to the asylum a year later secured the presiding doctor's permission to have Mân transferred to a hospital closer to home.[75] This sense of panic that suffused some letters meant also that psychiatrists would write to reassure families about the release of patients. In 1927, the director of Biên Hòa wrote to the governor-general in response to a request for a patient's release. "His family can remain calm, I'm trying to discharge as many patients as soon as their state does not present any danger for society or for themselves. Thirty-six patients were released since the first of January 1927 versus only thirty all of last year."[76]

Just as the inability to work secured the abnormal status of the patient on the way into the asylum, regaining the ability to work significantly paved the way for his or her release. In order to qualify for a sortie provisoire, the patients most often had to demonstrate that their symptoms of mental illness had gone away, which did not necessarily (and often did not) mean that they had been officially cured.[77] This was particularly true for those harmless or calm patients suffering from chronic diseases with no hope of a full recovery. Doctors writing in patient files would often associate the disappearance of symptoms with observations such as "he is calm, a good worker."[78] In Indochina, where asylum labor played a major role in patient therapy, the ability to work would constitute critical evidence of improvement in the patient's condition. Conversely, those who were unable to work were often found ineligible for release.[79] Wanting to leave also emerged as an important indication of a patient's cure. In the case of one orphan asked whether he would prefer to stay at the asylum or return to his sister, he elected to leave, revealing to his psychiatrist an "instinct for liberty" that demonstrated his readiness for discharge.[80]

The ability to labor fueled other practical concerns over the patient's capacity to "make a living by [his or her] own means" upon leaving the asylum.[81] This emphasis on self-support was not motivated solely out of concern for the patient's welfare. As the local director of health in Mỹ Tho province argued in 1920, "Many epileptics earn a living: this disease does not lead to hospitalization for life and perpetual care with costs to the Colony."[82] For those households who lost a principal breadwinner to the asylum, petitions for release were also linked to broader strategies concerned with the financial survival of the family.[83] In a 1921 letter requesting the discharge of her husband, Mai wrote to the director of the asylum asking for his "return home where he has left the heavy weight of eight children who have become very miserable since the absence of their father who is their sole support." She was successful, yet the asylum director underscored that her husband would never be able to provide for his family and must be kept preoccupied with household chores under the surveillance of his wife.[84]

In letters to asylum directors, family members offered their own opinions about the patient's condition and at times asserted that their loved ones had in fact improved enough to come home. Families would make claims based on either eyewitness accounts from asylum visits or written communications with the patient. The director of the Vôi asylum observed in 1934 how families closely monitored confinement in the asylum: "It is certain that families are interested in their patients. Since the opening of the asylum, 325 visitors have come to Vôi. What's more, a correspondence has been established between the asylum and families who frequently demand news. Even after they leave the asylum, families continue to write to let us know what has become of the patients and if they have readapted to normal life."[85] Rules around family visitation helped accommodate the demand. The chief doctor had to approve all visits, which would be supervised by a guard so that families could not attempt to hand illegal packages (including prepared food or alcohol, knives, cigarettes, or money) to patients. Only calm patients were permitted to receive visitors, while agitated patients could be seen only in exceptional cases.[86]

Exchanges of information, whether with the patients themselves or with the asylum staff, provided families with the opportunity to make their own determinations about the patient's condition. In 1921 a woman petitioned the release of her husband writing "my husband lost his reason suddenly after being sick for two months. The notables considered him to be insane and he was sent to the asylum in 1919. But as soon as he arrived . . . his reason came back to him. The proof is that my sister went to see him two times."[87] Others would rely on written accounts received from the patient, "Judging from the tone of letters that my husband sends to us, he has a lucid spirit and consequently harmless for his entourage. I must add that I will engage to assume all responsibility of the acts of my husband."[88]

These family assessments did not always square with those of experts and, at times, would generate significant conflicts. Rather than ignore family protests, doctors would instead incorporate them when defending their diagnoses. In this example, the psychiatrist at Biên Hòa actually cites verbatim the claims of the family in crafting his response, "Although it *actually appears* that he is in a normal psychological state, I cannot share the opinion of Võ T. N. (mother of the patient) when she writes ' . . . vì nó thiệt mạnh đã lâu rồi. . . .' [he has long since been cured] or that of Tran T. (husband of the patient) who writes: . . . 'now she is cured.'" He draws on language typically used in case files to accuse one of the petitioners, Trần, of himself being "incoherent" and of "presenting himself with an attitude that ripples with insolence demanding the immediate release of this patient."[89] In responding to challenges mounted by family members, doctors became exasperated and attempted to reassert their expert authority: "The petitioner writes in talking of her son, 'Nay nó thiệt mạnh rồi . . .' [he is now completely cured]. That is an assertion without foundation. Ky has received since his admission to the Asylum . . . only one visit, from his brother, and this happened nearly four years ago, that is, two months since his admission. I don't suppose that this visitor possesses the sufficient psychiatric knowledge for him to appreciate the cured or stabilized condition of our patients."[90]

By quoting the original Vietnamese in their replies, doctors demonstrated the extent to which they took seriously attacks on their expertise even as they skewered the conceit of the petitioners. Yet in translating these demands into French, and emphasizing the distinction between the appearance and the reality of mental illness, their responses underscore how these debates continued to be framed in Western terms that limited the scope for negotiation. Families thus engaged in forms of protest that ranged from challenging the decision to confine to questioning the knowledge upon which such judgments were made. Ultimately, however, it was asylum directors who held the authority to determine the risk of the patient to the community, making recourse to police powers in order to enforce their professional opinion. The spaces of overlap that emerged between experts and nonexperts therefore proved both shifting and profoundly unequal.

While psychiatrists faced opposition from families about their decision to prolong confinement, they also encountered resistance from colonial officials over the release of patients. For those with a dangerous history, even if their symptoms disappeared, local authorities feared that the disease would manifest at a later point and the lunatic would again pose serious threats to the security of the community. In 1925, the prosecutor general in Saigon used the case of one patient to warn of a broader pattern in which "the existence of these individuals is a vast cycle where prison and asylum alternate with phases of liberty when they commit minor offenses, misdemeanors and crimes which lead to a new confinement." The discharge of the patient in question would simply recommence "the conflict between the Medical Administration and Judiciary Service in another form."[91] Family demands for release must thus be situated within a broader constellation of concerns that included not only those of psychiatric doctors but also those of colonial authorities who sought to protect public safety.

These concerns over public safety surely responded to the growing political unrest of interwar Vietnam, which included increasing strikes as the result of worsening economic conditions and the massive repression that followed such incidents as the Yên Bái mutiny and Nghệ Tĩnh Soviet movement of 1930–31. These events perhaps explain why the colonial police force may have felt more eager and emboldened to maintain order in the streets, while institutional overcrowding and mounting financial pressure on asylum directors may have encouraged the release of patients before a full recovery. Communities, meanwhile, who had long developed their own mechanisms to preserve social order, became faced with a new set of social, economic, and political pressures to consider when determining whether to petition for the discharge of the mentally ill from colonial institutions.

These pressures impinging on the capacity of Vietnamese families and communities to take care of their own increasingly came to the attention of colonial officials. In a 1930 letter to Governor-General Pasquier, René Robin, the resident superior of Tonkin, reported that the custom of villages providing aid to the less fortunate had fallen into disuse in recent years. He observed that this communal custom, while not properly encoded in Annamite law, nevertheless formed an important part of oral tradition. In fact, the ethics of mutual aid and charity had long played a significant role in Vietnamese village life, particularly in the Red River Delta in northern Vietnam. Village covenants (hương ước), which date from at least the fifteenth century, lend proof of the power of these ethics of benevolence in shaping local customs. They found expression in the creation of mutual aid societies that allowed villagers to pool their resources—whether money, labor, or agricultural equipment—to protect themselves and each other in the event of death, disease, or disaster; to organize group celebrations like marriages and funerals; and to underwrite the costs of ritual ceremonies. Under the reign of Emperor Tự Đức (1848–83), the granary system also expanded. Inspired by Chinese models, the granaries provided a mechanism with which to regulate grain prices and feed the population in times of food shortages. While some French colonial administrators eventually tried to discredit and dismantle granaries as corrupt and inefficient, given their association with the ancien régime, others suggested resurrecting them as a model for food security well into the twentieth century.[92]

These mutual aid societies—which provided assistance to populations in rural areas and increasingly those in cities—critically helped to ease the pressure on colonial state resources, as Robin well appreciated.[93] Still, as he underscored in his letter to the governor-general, "This imprecision of charges of assistance imposed on the communes does not allow a clear discrimination between the respective duties of the family, village and the administration." Instead, Robin observed that villages had developed the tendency of discharging all obligations towards their "misérables" by directing them to the provincial hospital and even to the offices of the colonial administration. He conjectured that the recent upswing in vagrancy, especially in cities, could be traced to the negligence of communal authorities and the inhabitants themselves, and it would therefore "be convenient to remind them of their obligations toward the infirm and indigent, and to exactly spell out their responsibilities. . . . Still I do not think it's necessary to enact a new regulation. Simple respect for customs must suffice."[94]

How to allocate responsibility for the sick and unwanted, especially those perceived as mad, would require a complex readjustment in expectations that would tie families, communities, and the colonial state together in unprecedented ways. Perhaps Robin was correct that the social bonds on which the care of the mentally ill traditionally depended had begun to fray. Yet some families may have also come to see psychiatric confinement as a strategic resource and not only as a dumping ground.

Assessing Families as Caregivers

Doctors did not approve requests for patient release until they determined whether the family was in a position to take appropriate care of the patient. Family members were expected to look after the patients until they were cured and pledge responsibility for any violent acts that might occur in the event of a lapse in surveillance.[95] Those patients considered potentially dangerous would often still be released so long as their family took extra steps to ensure "a rigorous surveillance"[96] and to watch over them "day and night to avoid any sort of incident (fire, suicide)."[97] Some patients proved just difficult to manage: "I would like to signal that this is a cumbersome patient, difficult to feed and at times very loud. I doubt that his family can easily look after him."[98]

Given the burdens associated with guarding patients, psychiatrists investigated families, including their household income and personal habits, to determine if they were adequately equipped to provide care. Historians of colonial Southeast Asia have explored the ways in which the colonial state policed the intimate lives of families, especially in the realm of sexuality, but determining the capacity of families to meet the basic needs of their own sick responded to a different set of concerns about the social organization of Vietnamese family life.[99] As Hilary Marland argues in her work on insanity in Victorian Britain, this practice of assessing the quality of family care allows us to see how the state entered the entire household of the lunatic.[100] In 1922 the president of the municipal commission in Cholon confirmed that Nho, the brother of a patient, lived in a hut bordering a rice mill, where he earned 24 piasters per month. His salary was found sufficient to provide for the needs of his sister, who was subsequently released into their parents' care.[101] The location of the family home itself could play an important role. In 1924 the release of a woman to her daughter was approved as her "home is found just next to the police station, which allows us to believe she will be sufficiently guarded."[102] Scrutiny extended as well to the personal habits of family members. For example, in 1921, Etievant, the head of the security police in Saigon, described the brother of one patient as "35 years old, father of a family, a well-behaved and punctual worker at the Imprimerie Commerciale. . . . When summoned to my office he renewed his assurance to watch over his parent and to urgently warn the authorities if he notices any sort of relapse."[103] This case, however, illustrates the fears should surveillance at home fail and underscores how colonial authorities and doctors could hold different opinions on the fitness of family members for care. While Etievant approved the family, the director of Biên Hòa asylum nevertheless worried about the quality of care Sau, the patient, would receive at home. He approved the release under the condition that the family take full responsibility because, "mentally disabled, he will, without surveillance, rapidly begin to lead a life of debauchery, of laziness, and of vagrancy which will bring him again to either the prison or the asylum." The chief prosecutor also worried that given medical reports that the patient was not yet cured and still at risk for "excesses of all kinds," it was "to be feared that his brother would not be able to effectively watch him because of his job and Sau would commit serious violent acts."[104] Sau was consequently kept at the asylum under observation for two more years.

Refusals based on poverty were most often motivated by similar concerns: if the family proved unable to take adequate care of the patient, he or she would return to begging and vagrancy, risking relapse and a return to the hands of the colonial administration.[105] In a 1925 report to asylum officials, the administrator of Cần Thơ province described a set of petitioners as "very poor. They live . . . in a miserable hut of the value of 6 piasters. . . . May cultivates a hectare of rice belonging to Van-Dat-Lieng and only takes 60 units of paddy with which he feeds and takes care of his mother. Another brother of the lunatic, . . . Thau, is currently in Saigon, in the Medical Auxiliary Service, and his monthly salary is 4 piasters. It is therefore impossible for the family of Duong to come take the patient from Biên Hòa and care for him."[106] Only if Duong were found "capable of working and assuring his own existence" could he be released. This example demonstrates that not only wealthy families requested release. Families from a range of income levels would appeal for the return of patients, which, in certain cases, carried with it the assumption of a significant financial burden.

Home Care and the Competition for Clients

Doctors grounded their refusals not only in objections to the income level of the family but also in the type of care they thought the patient would receive at home. In one case, a psychiatrist determined that a patient, in the end, was "not a lunatic in the proper sense of the term." Yet the doctor worried that he was "a weak spirit, unfavorably influenced by mystical ideas and by the religious life that he has adopted over the last nine years. Will probably give release on a trial basis but he must return to his family and not the pagoda."[107] Indeed, French psychiatrists continued to compete with indigenous healers well into the 1930s, even as the colonial state worked to increasingly restrict the practice of traditional medicine and promote widespread and exclusive recourse to Western medical care.[108] In 1932, one psychiatrist worried over the "misdeeds of sorcerers in the psychopathic domains," noting that the "majority of the insane do not come to asylum until they have been dragged from pagoda to pagoda, sorcerer to sorcerer."[109]

In a 1928 article published in the French psychiatric journal *L'Hygiène mentale*, André Augagneur, the director of Biên Hòa asylum, and Le Trung Luong, a French-trained Vietnamese psychiatrist and the asylum's chief medical resident, described the local practices surrounding the treatment of mental illness in Indochina.[110] While contact with the Chinese over centuries may have, in the words of the article's authors, held "incontestable advantages" for the Annamites, they also inherited those "tenacious prejudices, ineradicable traditions and a complete ignorance for all that concerns mental afflictions." In Augagneur and Le's formulation, Chinese and Annamite doctors were the most to blame. They describe, for instance, how these doctors would continually relegate those diseases for which they were unable to explain the etiology or pathogenesis to the "immaterial world," noting, "It is infinitely practical for a man of the art of medicine, finding himself embarrassed, to chalk up his professional failures to occult powers. As doctors of the body, they can only master those physical sufferings which stem from the body, but they are powerless to annihilate the evil effects of spirits who are the vindictive and earthly manifestations of the wrath of gods and genies." Once a family witnessed one of their own fall mentally ill, they most often called upon the services of a practicing doctor, which invariably yielded no result. The authors describe a kind of "Asian politeness" whereby the family would insinuate that perhaps the disease was caused by spirits and therefore could not be cured by ordinary means. In this way the family and doctor would "mutually persuade each other" that malcontented spirits were to blame for the mysterious illness and that only one in possession of supernatural powers could counteract their evil effects.

It is here, as Augagneur and Le note, that the soothsayer "enters the scene." One apparently finds him "meandering in the streets, walking painfully with the aid of a cane, an indispensable accessory that serves as his guide, as this extra lucid clairvoyant is invariably blind. A very interesting detail which goes to show the naïveté of people who address themselves to an infirm person who makes oracles appear out of cold hard cash." The sorcerer goes on to perform a series of rituals, including the preparation of potions, and "continues in this matter until the patient is cured (this must arrive, at least sometimes?), or until his state declines following a debauchery of deafening noise, cries and vociferations, or what happens most often yet, until the capacity of families to pay is reached and they cannot afford to continue to follow the sorcerer on such onerous grounds."[111] The disdain here is palpable and mirrors the language often found in nineteenth-century medical texts in the United States accusing "quacks" of peddling misleading and, at worst, dangerous, misinformation. At the same time, the effort to create distance between clear-eyed European rationality and dangerous Vietnamese superstition also conveniently ignored the recent vogue for mesmerism, spiritism, and the occult among France's urban middle class, who hosted séances in their homes. At the turn of the century, the advance of secular medicine in the metropole had notably failed to erode French fascination with the mysteries of the other world and their potential for healing.[112]

Colonial doctors often accused these spirit mediums, or "sorcerers" (sorciers) as they called them, of not only promoting a spurious brand of medical treatment but igniting underlying forms of dementia and even inducing states of mental illness that did not exist before. One French psychiatrist suggested that these "superstitious instincts profoundly anchored in the spirit of the natives," especially tenacious in the countryside, would become surchauffé, or "overheated," by sorcery practices. The unfortunate subject, suspended in a kind of excited delirium, would then slide all too frequently into a dangerous form of insanity.[113] At special risk were the sorcerers themselves, who, in the course of their professional practice, would fall into a state of such "progressive excitation" and become "so strongly saturated that [they were] more or less under its influence." The craft of spirit possession was considered singularly ill suited to "maintaining the equilibrium of one's mental faculties" and the reason why so many of its practitioners often fell "victims to the demands of their profession" (in 1928 alone, seven sorcerers were reported to be confined at Biên Hòa).[114]

At the time of "possession," French psychiatrists would routinely describe sorcerers and their clients as "momentarily deprived of reason." What for colonial experts was taken as evidence of an underlying psychosis, for the families of patients seemed rather to signal a state of being taken over by a supernatural force. According to Vietnamese folk beliefs, this state manifests in a sudden and otherwise inexplicable change in character: wandering aimlessly, talking nonsense, claiming to be spirits, knotting hair, tearing clothes, and other kinds of unusual behavior. Designated as a kind of yin illness (bệnh âm), this condition is viewed as a punishment for sinning against or offending one's ancestors and can be cured only through ritual performance (whereas yang illness relates to physical or bodily disorders that can be cured by pharmacopeia). During this ritual, known as lên đồng, practicing mediums (themselves often former patients) allow the spirits to possess them or "install themselves as the seat for spirits to sit upon" (*bắc ghế cho các ngài ngự*) in order to honor the dead and exorcise the ghost from the afflicted individual.[115] Whereas colonial observers used the theatrics of spirit possession as a way to discredit mediums as insane and pursue their confinement in asylums, in Vietnamese culture, past experience with yin illness is taken as clear evidence of one's destiny to act as a bridge between the worlds of the living and the dead.

While colonial texts may have dismissed lên *đồng* rituals as superstitious and empiric, they nevertheless played an important function in bringing about healing for those who participated. As Nguyễn Thị Hiền explains in the context of contemporary Vietnamese practices, "Lên đồng spirit possession can be seen as a mode of therapy, bringing to its performers and audience a state of happiness as well as an *expectation* of healing." This expectation is based on what Nguyễn terms the "mythic model" of yin illness, which identifies the origins of symptoms in the supernatural world and promises healing based on the ability of spirit mediums to diagnose and cure through the use of rituals. In this sense, as Jane Atkinson points out, shamanistic rituals hold important similarities with Western psychotherapy, which itself makes use of rituals, impression management, and faith.[116]

In colonial-era discussions of spirit mediums and their clients, there emerged a shared notion of not existing as one's true self but with different explanations that demanded different responses. Psychiatrists would note in case histories that patients themselves would protest the terms of their confinement by explaining their irregular behavior as derived from genies or spirits and not from mental illness. In 1921, one patient claimed, "A genie (white tiger) had entered him and gave him the supernatural power to cure the sick and to supervise the notables."[117] The file of another patient noted that "Thai sees genies . . . from time to time in the form of men [doctors and nurses), these genies talk to him and declare that he will be liberated soon . . ." Thai was diagnosed as a megalomaniac, and the file reported his tales of great accomplishment, including curing a woman suffering from beriberi in just five days.[118] Psychiatrists in Indochina would use the diagnosis of *délire mystique* to describe this particular kind of insistence as evidence of mental illness. The French psychiatrist Paul Sérieux described this condition in a 1909 text under the designation *folie religieuse* to imply an abnormal preoccupation with supernatural.[119]

The medical language used in this case file is striking and suggests perhaps one reason French medical authorities felt threatened by sorcerers who continued to hold sway over local populations and why claims of medical expertise may have been taken as evidence of insanity in patients. Indeed, it is clear that despite French pronouncements to the contrary, families and communities continued to view sorcerers as an important source of cures for a range of ailments, from mental illness to epidemic disease. Jean Quang Trinh Lê, a native of Cochinchina, affirmed in his 1911 French medical thesis that sorcerers mostly intervene during "serious epidemics" and in "desperate cases, before which even the most renowned doctors are found powerless." These included, most notably, those "nervous and mental afflictions and all those diseases with indeterminate symptoms." While generally dismissive of the prospects for this kind of treatment, he nevertheless points out in a footnote that they have had some local success in curing hysteria.[120]

In 1928, an asylum patient case file described one patient, Cac, a father of three and the guardian of a small but well-trafficked pagoda, as possessing no intellectual capacity and in the grips of senility. Nevertheless he reportedly held a "certain influence" over other villagers among whom he had earned a reputation as a healer. During a violent outbreak of cholera one summer, one father delivered his child to him in search of a cure. Convinced that a demon had possessed the child, the patient determined the only recourse was to burn the child, dousing him with gasoline while the father looked on helplessly. Despite condemning his supposed powers as pure superstition, the French doctor writing in the patient's case file underscored the fact that this sorcerer trusted completely in his curative abilities and that he did his work with "conviction and fervor."[121] While colonial officials most commonly referred to sorcerers as charlatans who took advantage of a credulous and backwards population, it was those who truly believed in what they were doing that piqued the interest of colonial psychiatrists. In at least one instance, a French psychiatrist seemed almost seduced by the conviction of one patient whom he described as possessing "the allure of a prophet, with long floating wavy hair, piercing eyes, an aspect of 'freedom' but absent. . . . During the period of observation he presented no crisis or related symptom, spoke little but carried himself with an illuminated air, indifferent to what happened around him except for when we attracted his attention."[122]

Just over a decade later, the charismatic Huỳnh Phú Sồ — also known as the "Mad Monk" (bonze fou)—also relied on healing powers to convert peasants in the Mekong Delta to his popular new religion called Hoà Hảo (Peace and Harmony), which drew on Buddhist millenarian traditions. Like Cac, he also sported long hair, as well as a beard and long, light brown robes. His predictions for the end of French rule and his growing number of followers worried the colonial security police enough that they remarked in July of 1940, "His attitude appears more and more abnormal and leaves serious doubts about his mental equilibrium." In his security file, the chief doctor at the Cần Thơ hospital noted that he struck him as a *"petit maniaque . . .* poorly educated, even from the point of view of the Buddhist religion, infatuated by his supernatural powers to cure the sick and at times even by his descent from Buddha himself. This gossipmonger troubles public order by his proselytism. I don't think we can count on his promises of calm and silence, because his pride would prevent him from resisting the call to his religious mission."[123] From August of 1940, colonial authorities placed Huỳnh Phú Sổ under observation at the neuropsychiatric clinic at Chợ Quán, where he showed "no signs of agitation or dementia" during his ten-month confinement. His doctors nevertheless described him as "feeble-minded" and of limited intellectual abilities. Perhaps the most famous Vietnamese patient of French psychiatry in this story, his case underscores the extent to which decisions to confine and release were closely tied to concerns over mounting political unrest in the colony. I have been unable to verify the legend that he successfully converted his Vietnamese doctor, Tran Van Tam, who was later executed by the Việt Nam Độc Lập Đồng Minh Hội (or Việt Minh), to the *Hoà Hảo* cause. However, the mythology around Huỳnh Phú Sổ's powers of conversion, and specifically his ability to upend French psychiatric power, speak to the politically charged nature of these encounters as a site of colonial resistance.[124]

The Absence of Families

Upon his release from Chợ Quán, colonial officials required Huỳnh Phú Sổ to relocate to Bạc Liêu province, far from his home base of Châu Đốc and Long Xuyên. For psychiatric patients, this kind of provision was exceptional—indeed, this is the only such case I found—and reflects instead a common strategy adopted for policing ex-political prisoners. Rather, in the vast majority of cases, colonial psychiatrists explicitly relied on family resources to support the release of patients from overcrowded asylums. Indeed, while the relationship between doctors and families could prove problematic, the very absence of families generated a sense of crisis within Indochina's psychiatric assistance program. Families would refuse to take patients back, but more often asylum directors and colonial administrators were simply unable to locate family members even after multiple attempts and, in more desperate instances, after testing broader family networks. Some were sent to the Asile des Incurables in Hà Đông, for instance.[125] In many cases, abandoned patients were simply hired on to work as coolies at the asylum.[126] In a 1937 letter the governor of Tonkin, Yves Châtel, signaled the "serious in conveniences" posed by patients who occupied the place of those for whom more immediate internment was required. He cited the Vôi asylum, built to accommodate 300 patients, which in 1937 housed 424. In June 1938, a Commission charged with Vôi's oversight deplored the presence of "those abandoned, who uselessly encumber the rooms of the asylum and risk becoming human wreckage."

No legal text obligated families to take charge of patients ready for release. At the same time, it was unlawful to prevent patients from leaving the asylum after they had been certified as cured.[127] This posed a distinct challenge to asylum directors. In 1925, a patient approved for release could not leave because his wife was deemed unable to care for him. Legally, however, it was imperative he be released without any delay or, as the director of Biên Hòa warned, it would constitute "an arbitrary detention." Here we see the formal limits of the practice of assessing families' ability to care for their loved ones. The local director of public health also cautioned that the family could not be used as an excuse, "I do not believe that it is possible to argue the precarious situation of the family for keeping him at asylum." He feared "an eventual accusation of sequestering, for which, if I were to say nothing, would make me appear to be an accomplice."[128] The case was ultimately referred to the prosecutor general for review in order to absolve the medical service of any responsibility. As with confinement, fears of accusation over the refusal to release patients generated pressures that dictated changes in psychiatric practices. Psychiatrists became caught between the anticipation of pushback from nonexperts (whether from other colonial administrators or families themselves) and the very real problem of exactly what to do with the population of cured patients with no home to return to. Proposals for the creation of separate asiles colonies, or villages of mostly cured patients placed into makeshift "families," while debated seriously in the late 1930s, never came to fruition.[129]

Examining the complexities of the discharge process reveals how the decisions to release patients were grounded in judgments of both the patient's condition and the care he or she would receive outside the asylum. But even as the households of patients became objects of expert oversight, families also exerted their own judgments of French psychiatrists, in some instances by turning to traditional healers instead. Earlier we saw how areas of overlap between French and Vietnamese understandings of mental illness formed a common space for establishing the abnormal status of patients as the basis for confinement. In the context of discharge, a different kind of overlap between the spaces of the family and those of the institution succeeded in generating new opportunities for surveillance outside the walls of the asylum. Exactly how to police those recovering from mental illness in the community—what that oversight should look like and to whom it should be entrusted—and whether patients were ready to reintegrate back into normal social life continued to test the limits of expert authority.

Families and communities played a critical role in shaping psychiatric practices in colonial Vietnam throughout the interwar years. They provided information that assisted experts in forming their diagnoses, contributed to colonial ideas about what constituted valid grounds for patient confinement and release, and supplied crucial forms of surveillance and care in the community. The hold of colonial psychiatric authority was therefore far less hegemonic than one might think. The power to confine or seek treatment for those perceived to be abnormal continued to grow throughout the interwar years with the expansion of psychiatric services in asylums and major hospitals, including new forms of community surveillance. But rather than see this as a process that flowed inexorably from the colonial state, this chapter has illustrated how families and communities pursued their own strategies that shaped colonial ideas about the meaning of deviance and the therapeutic possibilities for addressing mental illness. A focus on the movements of patients and the role of families and communities in mediating these movements not only helps blur distinctions between asylum and society, the institutional and the familial. For historians of Vietnam, such a perspective also offers a new window onto the local dynamics of colonial rule and especially the social relationships among and between families, communities, and the French colonial state throughout the early decades of the twentieth century.

For historians of medicine, the relationship between the asylum and the community also offers an important site for examining the production of knowledge and power in colonial settings. As the symbol of colonial psychiatric authority, the asylum serves as the natural point of departure from which to examine what French doctors took to be their mission as well as the challenges they faced in realizing their ambitions in daily institutional practice. But such a perspective misses the emergence of those more fluid, dynamic spaces where doctors were forced to confront alternatives to the brand of care they offered. Everyday exchanges between French experts and Vietnamese families signal not only small erosions in the authority of colonial psychiatrists but also the emergence of a new, more diffuse kind of psychiatric power. This power tied the authority of European science backed by a repressive colonial state to the social norms of local communities that prescribed the bounds of the conduct of individuals, as well as the obligations and duties of families charged with their care. Grasping the full extent of colonial psychiatric power and the resistances it faced becomes possible only when we read patient case files for what they can tell us about life outside the asylum as much as life inside its walls.

The problem of what exactly to do with the growing numbers of abandoned patients would dog the asylum administration throughout the 1930s. Meanwhile, those mentally ill individuals who fell between the cracks of Vietnamese and French oversight would continue to surface from time to time in the pages of the popular press—wandering the streets, abandoned by their families, they served as a kind of warning about the dangers and pitfalls of a society in motion.

CHAPTER 5

Mental Illness and Treatment Advice in the Vietnamese Popular Press

In 1932, a colorful vignette about a "crazy woman" (*con rồ*) appeared in the Vietnamese daily newspaper *Ngọ báo*. Described as "skinny as a stick," her clothes in tatters, the woman is taunted by a ring of children who pursue her down the street until she starts to cry out. Her cruel treatment by the children makes her deserving of the reader's sympathy, yet her refusal to quit begging clearly opens her to the reader's condemnation as well. At one point she is likened to a kind of tumor in the neighborhood that will not go away.[1] Stories like these about vagrants, prostitutes, and criminals captured the imagination of the Vietnamese reading public during the interwar period. This journalistic genre, known as *reportage* and popularized in colonial Vietnam most famously by the writer Vũ Trọng Phụng, drew public attention to individuals on the fringes of mainstream society. Figures like the crazy woman—dispossessed, marginalized, often victimized—were features of a rapidly urbanizing landscape marked by deepening inequalities. Their stories provided a way for journalists to talk about social changes in the colony and to advocate for much-needed reforms.[2]

From the 1920s, Vietnam's popular press experienced explosive growth, fueled by a booming economy, growing cities, and rising rates in literacy in French, as well as by the romanized form of Vietnamese known as *quốc ngữ*.[3] In this chapter I use works from the *quốc ngữ* press in order to examine how ordinary people came to learn about mental illness: where it came from, what it looked like, and how it could be treated.[4] I show how mental illness emerged as part of the public discourse in Vietnam, and how it even provided a new language with which to frame critiques of contemporary society. For historians of Vietnam, the press has proved an important site for studying the formation of political parties during the colonial era and the exchange of new ideas about what it meant to be modern. Young intellectuals questioned the Confucian values of loyalty and filial piety on which Vietnamese society was traditionally based. They debated whether Vietnam should look either west to Europe or east to Asia for new models of what it meant to be "civilized" (văn minh). Some intellectuals pushed for a radical break with the past and "tradition," while others advised cautious compromise with their French colonizers. These publications addressed not only politics and current events but also a host of specialty topics including youth, business, fashion, sports, and cinema. Periodicals devoted specifically to women's issues such as Phụ nữ tân văn (Women's News) emerged as Vietnamese women, especially those from more elite backgrounds, enjoyed expanded opportunities for education and activism. Fiction and poetry reflected shifting views on ethics and morality. Together these texts paint a portrait of a vibrant and dynamic city life, characterized by new consumption habits and modes of sociability as well as growth in political consciousness.[5]

This public sphere also played host to a new marketplace for ideas about mental illness—from melodramas about suicide and broken hearts to translations of Chinese medical dictionaries that cataloged symptoms of mental illness. Families discovered recipes for home remedies and asked for expert advice in newspapers, as well as the dozens of popular scientific and medical journals that emerged in interwar Vietnam, to address topics ranging from the science of weather and electricity to the spread of epidemic disease and the history of Chinese and Vietnamese, as well as Hippocratic, medicine.[6] Whereas colonial French sources tended to dismiss traditional Vietnamese medicine as quack or "empirical"—that is, nonscientific—these quốc ngữ journals provided a space where French and Western-trained Vietnamese doctors could communicate with each other and the public.[7] Rather than cast aside indigenous explanatory models of illness, these authors explicitly drew on local conceptions of health and disease in order to reach a lay audience. I look in particular at medical glossaries, found in serial form in popular scientific magazines, to examine how doctors attempted to align Vietnamese explanations of disease with French psychiatric categories. Not only did these authors concern themselves with furthering the public's understanding of abstract scientific concepts; they also offered practical information and treatment advice about the rational management of mental disorders, organized around an ethos of self-help and prevention. These texts promoted certain Sino-Vietnamese understandings about health while rejecting others as backwards and antimodern, even as they incorporated new concepts from Western biomedicine.

Writers and journalists also used the language of mental illness to denigrate rural prejudice and highlight the hidden perils of modern urban society. Suffering from mental illness was at once a mark of civilization and proof of an inability to keep up with the fast pace of modern life. It was evidence of a weak spirit as well as its cause, which one could and should take steps to manage. What is perhaps most striking is the mobilization of mental illness to speak about a range of contemporary issues—urban poverty, rural superstition, gender roles, colonial corruption, excessive materialism, and romantic individualism. In this way, mental illness increasingly surfaced not only in the streets of colonial Hanoi or Saigon but also in the pages of Vietnamese newspapers, novels, and scientific journals. This chapter therefore sets out to capture what the Vietnamese reading public learned about mental illness during the interwar years and how these lessons may have shaped family decisions around psychiatric treatment.

Popular Perceptions of Asylum Care

One novella, published in Hanoi in 1933, presents a decidedly dark vision of life in colonial asylums. *The Secret Tale of the Asylum* (*Bí Mật Trong Nhà Điên*), a work of translation (most likely from French), tells the story of a "ruthless" (*vô lương tâm*) asylum director who kidnaps patients for profit.[8] Rather than use his medical expertise to help people, the author explains, the asylum director, Bảo An, only tries to get as rich as possible. The asylum over which he exercises a "constant supervision" is described as a vast place, countless rooms following one after another, housing hundreds of patients. While people at a distance may think he is only being helpful, the author cautions that this place has "buried alive" (*chôn sống*) countless numbers of "good people" (*người lương thiện*). Bảo An's evil plot is facilitated by those morally bankrupt individuals who want to dispose of inconvenient family members. The author describes one instance in which a son wants to force an early inheritance of his father's fortune and produces a significant sum of money in order to "whisper" (*nói nhỏ*) in the ear of Bảo An. Afterwards the doctor comes to visit the son's family and, pointing at the father, announces in just one sentence, "This person is crazy." In this way, an innocent person is "pulled" (*kéo*) forcibly into the asylum, where he will one day actually become mentally ill and die. This scene echoes frequent complaints voiced in patient case files that sending a family member to the asylum would only lead to mental illness that did not exist before or exacerbate a preexisting condition. In the popular imagination, asylums were reserved only for the most seriously sick. While personal enrichment served as the most common motivation for illegal confinement in this story, there is also mention of a wife who "whispers in the ear" of the asylum director in order to exact revenge on her cheating husband. This kind of abuse, asserts the author, is "the real face of the asylum."

The Secret Tale of the Asylum depicts the asylum not only as a site of rampant corruption but also as one of brutal treatment. At one point in the narrative, an asylum guard enters a confinement room after hearing a patient's violent screams. He goes into scold the patient and slaps him once. In response, the patient becomes angry and jumps up to hit him. The guard chokes him, and when he finally releases his grip on the patient's throat, his body has stopped moving. The asylum director, upon hearing the story of the patient's death, becomes extremely angry over the loss of money for the patient's monthly upkeep, a bribe from the patient's wife and her sibling. The story conveys a vivid sense of the vulnerability of patients—not to mention those innocent, prospective patients—as well as the distrustfulness of doctors. This sinister aspect is reinforced by the book's cover, which presents a stylized image of a person in the shadows, his body contorted, clutching bars in an attempt to break free (figure 21).

While it was plucked from a different cultural context, the publisher clearly anticipated that this story and its macabre portrayal of asylum life would resonate with its Vietnamese audience. Indeed, it seems as if Vietnamese readers had, by 1933, already become familiar with these kinds of representations. Asylum directors often complained in their reports to the colonial administration about the unfavorable image propagated in the local press that likened the asylum to a prison and the personnel to prison guards who were "preoccupied only with guarding as many patients as possible."[9] It was not a completely unreasonable claim—many asylum employees were in fact former prison guards.[10] Moreover, an adaptation of the narrative to fit the local context—namely, the portrayal of both the asylum director and guard as Vietnamese rather than French—is significant. This story functioned less as anticolonial critique than as condemnation of greedy Vietnamese elites.

With the asylum envisioned as a place of last resort, a 1934 article published in the popular weekly periodical *Phụ nữ tân văn* can be seen as an attempt to demystify the goings-on at the asylum. First established in Saigon in May 1929, the highly successful *Phụ nữ tân văn* reached a peak circulation

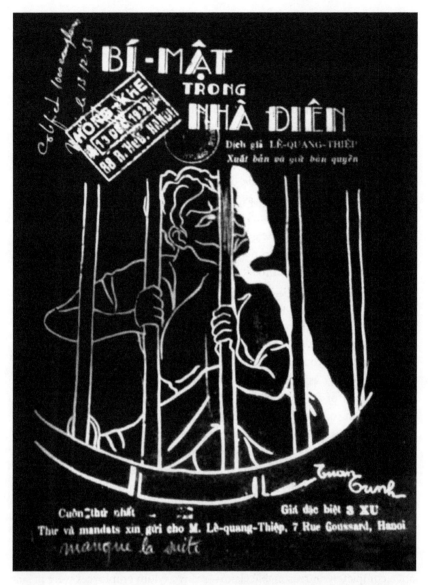

FIGURE 21.   Cover of *The Secret Tale of the Asylum (Bí Mật Trong Nhà Điên)*, 1933. (Bí Mật Trong Nhà Điên) dịch giả Lê Quang Thiệp. Published in Hanoi in 1933.

of 8,500 copies in 1930. It would shutter its doors just four years later in December of 1934. Despite the title's emphasis on women, *Phụ nữ tân văn* dealt with a range of social issues including religious practices, sports and hygiene, dialectical materialism, poor labor conditions in the colony, and the destitution of the Saigon's beggars and prostitutes. David Marr's description of the publication is instructive, "From beginning to end it was at once catalyst, conceptual testing ground, and disseminator of new ideas— indeed perhaps the best example of this type of journalism ever to emerge in Vietnam."[11] It is perhaps not a surprise then that concerns about mental illness surfaced within the pages of this journal.

The 1934 article took the form of an interview between the journalist Nguyễn Thị Manh Manh and the French-trained psychiatrist Nguyễn Văn Hoài, who would serve as Biên Hòa's first Vietnamese director from 1950 to 1955.[12] Nguyễn Văn Hoài was born in 1898 in Vĩnh Long province and grad- uated from medical school in 1919. After working at a hospital in Saigon, he left for Paris for further training at the Sorbonne before returning to Cochin- china in 1930. Bucking the popular attitudes of his peers that cast such posts as undesirable, he specifically requested an assignment at the Biên Hòa asy- lum. His unorthodox orientation to his profession—as unusually dedicated to a particularly undesirable class of patients—earned him praise but also a dose of humorous derision. Apparently those who knew or worked along- side Nguyễn Văn Hoài described the doctor as himself *gàn* or "eccentric."[13]

Framed as a dialogue between journalist and doctor, the article's language adopts a deliberately conversational tone, targeting an educated, if lay, audi- ence. Questioned about the risk factors for mental illness, Nguyễn Văn Hoài cites a range of "social diseases" including alcoholism, syphilis, and tubercu- losis. He is also asked about the numbers of patients treated at the asylum, the gender breakdown—twice as many men (420) as women (218)— as well as how many patients were released in the previous year (20–25), perhaps as a way to emphasize that confinement did not necessarily mean a life sentence. As for the causes of mental illness, Nguyễn Văn Hoài stresses that there is no absolute form of insanity or, as he notes in the interview, a *folie absolue*. Rather, he explains, it is composed of three elements: intellectual (in terms of loss of reason), emotional (or spiritual), and physical (determination or strength), which are present in varying degrees, therefore rendering mental illness individually specific. Drawing on local idioms that promoted the idea of health as humoral balance, he explains that when these three forces are distributed evenly, the body develops "like a seed or plant" (*nảy nở*).[14] Abnor- mality results from an excess or deprivation of one of these forces.

This emphasis on the individualized nature of mental illness also informed Nguyễn Văn Hoài's practice as an eager and dedicated observer who would routinely question both patients and families about their experiences. He reportedly approached the patient not simply as a "case" (*ca*) or "unit" (*đơn vị*) of an objective psychiatric category but rather as a "little galaxy" (*tiểu vũ-trụ*) that needs discovering.[15]

Nguyễn Văn Hoài also describes the kinds of treatment provided at the asylum, including the administration of medication, psychotherapy, and the use of labor. He explains the aim of treatment as a process of mental reordering away from the stresses of ordinary life, followed by a gradual reintegration back into society. In this sense, he notes, the pagoda can be seen as one form of treatment. Here Nguyễn Văn Hoài departs from the official line adopted by most colonial psychiatrists during the period who deplored the pagoda as at best, ineffective and at worst, detrimental to the mental health of patients. This is not altogether surprising in view of later characterizations of Nguyễn Văn Hoài as devoutly religious and extensively learned in Buddhist traditions. Apparently he saw his role as one of transforming the "hell" of asylum life into a kind of "heaven of the mind" (thiên đường tâm tính).[16] His background and training thus made him uniquely poised to act as an interlocutor between the Vietnamese and Western medical traditions.

Glossary Entries

Other articles discuss alternatives to asylum care in ways that demonstrate the eclecticism of Vietnamese beliefs about mental illness, and especially the influence of Chinese medicine on holistic notions of physical and mental health. This idea of health as humoral balance, for instance, draws on the precepts of Chinese traditional medicine, which state that all medical disorders, including various expressions of mental illness, arise from abnormal states of qi, or vital energy. The invasion by external forces (e.g., a sudden wind or temperature change) or internal imbalances (which include somatic or mental processes or both) may disrupt qi and prevent the heart (xin), which houses the spirit (shen), from functioning normally.[17] For some early twentieth-century Vietnamese writers and physicians, this environmental framework—stressing the balance among external and internal, physical and moral forces—was not necessarily incompatible with Western ideas about disease; instead they insisted on points of conceptual overlap.[18] Colonial-era medical glossaries, for instance, demonstrate how Western-trained Vietnamese doctors attempted to square Vietnamese understandings of mental illness with French diagnostic categories. Included as part of a popular health magazine published out of Hanoi, entitled Bảo an y báo, the glossary entries I examine here covered a wide range of chronic and infectious diseases, from mental illness to malaria, with short descriptions of common symptoms, origins, and treatment. Arranged alphabetically in Vietnamese, entries often included references to other comparable disease categories, resulting in an implicit ordering of related illnesses from the least to the most serious.[19]

In the typology of mental illness that emerged, what is perhaps most striking is the use of Vietnamese idioms of "weakening nerves" (*suy thần kinh*) and "poisoned blood" (*ngộ độc máu*) to describe various mental disorders while at the same time offering an equivalent French clinical designation (appearing in parentheses in the text, in italic font). Even as doctors made use of colloquial expressions and everyday experiences, they nevertheless sought to draw out in a more scientific fashion the distinctions between specific syndromes, often by making reference to more advanced French medical terminology. These French terms would act as temporary placeholders until satisfactory Vietnamese equivalents emerged alongside and would eventually assume their place in the scientific literature.[20] Glossary entries therefore served as a kind of compass that tacked between lay and expert, Sino-Vietnamese and French, understandings of mental illness and may have therefore helped the Vietnamese public navigate a complex therapeutic landscape. As one doctor put it plainly, one must first determine "exactly what type of craziness" and the reasons behind it in order to determine the correct course of treatment.[21] This was a project in which their readers were invited to participate.

When plotting the coordinates of mental illness in colonial Vietnam, the glossary entry for *điên* (or *folie* as the listed French equivalent) is the most natural place to start. Translating roughly as "crazy" in English, *điên* has its origins in Chinese, meaning literally "upside down" or "reversed." The entry describes *điên* as a common word used to identify a person who has "lost control" and is "therefore dangerous for both himself and for society." Noting the word's wide usage in everyday conversation, applied to any disease of the nervous system, the entry sets out to specify exactly which conditions qualify as *điên*. The author explains that there are two main categories. The first is attributed to the "weakening" of the nerves (*suy thần kinh*) and consists of several subtypes: those who are born with "under-average" mental capacity (*suy nhược* in Vietnamese or *débile* in French), those "eccentric" people (*gàn dở*) whose reasoning has "taken a wrong turn" (*délire systématisé*), and those whose brain has "degraded" gradually over time, losing all ability to reason (*điên rồ* in Vietnamese or *démence* in French). The second category belongs to diseases of emotion or excitement (*manie*), observed most clearly in people who dance, sing, or talk very exuberantly. While many make a full recovery, those who suffer from a more serious underlying disorder (*constitution maniaque*) may experience multiple relapses. Others may become frustrated or depressed, an emotional state conveyed here with the Vietnamese expression "no interest in anything" (*chán nản việc đời*). The entry cautions that this type of *mélancolie* is more dangerous because it may lead to suicide or even the murder of a relative. Throughout the entry the author makes multiple appeals to commonly held understandings about deviations from what is "ordinary" or "average."

The entry explains that điên occurs "when the disease of the nervous system is at its strongest" and individuals "lose their mental capacity completely." In this sense the term correlates most closely with the classic French definition of *aliéné*. The entry also points readers to a related but less severe disorder of the nervous system known as *dở người* (or *troubles mentaux*, as it was translated from French) listed under a separate heading in the glossary.[22] *Dở* (literally "unfinished" in Vietnamese) refers to an individual who has retained some level of mental capacity but who is nevertheless "mixed up" (*lộn trí khn*) or impaired because of "weak nerves." These individuals possess ideas "different from ordinary" that do not fit with reality or common knowledge, and their thinking can be best described as eccentric (translated as *gàn*). At special risk are women who are about to or have just given birth. In this case, *dở* is not necessarily the result of some underlying defect but instead tied to the condition of being pregnant. Whereas *dở* tends to refer to strange ways of thinking or using language, the term *cuồng* typically denotes the sudden loss of control of one's physical movements and actions. The entry for *cuồng* (translated as *délire furieux* in French) indicates that it may belong to the category of điên, but it may also refer to a disease of the tissue covering the brain resulting in a high fever and stimulated brain activity.[23] Symptoms include night sweats and nightmares, and recommended treatments range from covering the head with ice and washing the body with warm water to the use of pharmaceuticals such as chloral, bromure, and antipyrine for calming the patient down. It is important to note how glossary entries defined different mental illness categories by their underlying causes and characteristic symptoms as well as by their relationship to each other.

Weakening Nerves

These entries reveal understandings about the close relationship between the nervous system and mental illness. According to Vietnamese medical beliefs, the nervous system (*thần kinh*) is one of the four major bodily functions, alongside digestion, circulation, and reproduction. The nervous system is closely associated with the brain, which acts as the coordinating center that governs the functioning of all other organs. Along its various pathways, the nervous system also conveys emotions such as stress or sadness, which reflects the close intertwining of heart and mind in Vietnamese medical understanding. Observations about how Vietnamese people tend today to communicate emotional distress in terms of stressful thoughts (or thinking too much) reveal themes similar to those found in the colonial-era literature. As Tine Gammeltoft writes in her ethnography of contemporary health practices in northern Vietnam, "Talking about brains seems to be another way of talking about hearts, and intellectual capacities are about social/emotional capacities."[24] In everyday talk, the Vietnamese also tend to place their thoughts and feelings in their belly (bụng). The use of these idioms to communicate distress are therefore rooted in notions of the body as a single, integrated unit sensitive to imbalances emanating from within and threatening from without. They also reveal the extent to which negative emotions are expressed somatically.

During the colonial period, writers in the popular scientific press most commonly invoked the notion of "weakening" (suy nhược) to explain the strong relationship between one's physical and mental capacities. In 1938, the physiological connection between the nervous system and brain was explained to readers in an article published in the popular scientific revue *Khoa học tạp chí* entitled "What you should know about your nervous system," which opens with a page-sized image of a human skeleton. Here the nerves appear as a network of fibers that spread outwards from the brain.[25] Because of their association with the brain, nerves are perceived as directly responsible for the mental ability to control one's body and emotions. A "weak brain" (suy não) or "weak nerves" (suy thần kinh)—the two terms are often used interchangeably in many of these colonial-era texts—may lead to a host of both physical and psychological problems ranging from mild headaches or dizziness to full-blown madness (điên). The same article describes the weakening of nerves in terms of the depletion of lecithin, a natural chemical composed of phosphorous elements, which make up the fibers of the nerve. (In fact, lecithin is a building block of cell membranes that make up the majority of the protective sheaths surrounding the brain and nervous system. It helps the circulatory system transport fats and nutrients easily and works to protect cells from oxidation and hardening.) With a decline in the body's lecithin stores, the article explains, the nerve system becomes "poisoned" and the nerves "wear out." Calling this process "no different" from the moment when our bodies most need to eat, the entry draws the following analogy: just as "we keep rice in the house in case we are hungry, we also keep the chemical lecithin in the body in case our fibers require it." To this end, the author encourages the reader to eat fresh foods such as milk, eggs, raw vegetables, and rare meat, which contain the nutrients required to sustain lecithin levels and which, he further points out, are easy to find and affordable for most.

The concept of weakening also extends well beyond the physiological process of nerve degradation. Its use in the popular press to denote a distressed state reveals how physical strength is closely coordinated with emotional strength that can be compromised by a variety of social and environmental factors, from abrupt changes in wind and temperature to stress and bad luck in one's family. The weakening of nerves that results from these physical, psychological, and social imbalances puts one at special risk for mental illness.[26] Vietnamese discussions around the weakening of the nervous system also carry a clear moral valence that can be traced to Confucian notions of "self-cultivation" (*tu thân*), which stress the importance of reorganizing and internalizing one's emotions in order to lead a respectable life.[27] Whereas strong nerves are associated with highly desirable personal qualities such as self-restraint, determination, and intelligence, weak nerves imply a person's inability to control his or her body's physical movements and behavior, to conform to social rules, and to meet social obligations. Meanwhile, many colonial-era articles describe people with weak nerves as "cowardly," "not determined or decisive," and possessing a "weak spirit."[28] These attributes predispose individuals to mental illness, but they are also described as pathologies in and of themselves. Other authors draw explicit connections between mental illness and antisocial behaviors, likening alcohol and drug use, as well as sexually transmitted diseases, to poison for the nervous system, as further evidence of the inability to control one's desires.[29] In this way, the use of weakening to explain mental illness to the public carried with it the kinds of social judgments attached to ideas about one's ability to function in society, to weather adversity, and to prevent more serious forms of illness from developing. As an explanatory model, it looked to clues in the past, such as one's family history, while also making claims about the future in terms of one's responsibility to protect subsequent generations.[30]

What we see here is not an exercise in the straightforward translation, or even appropriation, of medical concepts across cultures. Instead the Vietnamese popular press became the site of a new assemblage of knowledge about mental illness, a composite or bricolage of different epistemologies. Glossary entries, for example, reflect the fundamental precepts of Sino-Vietnamese medical knowledge—itself a prior assemblage of Confucian, Taoist, Buddhist, and folk traditions—as well as the mobilization of French psychiatric designations in the elaboration and ordering of medical categories. The use of familiar local idioms like weakening to explain the relationship between disintegrating nerves and mental capacity also demonstrates the extent to which medical concepts traveled between Western-trained Vietnamese experts and lay readers. By playing host to a public sphere that brought new ideas to new audiences, the quốc ngữ press allowed diverse understandings about the provenance and progression of mental illness to be assembled in a way that was meaningful to its reading public. In so doing, it played a vital role not only in the circulation of knowledge but also in making a new kind of localized knowledge possible.

To Know, to Tell (*Mách Giúp, Bảo Giùm*)

Most texts eschewed medical theories in favor of offering practical advice on the detection of the symptoms of mental illness and tips on how to care for family members at home. Many articles open with a vignette about a particular patient whose story is used as an entry point for discussing the dynamics of mental illness more generally. A 1933 article in the popular scientific journal *Khoa học tạp chí*, for example, introduces the case of a student from Haiphong whose symptoms progressed from general forgetfulness and loss of focus and slurred speech to a more acute stage marked by delusions (mistaking a tree for the devil, talking about losing his spirit) and violently striking those around him.[31] His disease was attributed to weakening due to excessive mental strain associated with the stress of preparing for exams, as well as the bad luck experienced by his family and the pain, disappointment, and anger that it had caused. Students, in addition to business people, athletes, artists, and craftsmen were routinely cited as those people who faced especially high levels of stress in their daily lives and were therefore particularly vulnerable to mental illness.[32]

The student's case in 1933 serves as an illustration of the difficulty of treating mental illness because its symptoms seem to change all the time. The author cautions his audience, "You may think the patient is recovered when he is not." Readers here are also warned not to be too quick to romanticize the disease, "to attribute [it] to superstitious causes and wait for a miracle cure to arrive." Instead this author (among many others of the time) outlines concrete steps to take at home, especially making changes to the external environment, which was thought to impact mental health through the senses, in order to restore an individual's strength or inner balance. First, the mentally ill person should be removed from the noisy bustle of urban life to the quiet of home or the pagoda. Walls should be painted or covered in green or light blue, colors thought to possess soothing qualities, while red or black or dark blue was to be avoided. The author recommended inviting a monk to the house every other day, to look straight into the eyes of the patient and blink very fast for ten minutes in order to calm the patient's spirit. An abundance of flowers (especially Western roses—if they were white, all the better) was also recommended, for their aroma was thought to act as a kind of medicine that traveled through the nose to the nervous system. Listening to or playing music was also a common exhortation. People were also told what *not* to do. Rice and meat were to be avoided, as well as any salty, spicy, and sour foods. Alcohol was off limits, also coffee. Articles also cautioned against reading books, especially those to do with literature and science, and thinking too much in general. Sexual urges must be resisted, and brothel visits were prohibited.

Articles on mental illness also took the form of advice columns, which allowed concepts that in scientific language might be too difficult and abstract for the common reader to be recast into the form of confessions and "expert" responses.[33] They served as a kind of forum where the public was both addressed and enabled to talk, as in the case of one individual, Ông D. D. Nhit, who wrote to *Khoa học tạp chí* in 1934. He confessed that he was "crazy," violent and aggressive toward others, unable to control his actions but at the moment of recovery would grow very afraid and have nightmares. He described his heart and kidney as weak, a common trope among Vietnamese who attribute a decrease in vital energy and low bodily resistance to changes in these internal organs. In the answer portion, the column's editor, Dr. Nguyễn Văn Luyện, a Western-trained Vietnamese doctor, responded with recipes for various herbal remedies, including detailed instructions on their assembly and consumption at home. In one month the patient should recover, and he asks the gentleman to "let him know how it goes!"[34]

These advice columns in popular medical journals appeared alongside growing numbers of manuals that advised middle-class households on the principles of basic hygiene and preventive medicine. From the late 1920s books and pamphlets also began to tackle sensitive subjects such as sexual hygiene, pregnancy, childbirth, and venereal disease.[35] Together these texts allowed the public to troubleshoot problems at home and to self-medicate. The growth in networks of basic medicine stores, or *dépôts de médicaments*, run by the colonial health service, together with the rapid rise of the Western pharmaceutical industry in Vietnam, expanded the opportunities for taking care of basic health needs at home. Adjacent to an article on protecting the health of one's child, for instance, a Vietnamese woman might see an ad for Nestlé formula. Ads boasting the elixir qualities of syrups, balms, and pills to relieve the pain of arthritis or discomfort of poor digestion reveal the extent to which French, Vietnamese, and Chinese druggists worked to tap the urban population of colonial Vietnam as potential consumers.[36]

The reference to herbal remedies above also reflects the continued reliance on a vibrant and long-standing traditional Vietnamese pharmacopeia.

As the historian Laurence Monnais has argued, the availability and accessibility of both old and new medicines, as well as ideas about efficacy rooted in cultural beliefs about health and the body, themselves flexible and dynamic, determined the selective appropriation of treatments by the Vietnamese public.[37] In terms of treating mental illness, this therapeutic pluralism is clearly evident in observations of families bringing the mentally ill for care at hospitals and asylums, the dual use of herbal remedies and synthetic drugs at home, as well as the emphasis on diet and temperature which reflected more holistic understandings of the relationship between body, mind and environment. Sometimes nothing worked, and readers turned again to the pages of scientific journals for help. One women wrote to *Khoa học tạp chí* in 1934 about her younger brother, who suffered from a seizure disorder (*động kinh*), and described in close detail the typical progression of his episodes.[38] He had already taken many Western *and* Vietnamese medicines but had not yet recovered, and therefore, in an act of desperation she asked the medical doctor as well as the reading public for any advice. Her sense of helplessness underscores just how hard it was to treat mental illness and why there was so much of an emphasis in the press on prevention and the management of symptoms. These limitations extended to the colonial asylum, where an emphasis on older techniques of hydrotherapy and therapeutic labor prevailed in the absence of better, more effective alternatives. Drugs were typically administered in order to calm patients during acute psychotic episodes rather than for the purposes of long-term stabilization.

Advice columns served, in the words of historian Sabine Frühstück, as "spaces for choreographed interaction and exchange of knowledge between experts and the public," but they also demonstrate to what extent mental illness had become a topic of public interest.[39] The author of the advice column in 1934 cited above includes references to other stories about "brain disorders" and "disintegrating nerves" printed in the pages of the same journal and also discusses a number of cases documented in the newspaper *Đông pháp thời báo* from February of that year. What is significant is that the growing volume of articles on mental illness allowed the editorial staff of journals and their readers alike to start making connections and grouping together cases of those who seemed to suffer from similar symptoms. Here we see how knowledge about mental illness escaped the official channels of medical training and institutions in the colony. Alternative forms of expertise were staked on common sense and lived experience—on conversations with patients, on the correspondence they had with their readers, on direct and hearsay testimony of the relative success of different treatment methods.

In the eyes of their editors, advice columns also performed an important kind of public service. Writing in 1932, shortly after the appearance of the inaugural advice column "Mách Giúp Bào Giùm" in *Khoa học tạp chí*, the editor, Nguyễn Công Tiểu, reflected on the immediate popularity of the column, which paired those "who know and tell" with "those who don't know and ask."[40] According to Nguyễn Công Tiểu, the column performed multiple functions. It put experts into conversation with laypeople. It preserved family medical secrets handed down over generations by memorializing them in print, thereby making otherwise private knowledge public. Finally, and perhaps most important, it made knowledge free. For those who suffered from chronic disease but did not have the means to consult a doctor, the column had the potential to minimize individual suffering without also attempting to extract a profit. Nguyễn Công Tiểu offered a not-so-subtle critique of greedy doctors and insisted that the column, by contrast, was motivated by a sense of decency and social obligation, as well as a nascent nationalism, providing assistance for "all types of people who need to survive in *our* Vietnamese society."[41] While giving thanks for the deep enthusiasm of his readers "from all social classes," he also expressed dissatisfaction that the journal did not yet have the resources and power to reach everyone "nationwide." The 1920s witnessed the emergence in the Vietnamese language of new terms such as "citizen" (*quốc dân*) that reflected changes in political consciousness. An explicit goal of the advice column, therefore, was to democratize knowledge and to tailor that knowledge specifically for the needs of a nascent national Vietnamese community.

In this way, the promotion of new forms of self-medication during this period can be explained by the proliferation of health clinics, as well as by the growth of the quốc ngữ press, which connected expert knowledge with the reading public and an expanded consumer market for pharmaceutical drugs. In the context of mental health, the practice of self-medication was also an act of rational self-management: to prevent and manage disease meant avoiding certain foods, disciplining one's desires, exercising caution, taking control of one's life. To the extent these basic principles intersected with contemporary discourses about what it meant to be modern and Vietnamese, self-medication also entailed the performance of a new kind of subjectivity.[42] The ability to internalize and adhere to social norms offered evidence of one's sanity and moral virtue. For a society in flux, just what these norms should be were vigorously debated. Not surprisingly, the language of mental illness would be mobilized by experts and intellectuals to offer critiques of the past and prescriptions for the future, a blueprint for navigating modern life.

Breaking with the Past and New Ideas of the Self

The popularization of knowledge about mental illness reflected at once the new kinds of pressures confronted by members of Vietnamese society as well as new ways of talking about what that society should look like. It also revealed the extent to which mental illness had become mobilized as an instrument for framing social critiques. For an urban elite searching for new modes of social and moral order, the continued reliance on spirit mediums, especially in rural areas, was condemned as mere superstition, backwards and out of date. As one author remarked rather facetiously in *Ngày nay* in 1940, "Those with supernatural powers, don't worry at all: Vietnam still is the country of Vietnam, still the place of spiritual forces, ghosts, spirits and such sacred things."[43] He went on to tell the story of an elderly woman from Bắc Giang province who suddenly came down with a fever and began speaking continuously, almost in a dreamlike state. Her family hired a spirit medium, who proceeded to beat her in order to release the ghost and who was subsequently arrested by the colonial police for physical assault. The author complained that as long as people believed that ghosts hid in the bodies of patients, the arrest would have no effect at all on popular beliefs about mental illness. "The crime is in the way people think about ghosts—sorcerers will be out of a job if this kind of thinking changes; they will need to change occupations, learn to carry cargo, to plow in order to earn their living."[44] Superstitious beliefs were correlated with the lack of a work ethic and an unwillingness to take control of one's own life. They also served as a marker of the backwardness of rural society.

The inclusion of a caricature in the article—a small figure in profile, wearing traditional dress and walking blindfolded—provided a visual critique of a population that seemed content to follow in the steps of someone who was obviously lost (figure 22).

This use of satire to draw distinctions between old and new, tradition and modernity, was common in the Vietnamese press during this period. These distinctions also took on an important spatial dimension as the divide deepened between urban and rural areas. Satire found powerful expression in caricatures—often in the form of a simple, rural peasant attempting to navigate fast-paced city life—as a way to offer humorous critiques of rural prejudices, to affirm the status of the modern elite urban class, and to express ambivalence about the changes rocking 1930s Vietnam.[45]

For Vietnamese intellectuals, superstition (*mê tín*) was diametrically opposed to the scientific thinking that was essential for the development of a modern society. Science, based on rigorous and objective inquiry, would

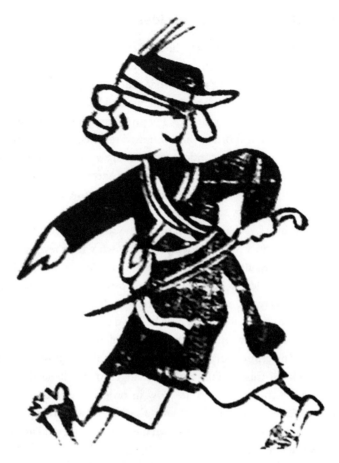

FIGURE 22. Caricature used in article critiquing superstition. "Chuyện: Ma làm," *Ngày nay*, July 20, 1940.

not only unlock the mysteries of the natural world but also liberate the Vietnamese peasant from the chains of superstition.[46] Yet the path to modernity was also marked by a profound ambivalence. In the 1920s, a new kind of pathology known as "neurasthenia" had begun to afflict a growing number of urban elite who suffered from symptoms of depression, anxiety, insomnia, and nervous and mental exhaustion. This clinical diagnosis was *not* applied to the Vietnamese population by French doctors and was instead reserved exclusively for white patients who suffered from "tropical" or "colonial" neurasthenia. Yet the disorder found its way into the pages of the Vietnamese popular press, including ads for pharmaceuticals and electrotherapy clinics to treat weak nerves. While neurasthenia sometimes appeared under its own designation in Vietnamese (*suy não*), more often authors used the French terms of *neurasthénie* or *surmenage*.[47] Considered a *malaise de civilisation*, neurasthenia served as a marker of modernity and therefore a positive measure of equivalence with the white colonial population. Vietnamese journalists insisted that, rather than displaying a cultural tendency to suicide as suggested by French colonial observers, this "fast-growing epidemic" of neurasthenia could be attributed to "disappointment, weariness of living, nervousness, and depression."[48] No matter one's station in life, maintaining physical and mental health would require more vigilance than ever before.

Neurasthenia's emergence spoke to deep anxieties shared by Vietnamese intellectuals about the disorientation that comes with social change.[49] These anxieties took an even more dramatic form in the spike of suicides during the 1920s and 1930s. In the space of twelve years, the number of suicides in Hanoi jumped from thirteen in 1927 to forty-two in 1934. These statistics include only reported deaths from suicide, not attempts.[50] One journal compared the frequency of suicide reports to a contagious disease spreading throughout the city, while another spoke of a "season of suicide" (*mua tự tử*) in its August 1935 edition. Meanwhile the weekly *Phong hóa* ("Mores") asked whether suicide, as the ultimate act of individual will, was not the "price of modern civilization."[51]

Interpretations of the suicide epidemic tended to link individual acts with social causes, from the oppression of peasants by the communal authorities to the disintegration of traditional family life to the effects of the economic depression, whose nadir coincided with the rise of suicides in the colony between 1931 and 1934. This is markedly different from the static culturalist frameworks employed by nineteenth-century French observers who explained suicide among the Vietnamese population as excessive expressions of nostalgia or the fear of dishonor.[52] In his 1937 doctoral thesis from the Hanoi School of Medicine, Vũ Công Hòe also establishes mental illness as a "somewhat frequent cause" of suicide. He cites the work of the famous nineteenth-century French psychiatrist Jean-Etienne Dominique Esquirol, who contended that all those who commit suicide are by definition insane. Esquirol reasoned that if the pursuit of life is a normal phenomenon, then any act that threatens its integrity is inevitably abnormal and hence pathological. Suicide is therefore an *aliéné* "of the moment." Vũ Công Hòe concludes that, in the Vietnamese context, these individual and social explanations "intertwine" to produce heightened vulnerability to suicide.[53] While suicide may be the act of an individual, society "cannot declare itself to be entirely irresponsible" and, by improving living conditions, it has the capacity to mount an "effective prophylaxis against this social evil."[54] He thereby absolves Vietnamese culture as the sole cause of suicide and instead, citing Emile Durkheim, insists on suicide as an inevitable byproduct of any modernizing society.

For concerned onlookers, the suicide epidemic also made visible the dangers associated with the decline in Confucian ethics, which generally condemned suicide as an act of weakness and as abandonment of duties toward one's parents. The worrying rise of romantic individualism was also to blame. Young people between the ages of twenty and thirty accounted for nearly half of the 242 suicides in Hanoi between 1927 and 1936. Young women, daydreaming and impressionable, seemed at special risk; their suicide rate exceeded that of men in 1931.[55] Vietnamese publications detailed the suicides of heartbroken young women in the lakes that dotted Hanoi, dubbed the "tombs of beauty" because of these premature deaths.[56] While some saw suicide as an explicit act of rebellion against cruel mothers-in-law and forced marriages, others blamed the popularity of sentimental novels like Pure Heart (Tố Tâm), which detailed the passionate love affairs between young men and women who met tragic ends. Pure Heart, published in 1925 by Hoàng Ngọc Phác, is an adaptation of the traditional "scholar-beauty" story (tài tử giai nhân) format that became popular in seventeenth-century China. It also drew inspiration from nineteenth-century French romantic literature, which emphasized the subjective experience of individuals and privileged emotions over reason and senses over the intellect.[57] This romanticist sensibility informs the main action of the novel, which can be found in the close examination of the interior lives of its two main protagonists, Đạm Thủy and Tố Tâm (after whom the story is named).

Hoàng Ngọc Phác later described his work as a "psychological novel" (tiểu thuyết tâm lý). Using first-person narrative and letters and diaries to give the reader entry into the thoughts and feelings of the two lovers, the novel marked a departure from the Vietnamese literary tradition, although the famous romance the Tale of Kieu (Truyện Kiều) is a notable exception. In a 1942 interview, Hoàng Ngọc Phác reflected on his approach to writing Pure Heart: "My goal was to write a novel (tiểu thuyết) completely different—in both form and content—from existing novels. In form, I followed the new French novels; the way of telling the story, the description of scenes—all this was according to French literature. In content, I brought in some new thinking; the psychology of characters was analyzed following the techniques of the well-known contemporary novelists."[58] Most notably, these included Paul Bourget, a member of Émile Zola's circle in Paris and a leading practitioner of the psychological novel. His 1889 work *Le Disciple* served as direct inspiration for some of the scenes in *Pure Heart*. These references to French romantic literature would not have been lost on *Pure Heart*'s readers, who, like the protagonists in the book, included members of Hanoi's elite; as part of their education in French schools, they would have read the works of Victor Hugo, Alexandre Dumas, and Alphonse de Lamartine. The novel caused a sensation, not least because it seemed to imply an attack on Confucian morality. While Tố Tâm ultimately sacrifices her personal happiness to marry someone she does not love, she nevertheless expresses initial reluctance to succumb to familial pressures. Her potential willingness to disavow her filial duty and the perceived injustice of her punishment, a slow death from tuberculosis (itself a major romanticist theme), made a deep impression on readers.

Hoàng Ngọc Phác, reflecting on *Pure Heart*'s tremendous popularity, remarked, "It seems to have appeared when we were waiting for such a novel."[59] Indeed, the novel's publication tapped into a growing fascination among interwar Vietnam's reading public with notions of the self as separate from one's social role, family ties, or place of origin.[60] The idea that it was possible to have a secret life, an interior space invisible to others, proved as destabilizing as it was liberating. Novels such as *Pure Heart*, in detailing the emotional lives of its characters from their own points of view, provided a welcome opportunity for readers to probe these previously uncharted psychological depths. Just as glossary entries in popular scientific magazines served as a kind of compass that helped the Vietnamese public navigate a complex therapeutic landscape, the psychological novel provided a compass for navigating complex emotions that accompanied the trials and tribulations of modern life. It did so not just in terms of exploring new themes around the individual's subjective experience but also by experimenting with new forms of storytelling. Freud, for instance, clearly influenced the prolific writer and social commentator Vũ Trọng Phụng whose protagonist in *To Be a Whore* (*Làm Đĩ*) recounts the history of her sexual life as a series of evolutionary stages in ways that resemble the confessional style of the psychoanalytical method.[61]

Readers learned how to read themselves not only in romantic novels but also in the "New Poetry" (*Thơ Mới*) where poets laid bare their inner fears and fantasies for the world to see.[62] The works of Western philosophers like Kant and Nietzsche, via interlocutors like Nhất Linh, provided novel concepts for organizing the self and its relationship to society while readers were introduced to Western psychological concepts like "the unconscious" and "the ego" in the pages of Southern Wind (*Nam Phong*).[63] In their explorations of the self, these popular works also cultivated a certain kind of "modern" reader: capable of self-reflection and self-doubt, skeptical of dogma and ideology, reflexive and flexible, balanced and insightful, even displaying a sense of humor.[64] It should be noted that these are all qualities explicitly *not* associated with mental illness.

The deployment of psychological concepts in popular culture—not just in the biomedical literature but in novels and poetry—provided new tools with which to know oneself in a rapidly urbanizing society. The alienation that resulted from city life could produce a disintegration of identity, even lead to suicide, yet it also allowed for the liberation and even reinvention that comes with living outside the confines of family and communal life. For some, the rise of individualism (*chủ nghĩa cá nhân*) marked a critical, and welcome, break with the Confucian past, while others warned of a descent into immorality and corruption. Radical intellectuals yoked the emancipation of the self to the movement for national liberation while also worrying about the social implications of privileging individual needs over collective goals.[65] These new aesthetic sensibilities and literary forms therefore allowed writers and their audiences to turn inward as they redefined what it meant to be both modern and Vietnamese.

Mental Illness as Social Critique

Stories of mental illness were also used to condemn new forms of consumption, to diagnose society itself as corrupted and weak. One article written in 1940 talks about a man who became crazy after winning the lottery as a kind of allegory about the dangers of wanting too much too fast and the importance of maintaining a balanced life.[66] What is interesting here is not the condemnation of excessive wealth per se but the pathologization of indulging in grandiose fantasies in the first place. The consumption of psychological theories themselves also served as a vehicle for skewering the bourgeois pretensions of urban elites as exemplified in Vũ Trọng Phụng 's 1936 satire *Dumb Luck* (*Số đỏ*). In the novel, a character named "Dr. Straight Talk," a misinformed quack, attempts to explain the sexual deviance associated with male puberty and female menopause by making reference to the work of Freud and Pierre Vachet, the famous interwar French sexologist. At a gathering of Hanoi's finest, for example, Dr. Straight Talk makes the following observation,

According to Dr. Vachet, during periods of sexual crisis, women often exhibit strange and unexpected symptoms. The interruption of menstruation coinciding with the shortening of the temper signifies the onset of physical and spiritual changes that in turn may trigger a complex and intractable desire for sex. . . . The crisis is virtually unavoidable, but, fortunately, it lasts for only a limited period of time. Ultimately the cause lies in the sex organs themselves: the fact that the eggs lack blood and the uterus ceases to menstruate. This gives rise to a kind of physical chaos that Vietnamese women often refer to as "the end of the guilt."[67]

The author, as if to express his own skepticism, makes several references to the crowd's "roars of approval." He also notes the kind of shallow comfort these mangled scientific pronouncements provided, as evidenced by the adulterous Mrs. Deputy Customs Officer, who "was glad, in fact, to know that she had misbehaved in such a scientific way."[68]

One article published in 1938 concerns itself with a different kind of social pathology.[69] The author, Tân Thạch, writes in the first person about a recent visit to the asylum. Tân Thạch describes entering the area where they keep the "crazy people" (người điên). First he directs his gaze through an opening no bigger than his open hand into a small, locked room, so dark that you cannot see in from the outside. The world of these real "flesh and bone" patients, he marvels, "stops at these four walls." But before we start to pity crazy people too much, he reminds his readers that they have their own profound, interior worlds and just as with Molière's comedies, we should not make inferences based on hasty impressions. The article then proceeds as a series of encounters with individual patients—a man who had fallen into a deep depression at the end of a relationship, another who had lost his entire fortune, and a young woman, a spirit medium, accused of insanity in the course of her professional practice. As we saw in the previous chapter, this was not an uncommon occurrence; French psychiatrists considered sorcerers to be at special risk for mental illness.[70] The author demonstrates a deep sympathy for these patients. He insists, "I don't want to be like the doctor" in search of the reasons behind their insanity. Instead he argues that the doctors have got it all wrong, that they "keep confined the happiest people, they are not crazy."

Up until this point, the article is written from the perspective of an outsider literally looking into the darkness of the asylum cell, a metaphor for the disorientation of the confined patients and their segregation from society. Here, however, the piece dramatically reverses perspective and instead looks inside out. Rather than those confined, removed from society, it is we, Tân Thạch insists, who "are the crazy people" for continuing to allow fascist leaders like Hitler and Mussolini their freedom. He notes that on the doctor's certificate prescribing confinement, "it says this person is dangerous and harmful for other people. . . . It's meaningless!" At the same time, these leaders are clearly crazy (điên đồng bóng) and pose a real threat to millions of people, and yet nothing is done. He goes on, "If anything, we should be locked up for pretending not to know and for flattering world leaders who are dangerous for society," for we are "crazy in spite of ourselves" (here using the French term aliéné malgré nous). One interesting aspect of the article is the play on the theme of light and shadow. Tân Thạch begins and ends the article with the same scene: "One day at noon in the summer I was looking for shade." In other words, at a time of intense direct light, he sought relief in the darkness. He continues, "I see myself wanting to be crazy, in order to quietly smile, even though my heart is full of pain and bitterness." This statement can be interpreted to mean that there is a happiness and peace that comes with ignorance or even insanity. Understanding the world too much, a world that has itself gone crazy, only brings hopelessness and despair.

One last set of articles shows how mental health intersected with ongoing debates over the place of women in Vietnamese society. An especially fractious divide can be found in the coverage of a sensationalized murder trial that rocked the pages of Trung bắc tân văn in 1940.[71] A woman named Vũ Thị Cúc was accused of killing her lover, Nguyễn Xuân Trường, a mandarin from Bắc Giang province, out of jealousy by stabbing him thirty-eight times. The court case boiled down to a question of motivation: was Vũ Thị Cúc a "victim of love," which drove her to momentary insanity, or a "criminal of civilization" who knowingly committed a brutal act? The case attracted intense public and media interest due to the high rank of the male victim, the beauty and youth of the accused woman, and the intense passion that fueled her crime. Reactions to the trial also served as a barometer for shifts in perceptions of gender roles, about what counted as normal or acceptable behavior as the measure against which claims about insanity could be measured.[72]

According to one newspaper that documented the proceedings, the court's audience divided into two camps. The first, described by the author as "old-fashioned" (cổ phái), condemned Vũ Thị Cúc for killing her lover in such a brutal fashion. According to this point of view, if a woman is abandoned by her husband or even if she is subjected to cruel treatment, she should bite her teeth (cắn răng) and bear it. They expressed nostalgia for older times when wives, thrust to the side in favor of younger concubines, nevertheless respected the moral duty to reconcile themselves to their husband's wishes. To present a gentle, submissive face was a priority. This position clearly embraced a traditional conception of women's role based on orthodox Confucian texts that stressed the three submissions (to father, husband, and eldest son), as well as the embrace of the four feminine virtues of labor, physical appearance, appropriate speech, and proper behavior. In this rigid formulation, women's lives were subordinated entirely to the preferences and comforts of men. It should be emphasized that in general, but especially at an earlier stage of Vietnamese history, male and female roles were far less differentiated and much more flexible in reality than the kinds of idealized relationships promoted in scholarly texts.[73]

Meanwhile, the second faction, the one belonging to "new ideas," expressed pity and hope for Vũ Thị Cúc that she not be judged too harshly. This group stressed the love and honesty of Cúc, who sacrificed all of herself, including her virginity, for this man who ultimately betrayed her. While they conceded the shocking violence of the crime, a different version of womanhood is nevertheless presented here, one in which the woman has an identity separate from her partner's and whose actions are motivated by romantic affection. This position, challenging the predominant social norms about female weakness and dependency, intersected with broader attempts in the early twentieth century to rehabilitate the position of women in society. Heroines like the Trưng sisters, for instance, saw their prominence elevated during the colonial period as part of efforts to tap into a long revolutionary tradition and bolster a nascent Vietnamese national identity. This camp of new ideas also included those who saw women as a social group with their own specific interests and demands, a need that materialized in the form of women-specific organizations during this period.[74] Some Vietnamese intellectuals, men and women alike, advocated for expanded opportunities for education and employment, while others went further to condemn Vietnamese family and social systems as a whole and insist on the rights of women to share political power with men. In the context of the Vũ Thị Cúc trial, her supporters adopted a moderate position, which was perhaps seen most clearly in the discussion of Cúc's chastity. Chastity—the mandate to preserve one's virginity before marriage and to be faithful to one's husband, even after death—was an important cultural precept guiding expectations for marital relationships. By ignoring sexual desires, it also implied a kind of purity of spirit that was highly valued. Cúc's supporters argued that women who had been badly treated by men deserved sympathy and not social rejection. The fact that she sacrificed her virginity to her husband demonstrated the depth of her attachment and consequent jealousy, as well as the injustice of the dual standard of the chastity principle that applied to women only.

The language of mental health suffused the coverage of the trial. Vũ Thị Cúc's lawyer, a Frenchman, argued that because of overwhelming emotions and disappointment, she had lost consciousness and in a moment of insanity committed this terrible crime. He recommended that she be sent to the hospital for treatment rather than to prison for punishment. The fact that she was so young and weak lent fuel for her defenders, who argued that insanity provided the only reasonable explanation of how she had the strength to stab her lover so many times. Furthermore, the papers reported that whenever she was asked about the case, Vũ Thị Cúc would cry hysterically and shiver terribly "like people with a mental health problem" (*bị bệnh thần kinh*). Her supporters took this behavior as a significant indication of her remorse and relative innocence. An editorial written about the trial, which posed the question "Is Cô Vũ Thị Cúc crazy or not?" stressed the importance of looking at the "psychological" aspect of the case.[75] According to the editors, this aspect was important not only for understanding her motivation but also, in so doing, for generating sympathy for her humanity. In order to reach a verdict, the editors explained, the court would have to consider whether she had retained consciousness under the power of extreme emotions and very strong "sexual desires" (*dục vọng*). This reference to sexual desires is not altogether surprising given the increasing interest in Freud among Vietnamese intellectuals from the mid-1930s.[76] In the case of Vũ Thị Cúc, the power and intensity of her sexual instincts were suggested here to have overwhelmed her sense of right and wrong. Unfortunately for Vũ Thị Cúc, expert medical opinion did not find her to be insane either in general or at the moment of the crime.

While the judge would be the ultimate decider of Vũ Thị Cúc's fate, it is the court of public opinion that holds special relevance here. Among the trial's eager bystanders, assessing Vũ Thị Cúc's criminal responsibility was tied not only to judgments about her motivation to violate social norms—whether she was sane or not—but also the legitimacy of those norms. It is clear that for some of her supporters, a momentary lapse in sanity was understandable, permissible even, given the unfair and desperate situation in which she found herself. In a dramatic and very public way, Vũ Thị Cúc's trial exposed the shifting and conflicted cultural terrain upon which popular assessments of mental illness were made. In particular, her deviation from gender norms—indeed, her violent refusal of them—was taken by some as true madness and by others as evidence of the injustice of the patriarchal system itself. It was this flexibility to tack back and forth between the individual and the social, between what was and what ought to be, that helps explain why discourses of mental illness were so often mobilized in colonial Vietnam to make claims on the modern world.

Lessons from the Popular Press

Throughout the interwar years, colonial psychiatrists enjoyed a widened scope for their expertise as the asylum system expanded in Vietnam. Yet faced with the twin pressures of spiraling costs and severe overcrowding, they came to rely more than ever on the participation of the public. The formalization of family care in the form of "trial leaves" succeeded in generating new opportunities for surveillance outside the walls of the asylum. This extended not only to patients but also to the households of patients, which themselves became the objects of expert scrutiny. Families, meanwhile, pursued their own strategies for dealing with troublesome or abnormal family members in ways that reflect the historically complex and dynamic patterns of therapeutic pluralism in Vietnamese society. Families sought the care of both local and foreign experts, but they also asked for advice on home remedies in the pages of popular medical journals that emerged in the 1920s and 1930s as part of Vietnam's vibrant press culture.

Sources from the quốc ngữ press provide a unique glimpse into how popular understandings merged with expert knowledge to produce a distinctive Vietnamese discourse around mental illness in the 1920s and 1930s. This discourse, which drew from both Sino-Vietnamese and Western medical traditions, found practical application in medical glossaries and advice columns that provided families with specific instructions on how to care for the mentally ill at home, including tools for prevention and prescriptions for self-management. The failure to avoid mental illness usually implied a bad family history, weak nerves, or an inability to cope with the stresses of modern life. Suffering from mental illness made some the objects of derision and others the objects of pity. The difference depended in large part on one's status in society and the cultural expectations, themselves in flux, attached to one's position in society as a woman, student, beggar, or mandarin, to name just a few. The likelihood that one would find oneself at an asylum also depended on preexisting hierarchies of vulnerability, with rural poverty as the surest predictor. Families played an important role in shielding patients from the outside world or giving them up to experts, whether local or foreign, as well as initiating changes to diet and the home environment. What they learned from the popular press may have shaped their expectations of what asylum care might look like and whether it was even necessary. It may also have reinforced a sense of how the practice of vigilant self-discipline, and even the performance of caregiving itself, could be considered a vital part of what it meant to be modern and Vietnamese. These lessons mostly reached an urban reading public composed of shopkeepers, artisans, clerks, teachers, and journalists. For the rest, narratives of punishment and neglect were more familiar story lines.

CHAPTER 6

Psychiatric Expertise and Indochina's Crime Problem

This chapter examines the interplay between the emergence of a new medical-legal category, the delinquent child, and the professionalization of psychiatry in colonial Vietnam. Until the 1930s, psychiatrists played only a limited role in the criminal justice system, charged with delivering judgments of insanity after a crime had already been committed. These medical-legal opinions quickly became a flashpoint of bitter controversy between the colonial medical establishment, the prison system, and the criminal courts, each of which sought to specify the nature of Vietnamese criminality and the appropriate service to be charged with providing oversight. Battles over the bounds of professional jurisdiction challenged assumptions about the neat alignment of psychiatric knowledge with the goals of a unified colonial state. Instead they exposed the competing priorities of prosecutors tasked with the protection of public safety and those of psychiatrists who sought to safeguard their professional autonomy. These contests also generated new opportunities for the elaboration of psychiatric expertise itself.

Frustrated by their lack of influence, colonial psychiatrists began to carve out an expanded role for themselves that went beyond individual determinations of insanity. They came increasingly to focus on the problem of juvenile delinquency as a way to redefine their role as experts and enhance their professional status within the colonial administration. By locating the problem of adult criminality in the abnormal instincts of children, they increasingly pitched their expertise as helping to answer the social question of crime prevention. Their professional claims found new traction amid the rebellions, strikes, and generalized political insecurity of the 1930s. In drawing attention to the failure of the state to protect children from those conditions that predisposed them to criminal careers, they worked to reposition themselves at the center of debates about child welfare reforms and the moral responsibilities of the colonial state during the interwar period.

Scholars of children and childhood in colonial Vietnam focus almost exclusively on the figure of the métis, or mixed-race child. Juvenile delinquents, meanwhile, rarely surface in these histories. When they do, they typically appear as a way to illustrate the shortcomings and premodern character of the colonial prison system.[1] That children continued to be found in adult prisons throughout the 1930s implies more than just a general failure of Indochina's penal system. The notion that children were different from adults, and therefore required a distinct set of laws and forms of punishment, signified not only their special status encoded in French legal tradition but also an increasingly sophisticated field of expert knowledge and practice. Throughout the 1920s and 1930s, the gap between metropolitan discourses and colonial practices around juvenile delinquency appeared all the more striking to colonial administrators and experts concerned with the rise of youth criminality and the limits of reformatories that looked more like penal colonies than "houses of reeducation." Debates over how to reform the system drew on the work of metropolitan reformers to elucidate new ideas about childhood and the origins of deviant behavior. Rather than locate the history of juvenile delinquency within a history of the colonial prison, this chapter situates its development in the context of an emerging child health movement in Indochina and the proliferation of state institutions dedicated to the protection of children. While scholars have largely insisted on the absence of a rehabilitative impulse in the colonial penal literature, I suggest that this absence may be ascribed to an increasing division of labor among a new class of experts during the interwar period.

By situating the history of psychiatry within a wide institutional context—one that looks beyond the strictly medical realm—this chapter argues that psychiatric expertise was produced locally in cooperation and competition with other actors, particularly members of the colonial penal administration. Battles over jurisdiction in cases involving the mentally ill expose the complex alliances and fractures that characterized the everyday administration of empire.[2] In this chapter, I examine the role of an emergent class of experts in promoting new ideas about criminals and their management, particularly in terms of identifying "abnormal" children as a reservoir of potential future offenders who required oversight from an early age. Here I trace their efforts to promote the delinquent child as its own kind of medical-legal category, one that required special forms of expertise and special forms of protection modeled after those in the metropole. More than a shift in emphasis, this chapter shows that psychiatric experts were often at odds with the policing structures of the state, and that criminals were often shuffled back and forth between prison and asylum systems in highly contested exchanges.

Certifying Insanity

The first asylum law introduced into colonial Indochina in 1918 marked the first attempt to routinize psychiatric expertise as part of the internment process. To briefly recap, in Indochina as in France, there were two principal ways people could find their way into the asylum. A *placement ordonné*, or mandated admission, was requested by the administrative authorities, while the other, a *placement requis*, or admission request, was initiated by the patient's family, relatives, or friends. Each required a medical certificate confirming an insanity diagnosis and issued only on a temporary basis. At the end of six months, confinement could become permanent depending on the medical progress of the patient. Psychiatric experts were also tasked with assessing the criminal responsibility of accused individuals and, after a period of observation, to recommend or advise against punishment. According to the decree's authors, the formal establishment of the medicolegal opinion was designed to protect the public's safety as well as the rights of patients against abuse and wrongful confinement. In Indochina, it was framed as a vital improvement over prior measures where expert opinions were either provided ad hoc or rendered meaningless given the lack of clinical services at the administration's disposal.[3] The 1930 law also extended the grounds for confinement under a mandated placement from disturbing public security, tranquility or decency (as explicated in the 1918 regulations) to include more medically grounded justifications for those who risked their "own security or possibility of cure."[4]

Criminals suspected of mental illness submitted to a special set of procedures. They were to be transferred from their holding cell to special sections of hospitals (or prisons), where they submitted to psychiatric observation. In urban centers, these exams would be performed by specialists in major hospitals, which by the 1930s also housed mental health clinics, and in rural areas by doctors with basic psychiatric training at best.[5] In the course of the criminal trial, experts were required to produce medicolegal reports that addressed the following two questions: Is the individual dangerous to himself or to others? If so, should he be held accountable for his actions and punished or should he be acquitted and confined in an asylum for treatment and care?[6] Doctors based their medicolegal reports on a period of direct patient observation as well as interviews with the patient's family and neighbors. Reports included crucial information such as age and gender, profession, and place of birth. They also detailed the patient's family medical history, usually indicating the presence or absence of alcoholism and other disorders associated with "degeneracy," as well as the motivating circumstances that led to the patient's arrest. Reports tended to merge this background information with remarks on the patient's physical symptoms and demeanor, as well as impressions of the patient's degree of socialization, observing for instance how she would respond to questions and how she related to other people or objects in the room.[7]

An important aspect of diagnosis and determination of criminal responsibility also included assessments of whether the patient was aware he or she had committed a crime and risked imprisonment and, if so, whether he or she felt at all guilty or repentant. Diagnoses also relied on moral determinations derived from the nature of the crime itself: "This criminal act which we have just related seems to be the act of an individual momentarily deprived of all reason because if not it would have to be considered the crime of a sadist. This latter position is too difficult to grasp if we consider this elderly person, partially disabled and infirm, timid and mostly sweet during his normal state, such is the accused."[8] The language of these reports varies between highly technical, scientific terminology, affirming the special status of psychiatric knowledge, and more colloquial expressions, perhaps as a way to more directly address the lay audience of the courthouse: "In one word, this is a peasant who will always be primitive and whose minimal intelligence is in the process of deteriorating as much as possible under the influence of senility."[9]

Following a mental illness diagnosis, the medical expert would then issue an *ordonnance de non-lieu* and recommend to the courts the patient's removal to the asylum for treatment. While the 1930 law called for a pavilion designated for the criminally insane, to be named after the famous French theorist of degeneration Benedict Morel, plans for its construction remained plagued by delays. In the meantime, criminals found themselves temporarily in the wing for agitated patients regardless of their diagnosis. To give a sense of the numbers of criminals sent to asylums and the kinds of crimes for which they were accused, in 1926, out of 600 patients residing at the Biên Hòa asylum,

56 were criminals (or approximately 9.3% of the total asylum population), described by their doctors as "alcoholics and degenerates . . . who comprise the majority of simple delinquents."[10] In 1931 alone, 19 criminals entered Biên Hòa out of a total 165 patients, or 11 percent of all those newly admitted. This figure included an uptick of patients charged with more serious crimes like theft and violence. In his annual report to the administration, the asylum director attributed this increase to the consequences of the "troubling economic situation," which had resulted in a rise in crime, as well as the dangers of alcoholism, which he warned had "made serious progress in the colony over the last five years."[11]

In 1928, the Chợ Quán Hospital in Saigon opened a psychiatric service alongside a special section of the hospital reserved for those accused or convicted of crimes. This "psychiatric annex" allowed for the surveillance and clinical supervision of criminals and delinquents suspected of mental illness. This coordinated service represented a significant improvement over the metropole, which had yet to implement similar measures, as doctors at Chợ Quán pointedly highlighted in their official correspondence. Not only did the service offer a place to conduct psychiatric observation and therefore provide an important legal role in terms of diagnosis, but its future expansion also promised to help prevent serious crimes before they were committed. In 1934, the service received a "countless number" of "mentally disturbed delinquent minors" picked up for "theft, scandal, rebellion and minor injuries." Eleven criminals, accused of murder or attempted murder and arson, were diagnosed with a range of mental disorders including idiocy, mental confusion, epilepsy, melancholy, dementia, mania, and "mystical delirium" (délire mystique). Following a study of the records of these criminal patients, the director of the service determined that ten out of the eleven cases had previously shown signs of mental problems, but because of ignorance or the inability to cover the costs of hospitalization, families or villages had elected to keep the sick at home.[12]

For colonial psychiatrists, providing medical-legal opinions represented an important opportunity to publicly elaborate their knowledge base and expand the legal basis for their authority into the criminal courts.[13] For that same reason these opinions also faced frequent challenges from other members of the colonial administration. For those officials increasingly concerned with preserving social order, the ability to send disruptive people to asylums emerged as a useful public security strategy, as well as serving to divert traffic from prisons to asylums. Prosecutors would therefore often contest the conclusions of psychiatrists on the grounds of public safety, especially when they recommended the release of patients back to society or their return to the prison system, which imposed significant financial and administrative burdens. Psychiatrists, meanwhile, deplored the wrongful confinement of patients as they also grappled with the errors committed by generalist doctors. Sloan Mahone argues that the process of lunacy certification in Britain's East African colonies provides a snapshot of the medical and political tensions that existed between the medical establishment, the prison system, and the criminal courts.[14] In the following section, I take Mahone's claim a step further and argue that these tensions were actually constitutive of psychiatric expertise itself.

Conflict over Medical-Legal Opinions

When colonial experts issued judgments that appeared consistent with the wishes of the police and judiciary, an easy working relationship followed. But this was not always the case. Rather, the medical-legal opinion became an important source of conflict among the different branches of the colonial administration throughout the interwar years. In 1928, for example, a patient named Dung was accused of killing his wife. Suspected of mental illness, he was put under the observation of the director of Lạng Sơn Hospital, who determined that Dung was insane and therefore should not be held responsible for his crime. The prosecutor general in Hanoi subsequently registered his opposition to this *ordonnance de non-lieu* with the president of the provincial tribunal of Lạng Sơn, claiming that the medical-legal exam "did not appear to him to be sufficiently in depth and the conclusions only hypothetical."[15] In a letter challenging the expert opinion, the prosecutor drew on additional information he had obtained from Dung's neighbors and village notables with whom Dung apparently enjoyed friendly relationships. Evidently "nobody suspected that he was . . . mad." Indeed Dung's psychotic periods, as described by those who knew him best, seemed largely unremarkable; he did not dance or sing, did not destroy any objects or hurt anybody. These periods reportedly occurred only once or twice a day and would not last long, immediately after which he would return to his normal behaviors and routines. The prosecutor concluded with a request for a second opinion by a Dr. Naudin, specifically citing his "specialization in these types of questions," and requested the removal of Dung to the Indigenous Hospital of Hanoi (for which Naudin served as the director) for further observation.[16]

This episode provides two critical insights. First, it demonstrates a reliance on indigenous knowledge and experience (privileged even above the expertise of the French doctor), which here is mobilized by the prosecutor general to build his own narrative in the pursuit of the prosecution of Dung.

Indeed, it serves to illustrate an important point: the certification of insanity in Indochina did not result in the straightforward, progressive medicalization of the confinement process. Rather medical-legal reports were marked by the use of increasingly sophisticated and technical language alongside more generalized impressions of patient appearance or demeanor, including lay observations of behavior gathered from family members and neighbors. Second, the episode reveals the distinction increasingly drawn between specialists and nonspecialists. It was those opinions, however, in which psychiatrists found the accused to be sane, that drew the most fire. This included opposition over expert medical decisions to send patients back to the judiciary for sentencing or to release individuals, previously charged with crimes and sent to the asylum, who had since recovered from their mental illness and were deemed fit for social life. According to the law, special procedures applied to the release of criminal patients. If a patient was cured before the length of his prison term had elapsed, he was to be delivered back to the penitentiary, where he would serve out the remainder of his sentence. If a cure did not arrive until after the term had expired, she was to remain at the asylum until she was deemed healthy enough to return to society. In practice, most criminals had long since transferred to pavilions with calm patients and were treated like the others. This meant, in actual practice, that once declared cured, these patients were eligible for immediate discharge.[17]

Security and police forces most often articulated their challenges to expert opinions in the name of public safety, typically by underscoring the possibility that an individual's mental illness could come back. A long stretch between bouts of mental illness, in the words of one prosecutor, "proves that the mistaken appearance of current calmness" has actually little to do with the underlying foundation of mental illness. He continued, cautioning, "Recent examples taken from the judicial records in France demonstrate the inconveniences that have resulted from giving freedom to criminals due to short periods of mental disorder."[18] These scenarios warning of the potential return of mental illness raised the difficult question over how to balance individual liberty as guaranteed by asylum laws against risks to public security. As signaled by the police commissioner of Hanoi in 1939, "It is to be wished that [the released criminal] does not make poor use of his recovered freedom and that he does not prove to be a future danger to the public."[19] There was also the question of what to do with those who were perceived as threats to the public's safety on account of mental illness but whose condition was not serious enough to merit asylum care.[20]

Debates between doctors and the police were not only framed by the competing imperatives of individual freedom and public safety but also pitched at the level of efficacy. Were accused individuals more likely to respond to the sanction of punishment or to care in an asylum? For psychiatrists, answering this question required distinguishing simply abnormal or deviant behavior from true mental illness. Making these distinctions proved to be the bread and butter of psychiatrists' efforts to expand their expertise in the criminal courts. In May 1925, André G., a twenty-two-year-old métis guard of the public works in Kampot, after he was found wandering the streets, demanding aid, and making violent threats to kill others, was confined at the Biên Hòa asylum. Dr. Levot, the medical expert with the assistance médicale in the city of Cần Thơ who was charged with his initial examination, concluded in his report that André was "antisocial" and could, given the occasion, commit a serious offense. He therefore argued, "In my opinion, prison is illogical because this is someone who is of weak or rather infirm mind and any sanctions will therefore be ineffective as can be proven by his resistance to the numerous previous sanctions for which he has been the object."[21]

Two weeks later, after his transfer to Biên Hòa, Dr. Roussy, the asylum's director, concluded that André's mental illness was no longer "sufficient" to require his continued stay in the asylum. While admitting that he would likely continue to commit crimes after his release, Roussy argued that "imprisonment should be required rather than confinement," determining that his "responsibility seems only slightly diminished."[22] After months of protestations, from both André himself and the asylum management, he was finally released from Biên Hòa in February of 1926. A couple of months later, however, André once again returned. When Dr. Augagneur, the new director of Biên Hòa, pressed for the details of the circumstances motivating André's recommitment, he was presented with a laundry list of various "eccentricities": living by himself in a grass hut near the local theater, shouting calamitous warnings in the street, forcing coolies to pull him around in rickshaws for hours, and demanding money from passersby, including 49 piasters from the governor of Cochinchina, a request personally made in the governor's own office. Augagneur contested the grounds for confinement in a letter to the governor-general arguing, "From these reports one can only affirm the conclusions of both my predecessor and myself that André G. is mildly mentally retarded, amoral, lazy, perverted, violent at times, and perfectly capable of injuring those who refuse his demands. But he does not remain less than perfectly responsible for his acts, this is not a mentally ill person, his place is not in an asylum. If André G. finds himself accused of any crimes, he must respond to the tribunal."[23]

The difficulty in resolving the disagreement between psychiatrists and the police had its practical effect in the itineraries of patients who seemed to endlessly cycle in and out of asylums, prisons, and family homes. The story of one patient named Sau—which opened this book—provides a striking example. As noted in his 1921 case file, when Sau first entered the asylum, "His exit can be envisioned, but under the condition that the family can take care of him because, mentally impaired and without surveillance, he will start again to pursue a life of debauchery, laziness, and vagrancy which will lead him all over again to the prison or asylum."[24] The observation proved prescient. Two years later, in June 1923, Sau found himself back at the asylum after being accused of murdering a Chinese man. Dr. Baudre, of the Hôpital Principal in Saigon, charged with providing an expert opinion in the case, found Sau to be insane and recommended his confinement. As a reminder to readers, the doctor used Sau's case to warn of a broader pattern in which "the existence of these individuals is a vast cycle where prison and asylum alternate with phases of liberty when they commit minor offenses, misdemeanors and crimes which lead to a new confinement."[25]

Yet almost six months later, Sau had yet to present any symptoms of mental illness. His continued presence at the asylum, however, was justified on the grounds of a prolonged observation. Eventually Dr. Roussy, the director of Biên Hòa, recommended his release, stressing above all his qualities as an inveterate alcoholic, lazy and libertine. Roussy argued that Sau was "much better suited to prison than to the asylum; in my opinion he should only be brought to justice at the prison; intoxication and alcoholism should never be considered attenuating but rather aggravating circumstances."[26] He opposed the conclusions of Dr. Baudre, even going so far as to accuse Baudre of allowing his knowledge of Sau's first stay at the asylum to bias his expert opinion in favor of confinement.

While Roussy expressed concern over the legality of retaining a patient once he or she was cured, the prosecutor general mounted a vociferous objection to Sau's release, warning of his danger to society. He too cited the earlier medicolegal report provided by Dr. Baudre but argued that a consideration of early violent episodes was an act of common sense, not bias, noting "in the future, one should not lose sight of earlier precedent." In any event, he warned that even if the advice of the asylum director were followed and Sau was tried at court, the defense would not fail to establish the insanity of the accused, and he would be sent again to the asylum, from which he would again be released. The discharge of Sau would therefore simply recommence "the conflict between the Medical Administration and Judiciary Service in another form."[27] As a result, in this particular case, the prosecutor wrote, "These considerations exposed, I can only give advice to the Director of the Health Service while clearing, for the future, the responsibility of my service."[28]

For both doctors and prosecutors, the concern to establish clear jurisdiction over these cases also required determining the limits of responsibility, as a way to protect themselves and their service from potential accusations of negligence. Take, for example, the case of Cuu, who murdered and proceeded to cannibalize his young victim.[29] A couple of weeks before the incident, the prosecutor of Cần Thơ had released Cuu to his family without pressing criminal charges, in spite of a medicolegal report that confirmed his mental illness and need for confinement. In this case, the prosecutor's office did not mount a challenge to the expert diagnosis but had instead completely disregarded it and as a result, failed to prevent the murder. The burden of negligence therefore fell on the prosecutor's department as well as that of the provincial chief. The case also proved to be a local sensation in the newspapers, generating considerable public pressure on the colonial administration to take accountability.[30]

Colonial psychiatric services also came under fire from the prosecutor's office itself. In the summer of 1933, a patient named Vu died while receiving treatment as a patient in the psychiatric ward at the Hôpital Indigène du Protectorat. In the words of a nurse who was present the day of the incident, "Events similar to this are perfectly possible in a space where fifty individuals of more or less 'turbulent' nature are installed and quarrel at every instant with different motives. Whatever kind of surveillance is exercised, however vigilant, one cannot prevent these quarrels. It is therefore very likely that Vu, finding himself at the edge of the bed, had an altercation with his neighbor and that he was pushed by this person, causing him to fall on the ground. The fall, even from not a great height, may have caused the rupture to an already fragile spleen."[31] Naudin, the presiding doctor of the psychiatric ward, also blamed the incident squarely on conditions marked by a "precarious installation," noting, "It would be difficult to make it more efficacious given the actual conditions. As a result, one cannot attribute the cause of death to the negligence of the surveillance. It must be thought of as an act of fortune that could not be avoided." Even by 1933, Naudin remained waiting for the opening of the Vôi asylum, which would relieve some pressure on his service to care for all the mentally ill in the region.[32] Yet despite Naudin's best efforts, the prosecutor general tasked the police commissioner in Hanoi with an investigation in order to ascertain the possibility of a "certain negligence in the surveillance of the mad which may motivate in this instance an intervention and administrative sanctions."[33]

Doctors also hit back at the judicial service. They accused their colleagues of imprisoning convicts who presented signs of significant mental disability without bothering to solicit the relevant expertise. Even prior to his first conviction, "the author of a crime is often known as a violent or dangerous person or presents anomalies of behavior. Sometimes, he is the object of simple police investigations, other times, he is admonished by the authorities, but always the most rational measure, the psychiatric exam, is not practiced."[34] Bouisset, a French doctor at the René Robin hospital in Hanoi, cited multiple cases of symptomatic prisoners as evidence of a "systematic refusal" to gain information about the mental state of the convicts.[35] Raymond, the head of the health service in Tonkin, also blasted the judicial service for lagging behind in regularizing the confinement of patients from temporary to permanent stays after an initial observation period of six months. What proved more worrying, however, was the delay in approving patients for release after they had been deemed cured. Not only was it illegal to keep these patients in custody, but it was also a real nuisance to the asylum, which remained overcrowded enough. Of the 122 patient case files sent for judicial review in May of 1938, by August about half still awaited a formal response.[36] Psychiatrists thereby grew increasingly frustrated, complaining that their expertise was underappreciated or simply bypassed. These frustrations were born of the challenge of working within a justice system concerned with punishing criminals rather than framing crime as a social and medical problem whose management required a special set of skills and expertise.

Generalists Making Trouble

Generalist doctors further complicated the efforts of experts to consolidate the authority of psychiatric knowledge by offering conflicting medical opinions that could then be mobilized by a dissenting judiciary. Experts complained that even when a psychiatric exam was performed, generalists, noting some sort of mental disturbance, would affirm a diagnosis of insanity without paying attention to distinctions between those *demi-fous* who commit criminal acts and those "truly mentally ill" (*vrais aliénés*) who should be found completely irresponsible for their actions. For Henri Reboul, a trained psychiatrist and director of the health service in Annam, this meant he was often called upon to "attenuate" the conclusions of his poorly trained colleagues who interpreted any symptoms of mental illness as evidence of true insanity; in his view, the knowledge to perceive gradations of insanity distinguished the true expert from the "improvised expert."[37] Even then, experts did not always agree. In 1927, the local director of health in Saigon had to resolve a dispute between two conflicting expert opinions over the readiness of a criminal patient to leave the asylum, "Both have a real competence in psychiatry, a particularly delicate science where divergence in the interpretation of symptoms is far from being rare even between the most qualified specialists."[38] For him, the difficulty lay not just with the generalists but with the particular nature of the field itself, which opened itself up wide to interpretation.

Medical-legal opinions provided by generalists also signaled the more fundamental problem of the lack of expertise in the colony. As one psychiatrist noted with clear frustration, "The magistrate is left with the responsibility of calling on experts, who [in the provinces] does not always possess the psychological rudiments necessary for his profession. It is thus how we have examined several criminals who have already been convicted and how, in a province in the delta, the judge received an order to not use mental expertise or autopsies because the provincial budget would not support the cost."[39] From the perspective of the patients themselves, the lack of available experts could hold disastrous consequences. A 1912 report by Reboul recounted the experience of one Vietnamese patient, a "degenerate and epileptic," who was fired from his job in the local colonial administration and "repatriated" to Marseille.[40] Rather than present for treatment, he instead joined the French Foreign Legion, which eventually brought him back to Tonkin several months later. Once returned to his home soil, he entered into medical treatment at least twelve different times with no paper trail allowing doctors at various institutions to connect the dots. Only after a criminal arrest was the patient put under expert observation for four months. This example not only demonstrates the structural deficiencies of psychiatric expertise in the colony but also shows how the movements of patients traced the expanding geographies of the French empire in the early twentieth century. It is also important to note that it was only at the moment that the patient entered the court system that his medical case was finally resolved.

Reboul wondered how those practitioners who had most likely never seen an aliéné in their life—meaning one so severely ill that he required confinement—could "hope to offer a precise diagnosis and to discuss this diagnosis with lawyers." For Reboul, the fault lay not with the doctors but with the organization of medical education in France, which tended to sideline psychiatry as superfluous or redundant. While young doctors tackled questions of "pure science" or studied that "rare operation which they would almost certainly never perform," the everyday demands of psychiatry continued to grow apace.[41] Beyond the ready stream of patients, the field itself was rich and expanding, rife for discovery and innovation. As Reboul wrote in 1912, "All is to be done: what's missing are scientifically armed observers." After World War I, psychiatrists would content themselves not as mere observers but as key players in the colony's medical and judicial worlds.

Turning to Juvenile Delinquents: The Move Toward Prevention

Colonial psychiatrists, frustrated by their lack of influence, soon began to carve out an expanded role for themselves that went beyond individual determinations of insanity and instead focused on the social question of juvenile crime. By locating the problem of youth criminality in abnormal instincts that could be identified and managed by experts, psychiatrists worked to reframe the problem of juvenile delinquency in Indochina around the twin imperatives of prophylaxis and rehabilitation. Throughout the 1930s, psychiatrists increasingly turned their attention to identifying and treating abnormal children before they became fully pathological, emphasizing early screening and treatment that would reroute the movements of juvenile delinquents through their expert care. By offering new explanations for the patterns of youth criminality that tied social circumstances to individual pathology, psychiatrists worked to align themselves with a broad reform movement that included prosecutors, doctors, lawyers, educators, and social workers. Rather than simply affirm or dismiss the criminal responsibility of offenders, psychiatrists located the problem of adult criminality in the abnormal instincts of children that could be identified and managed under their expert care.

The impetus behind reforms in Indochina must also be understood as part of metropolitan changes during the first half of the twentieth century, when reformers in psychiatry, social work, and law transformed France's punitive juvenile justice system into a profoundly therapeutic one.[42] In France, the notion that incarcerated minors should be separated from adult prisoners and receive education in specialized institutions was established in 1810 by the Napoleonic Code. The code also first introduced the concept of discretion—or determining a child's criminal responsibility based on whether he or she understood the difference between right and wrong—as a way to reconcile notions of punishment with protection for minors. But how to distinguish the guilty from the innocent, and increasingly to question if that distinction was relevant at all, animated debates over juvenile justice reforms between France and its empire.

Psychiatric expertise played an important part in metropolitan discussions over juvenile justice reform. By introducing new medicalized understandings of childhood and deviance, psychiatrists worked to shift the focus of juvenile justice from the criminal act to the characteristics of the child himself.[43] Georges Heuyer, a founding figure in child neuropsychiatry in France, assumed a major role. He argued that recidivists (who, he wrote, incidentally comprised the majority of the prison population) most often demonstrated evidence of antisocial tendencies from their childhood or adolescence. In pronouncing "the problem of guilty children is that of adult criminality," Heuyer called for a broad collaboration between judges *and* medical experts in reorienting the juvenile justice system around the principle of prevention.[44] The transformation of the metropole's juvenile delinquency establishment from a punitive system to a profoundly therapeutic one occurred as part of what Marc Renneville describes as a progressive, if uneven, "psychiatrization of the carceral system" in France during the early decades of the twentieth century.[45] That psychiatrists were most successful in the realm of juvenile delinquency was a point that they themselves often remarked on and took for an important lesson as they sought to expand their influence into other domains of the criminal justice system.[46] For psychiatrists in Indochina, the work of Heuyer and others would serve as an explicit model for practice in guiding their own reform efforts. One Vietnamese reformer, Lê Vân Kim, echoed the words of Heuyer when he wrote in 1934, "The criminal adult was almost always an unhappy child."[47]

Juvenile Justice in Disrepair

These psychiatric calls for reform emerged against the backdrop of a juvenile justice system in serious disrepair. Following the famous model of Mettray in France, colonial administrators in Indochina had established two youth reformatories to address the problem of juvenile delinquency. These reformatories were designed as large agricultural colonies where young Vietnamese male delinquents would learn labor skills and principles of moral discipline that would rehabilitate them into "honest workers."[48] In 1904, the colonial state established the colony's first house of correction for delinquent youths adjacent to the Ông Yêm agricultural station in Thủ Dầu Một outside Saigon. A second reformatory, named Trí Cụ, later appeared in Bắc Giang province in Tonkin in 1925.[49]

Within the institution's walls, the attempt to formally segregate the guilty from the innocent, and young children from older, more seasoned delinquents, reflected the ambiguities of the mission of the reformatory both as penitentiary for child criminals *and* as refuge for the indigent and abandoned. Indeed, the majority of children ever sent to Trí Cụ reformatory ended up there by an administrative decision alone. In practice, however, the enforcement of different regimes of children failed to hold. Colonial reformers grew alarmed at the possibilities of corruption, with one warning that the reformatory, "far from giving the hoped for results . . . is a center of contamination of the first order because of the presence of incorrigible wrongdoers of an older age."[50] Others insisted that even if physical separation could be achieved, the threat of an "inevitable promiscuity" remained ever present. Keeping children separate from each other formed only one of many everyday challenges that seemed to overwhelm the system: dormitories "falling into ruins," lack of potable water, the malnourishment of children compelled to labor, and the ineptitude of those tasked with their reeducation. According to one colonial official in 1931, nearly 90 percent of children left the institution completely illiterate.[51] The population of Trí Cụ jumped from 165 children in 1929 to 571 eight years later, almost twice its original capacity.[52]

Institutional deficiencies were compounded by the worrisome rise of youth criminality in the colony. Throughout the 1920s, children from the countryside began arriving in Hanoi with such frequency that one police commissioner complained they were "infesting" the city. Aged mostly between eleven and seventeen, with no family or home, these young vagabonds "proliferated" in the streets and committed petty crimes for which they were either acquitted because of their young age or condemned to prisons and the corrupting influence of adult offenders. As the police commissioner of Hanoi protested in 1927, "Very frequently, I will send these young hoodlums back to their own country, without escort, which cannot but cost the administration. It is, in any event, pointless because we see these undesirables reappear some time later."[53]

Yet children's stories, gleaned from official interrogations following their arrest, also served as sobering reminders of the crushing poverty of children in the colony. Almost all had at least one deceased parent. The fact that so many children reported their parents abandoning their home villages entirely gives a sense of the limited prospects that drove peasants (and their children) to seek opportunities elsewhere. It also yields insight into their own heightened sense of precariousness. One child confessed, "I have no one else in the world than my older brother," while another, orphaned at fourteen, told authorities that he not only had lost his parents but had "no uncle, no aunt, no brother, no sister" either.[54] In 1929, in a letter to the mayor of Hanoi, the commissioner of police offered an explanation for the rising tide of daily arrests of children, noting that "almost all have fled their villages, chased by the flooding and finding refuge in Hanoi where, without shelter, without resources, they roam the streets surviving only by begging and theft."[55] In fact, the majority of children testified they held jobs or at least intermittent forms of employment which had allowed them to survive on city streets for several months. They guarded bikes and cars, sold bonbons and tea on the streets, and ran errands for various businesses. At night, they slept in pagodas or shelters (*asiles de nuit*) or simply on the streets "wherever" (*n'importe où*), in the words of one boy.[56] For colonial officials, how to rid the city of young delinquents while also acknowledging the social circumstances that led them there—how to navigate between the different impulses of punishment and protection—presented a distinct challenge that distinguished the legal regime of children from that of adults. These stories also highlight the ambiguities of a legal order where being guilty of nothing more than finding oneself alone and poor in a new city, at a young age, meant falling within the purview of the colonial carceral system.

For an overburdened criminal justice system, reformatories represented an improvement over the transfer of children to adult prisons, the *dépôts de mendicité*, or simply back to their parents. One child, who counted six previous arrests, reportedly requested admission to the Trí Cụ, "so that I can work and have a regular occupation."[57] While one must take these kinds of declarations with a grain of salt, given the highly coercive setting in which they were made, it is not unreasonable to think that when a child was faced with a tiresome wheel of arrest and release, the prospect of regular food, steady employment, and a place to sleep would have appeared a welcome alternative.[58] Yet as children's testimonies and official statistics make clear, many continued to be sent home to their families or villages, if at all possible, or absorbed into other wings of the criminal justice system, including adult prisons, well into the 1930s.[59] Indeed, children increasingly found themselves caught up in the wider web of state repression that accompanied the explosion of political protests, peasant demonstrations, and strikes among workers on rubber plantations and in urban centers, which spilled an unprecedented number of people into colonial prisons. The failed insurrection at the French garrison in Yên Bái in Tonkin in 1930 only intensified the use of colonial violence in the region and spelled the death knell for the Việt Nam Quốc Dân Đảng (VNQDD, the Vietnamese Nationalist Party). Meanwhile, the nascent Indochinese Communist Party worked to channel rural discontent into peasant revolts in Nghệ An and Hà Tĩnh provinces and organized a dozen soviets along the lines of those developed in China. The poverty brought on by the Great Depression also triggered a crime wave that contributed to higher incarceration rates. The prison population in Annam, Tonkin, and Cochinchina grew from 16,087 in 1929 to 28,097 by the end of 1931.[60] As Peter Zinoman has argued, this rapid influx of thousands of communists and nationalists, members of secret societies and anarchist groups, peasants and urban laborers transformed the prison into a site of political organization and anticolonial resistance that transcended boundaries of class and geography.[61]

Between 1926 and 1930, the number of juvenile delinquents tried before tribunals in Saigon tripled, from 406 to 1,263.[62] Those charged with threatening the security of the state found themselves at adult prisons, where colonial officials expressed concerns over their physical safety and the threat of moral and political corruption by older offenders.[63] Others, meanwhile, ended up in youth reformatories where colonial officials likened them to an "oil stain" (tâche d'huile) that menaced those younger, more innocent detainees. An attempted mutiny by about thirty children who had been previously sentenced for "manoeuvers against state security" and dispatched to Ông Yêm in 1931 also exposed the woeful inadequacy of safety precautions at the reformatory, which included the lack of isolation cells, the worm eaten walls of the dormitories which made for easy escapes, and the absence of a staff large enough to subdue a genuine insurrection. In particular, the reformatory's director worried over those "mineurs communistes" who continued to be sent from different provinces all over the colony and requested their removal (twenty in total) to a dedicated alternative establishment (that did not yet exist).[64] To make matters even more difficult, once delinquents reached the age of twenty-one, the legal upper age limit of the reformatory, the question became, Should they be sent to the provincial prison to ride out the remainder of their punishment and risk corruption by older criminals or should they remain at the reformatory, where they risked corrupting younger children? Neither seemed all that desirable. Some colonial officials rejected both solutions by selectively granting early release (liberté conditionnelle) to children who expressed remorse and whose parents agreed to closely monitor them at home.[65] Others proved more unruly. A child named Dac, for instance, persisted in distributing political tracts after his internment and tried to provoke all sorts of "disorders," even trying to get the children to rise up against their Vietnamese guards. He was eventually removed to the central prison in Hanoi.[66]

Because youth reformatories accommodated only boys, delinquent girls (filles mineures) found themselves routinely sent to the female wings of ordinary prisons to serve out their terms. Justice officials complained that such a practice negated the entire spirit of the law, "which is the moral uplift of the minor," and transformed what was supposed to be a rehabilitative measure into a "true punishment."[67] Not only did adolescent girls suffer the same conditions as adult female prisoners and their young infants, who were kept in separate, cramped dormitories, but they also tended to serve longer sentences in view of their "rehabilitation," even for the same crime.[68] A young girl named Nuoi, for example, was convicted of theft at thirteen years old and sent to Hanoi's main prison, the Maison Centrale. While her sentence was eventually reduced to six years, her adult accomplice served only a total of three years behind bars.[69] To remedy similar situations, as early as 1918, colonial administrators in Saigon asked for a girls' section to be added to Ông Yêm, and administrators in Tonkin joined the chorus after the opening of the Trí Cụ reformatory. They were repeatedly turned down because of the small numbers of girls (as of October 1926, only four delinquent girls were counted at Hanoi's central prison) and the usual budget constraints.[70] Justice officials began to cast around for alternatives: convents or other private charitable institutions, extended family networks, or simply giving girls their freedom once these other options had run out.[71]

Calls for Reform

The mounting pressure to overhaul Indochina's juvenile justice system also coincided with a broad reorientation of colonial health policy toward child and maternal health during the interwar years.[72] Throughout the 1920s and 1930s, a growing interest in child welfare joined with fears over rising criminality to prompt discussions about the need to revamp the colony's juvenile justice system. From the late 1920s, the collaboration between religious, private, and public institutions in Indochina grew stronger as those concerned with child protection saw their mission as too important to not overcome any differences of opinion or principle.[73] This collaboration was overseen and coordinated by the Service of Social Assistance from 1929 onward; the service assumed oversight of youth reformatories that same year.[74]

In 1934, a meeting of the Conference of Childhood in Saigon brought together educators, doctors, lawyers, and administrators dedicated to the promotion of child welfare. The meeting was organized alongside the public launch of the Semaine de l'Enfance, or Childhood Week, an event that would be repeated in 1936 and again in 1938. In his opening speech to kick off the week, the organizer, Edouard Marquis, declared the ultimate purpose of the week was to "give the child truth, happiness and justice."[75] This responded to a bleak picture of childhood in the colony. "Carried along the muddy torrents of cities," Marquis wrote in 1936, children could be found "prowling through markets, in front of stalls, everywhere crowds are dense, pilfering here, begging there, wallowing in filth and vice, from one fall to the next, only to wash ashore at the banks of Corrections." Yet he also described children

"in Cochinchina, like everywhere" as victims of "odious parents," "con artists," "disastrous circumstances" as well as a "general indifference against
which they are powerless to fight." The organizers of Childhood Week,
drawing on metropolitan precedents, set out to combat this indifference by
arming native mothers with brochures detailing proper maternal and infant
health care. Healthy babies were put on public display, and doctors gave pre-
sentations on declining child mortality in order to showcase the benefits of
modern, state-directed public health initiatives in the colony.[76]

The 1934 meeting signaled mounting concern about the health of the
Vietnamese child but also growing attention to questions about the juridical rights of children, especially the failure to reform Indochina's juvenile
justice system that continued to operate under the 1810 French penal code.
France had since instituted a major set of reforms to the juvenile justice
system in 1912. Psychiatrists had played a major role in these metropolitan
reforms; by introducing new medicalized understandings of childhood and
deviance, they had worked to shift the focus of juvenile justice from the
criminal act to the characteristics of the child himself. Among other innovations, the 1912 law raised the age of legal majority from sixteen to eighteen and recognized adolescence as a distinct stage of child development,
stipulating that all minors between thirteen and eighteen years old submit
to an obligatory medico-psychological exam. This exam would serve as the
basis for determining which outcome would be best for the child (returning to the parents, placing under psychiatric observation, or sending to a
reformatory).[77]

The question over whether to extend the 1912 reforms to the colony
included discussions about the similarities of delinquent populations of
France and Indochina and to what extent the law's provisions needed to be
adapted to local conditions. At the 1934 meeting, colonial reformers debated
the creation of special tribunals for children, raising the age of legal majority from sixteen to eighteen, and the reinvention of the penitentiary as a
"house of supervised education" where children would be transformed from
troublesome wards of the state into productive laborers.[78] For a system that
had fallen into profound disorder, where those children who had been abandoned by their parents were sent to reformatories alongside others convicted
of crimes, the push to rationalize the legal regime for children raised some
critical questions: To what extent were these populations actually distinct
or the same? Were they criminals who needed to be punished or vulnerable children in need of social assistance? Who was the juvenile delinquent?
Answering these questions required a deeper understanding of the social
causes of delinquency, its physical and psychological manifestations, as a way

to assess not only the criminal responsibility of children but also the moral responsibility of the colonial state for their rehabilitation.

The modernization of Indochina's juvenile delinquency establishment would require new kinds of data that quantified the pressure on the reformatories to expand and specified the origins of children sent to the reformatory and what happened to them after they left. A commission specifically charged with advising the colonial administration on the reorganization of youth reformatories found that the growing numbers of children at the Trí Cụ reformatory could be attributed not only to an overall rise in juvenile crime but also to the fact that judges, knowing a special institution for minors now existed in Tonkin, "did not hesitate to pronounce convictions."[79]

Whereas judges previously had little choice but to send delinquents back to their parents or village, the establishment of youth reformatories generated a reality of juvenile delinquency in the colony that did not exist before. These institutions allowed judges to hand down convictions and recommendations for confinement that could now be captured in crime statistics, and the institutions themselves served as spaces for the study of delinquency through the systematic collection of information on child backgrounds.

Following their metropolitan counterparts, colonial experts discarded the notion of discretion (or criminal responsibility) in order to address the more important question: What had caused the minor to misbehave? Reformers, including psychiatrists, worked toward building a taxonomy of social conditions that predisposed children to delinquency as a way to stress the universality of childhood between France and colony. Comparative statistics were marshaled to demonstrate that delinquency, contrary to what might be expected, was not a more pervasive problem in the colony than it was in France. Lê Vân Kim, a Vietnamese reform advocate, extrapolated that if France's 40 million residents produced forty thousand abnormal children, then the same proportion for Cochinchina's population should hold at four thousand. He defended this "borrowing" of French statistics to paint a picture of delinquency in Vietnam by declaring, "The painful question of race has nothing to do with it." Just as "microbes, most particularly Koch's bacilli and Schaudinn's spirochetes, don't have a nationality," the social conditions that bred delinquency—the disorganization of family life, immorality, urban slums—could be found anywhere.[80] Dr. Grinsard, the Trí Cụ reformatory's chief doctor, as well as the director of the neighboring Vôi asylum, similarly concluded, "We have observed young children whose first offense was nothing but the consequence of the profound misery which confronts the Tonkinese people. Their history is common with all juvenile delinquents: a deficient heredity, abandoned by family and society, promiscuity."[81]

Vietnamese children, by virtue of their poverty, were also thought to suffer developmental delays rendering them *less* precocious than those in France. Habert, the director of the justice system in Indochina, concurred but offered a different kind of explanation rooted in Vietnamese culture: "The indigenous child does not acquire earlier than the European child a maturity of spirit, the notion of good and bad, and a sense of responsibility for his acts." If anything, his character was marked by an "atavism" and his moral sense developed even more slowly, the result of years of "submitting passively to the will of his parents or whoever he is dependent on" which delayed "the full blossoming of his personality."[82] Rather than suggest important differences between colony and metropole, colonial reformers tended to stress similarities in the psychology of children and child development as the basis for extending provisions of the 1912 French law (especially fixing eighteen years as the age of penal majority) to all of Indochina. Here the specificity of the colonial context was offered up not as a way to cast a fundamental difference between European and Vietnamese children but rather to highlight the need for similar if not greater protections for children in Indochina relative to the metropole.[83] By comparing European and Vietnamese children, colonial reformers tested notions of the universality of childhood itself.

In a 1938 study, Grinsard merged anecdotal evidence with physical and psychiatric exams of children at the Trí Cụ reformatory, collected over a ten-year period, to provide a more scientific study of juvenile delinquency in the colony. Drawing inspiration from the work of Georges Heuyer, the study attributes delinquency primarily to psychopathological causes, including infectious diseases and heredity, and their interactions with the social environment. Grinsard describes the Vietnamese juvenile delinquent population as "made up of a majority of children on which weighs a heavy heredity of backwardness and perversions. . . . They are undoubtedly abnormal beings."[84] The study found that most suffered from a state of "simple degeneration (*dégénéré simple*), which, barring early intervention, threatened a gradual devolution toward either criminality or madness. Grinsard proceeded to chart the typical development of perverted children, from "anomalies of conduct and character (persistence in the accomplishment of forbidden acts, lying, lack of affection and emotion, excessive development of ego)" through to puberty, when they began to engage in illegal activities of vagrancy, gambling, and theft. Grinsard drew on his experience as an asylum director to warn of the potential consequences of high rates of degeneracy among Vietnamese children, remarking on the example of one child who "presented problems of character with perverse instincts who was interned three times at the Vôi asylum and who escaped each time."[85] In 1938, the same year that Grinsard published his study, eight children were confined at the Vôi asylum, enough for the asylum's surveillance commission to recommend the creation of a pavilion dedicated specifically to children.[86]

Warning of the dangers of those children who had been left to themselves, Grinsard tended to emphasize the exacerbating conditions of social life rather than the inevitability of biological inheritance. As another psychiatrist wrote in referencing one adult patient at the asylum, "But I believe that his perverted instincts originate not only from possible hereditary predispositions, but also the abandonment to which this young man was left at a certain age. We have often witnessed that these perversions can be created by certain social conditions, these abnormal children are recruited among abandoned children left to their own devices in a milieu favorable for the development of base instincts."[87] The first step was therefore to remove children from their harmful environment and deliver them into the hands of experts.

Grinsard reported that 55 percent (or 68 out of 151) of all youth at Trí Cụ given a psychiatric exam displayed evidence of "social inadaptation" and displayed symptoms of a "more or less primitive" degeneracy. While he noted that certain delinquents, upon leaving the reformatory, could return to a more or less normal life, Grinsard warned that the majority of those suffering from degeneration possessed the form most commonly found among recidivists. That said, mental disability among children was typically mild; more extreme cases, Grinsard noted, would be destined for the asylum as opposed to the prison. Fourteen children suffered from intellectual disability and formed the unfortunate "punch bags" (souffres-douleurs) of their "more healthy comrades who use them to satisfy the slightest whim."

Alongside the psychiatric exam, a physical exam was also performed, revealing a variety of anomalies of development, including the form, dimensions, and volume of a certain number of organs (head, ears, teeth, limbs, genitals, skin, etc). Each organ corresponded to a different point of psychiatric interest. Grinsard demonstrated a particular fascination with the phenomenon of tattooing at the reformatory (an older child would administer tattoos using a needle and a mixture of ashes and water for coloration.) Apparently 35 percent (or 60 out of 142) children were tattooed, although the custom was apparently thought to be quite rare in the rural areas of the delta from which most of the children came. Tattoos, read on children's bodies as evidence of a "manifestation of individual vanity" and a desire to "externalize," also paradoxically revealed a lack of imagination. Eighty percent of tattoos were of Chinese characters, followed by roman numerals, quốc ngữ characters, and only rarely images. Grinsard also described children's sexual organs and sexual behavior at length, noting, however, that sodomy was "not a unique sign of disability" but a fact of prison life. It was no different at the agricultural colony, where "almost all *colons* engage in anal sex."[88]

At the conclusion of his study, Grinsard remarked, "The State must substitute for the father of the family: he must, at the prison, materially and morally educate the young delinquent; and upon his release from prison, he must allow him to honestly make a living. We no longer live in an outdated time when the young delinquent is considered a pariah, but in a time when we see in him nothing but a 'sick person' that society must, if not cure, at least improve, with a goal that is as much altruistic as egoistic." Rather than blaming children for the "multitude of defects, deficiencies, social and moral errors" that drew them into a world of crime, society should view delinquency as equally rooted in "their abnormal constitution and the abnormal circumstances of their life."[89] Even Jules Brévié, the governor-general of Indochina, in 1938 began to suggest that there were no significant differences between "young delinquents, abandoned children, and little beggars."[90] All required a "regular surveillance of their mental state."[91] While growing attention to the psychiatric designation of children as abnormal seemed to provide a more humane basis for reform, this new scientific language also worked to root delinquency even deeper into child natures and reinforce the perception that a tiny minority remained "incurable perverts" who should be punished.[92] Drawing these kinds of distinctions was useful, not just in terms of establishing a broad remit for the exercise of expert authority but also in sending a clear message to delinquents themselves. As Lê Vân Kim warned, "If we absolve all delinquent children, they will bring themselves to think that they are all abnormal or sick and there will never emerge among them a sense of responsibility."[93]

More Sick Than Criminal

If delinquents were assumed to be more sick than criminal, it followed that the state should adopt a more protective attitude vis-à-vis delinquent children. In debates over reforms, moral imperatives joined with more practical concerns that addressed whether reformatories could effectively rehabilitate children and prevent the emergence of a future class of criminal adults. For many colonial administrators, the reformatory was at its most valuable in its capacity not as a site of rehabilitation but rather as a kind of warning sign, a threat to potential delinquents that they would suffer the consequences of their criminal actions. Yet with growing attention to the social and psychiatric causes of delinquency, colonial reformers increasingly dismissed repression as a viable deterrent and instead insisted on more expansive reforms that included new kinds of pre- and postpenitentiary prophylaxis to be rolled out under expert supervision, including campaigns against alcohol and drug abuse and the protection of pregnant women and early childhood education, as well as unemployment.[94] This language found its way from conferences and the pages of medical journals into the reports of the colonial administration, signaling a broader shift in thinking around the aims and forms of juvenile reforms. A 1927 report on Indochina's justice service emphasized that internment for minors would no longer be considered punishment but would be reframed as an "administrative order," one that was more "preventive than repressive. . . . Modern society should less enforce the punishment of crimes than amend the ready instincts that lead astray."[95]

A series of reforms was proposed. Following the metropole, these proposals envisioned a "close collaboration of the psychiatrist and judge"[96] and fell within two broad camps: the first called for the medicalization of delinquency by routing those children who had already fallen within the purview of the criminal justice system through the care of psychiatric experts. Dr. Pierre Dorolle, a psychiatric expert and director of the Chợ Quán Hospital, recommended the creation of a neuropsychiatric service charged with examining these "abnormal and delinquent" children *before* their transfer to the reformatory (of which he estimated there were between four thousand and five thousand in all of Indochina). This new service would respond to the deplorable lack of screening and treatment for children, especially "in a service through which practically all psychiatric expertise passes in Cochinchina, not a single juvenile delinquent has been examined in two years."[97] Only the most acute cases found their way to the offices of the provincial doctor and then onto the asylum at Biên Hòa, all other children completely escaping expert observation. Dorolle also called for the creation of a special children's wing at Biên Hòa for those requiring long-term treatment.[98]

According to Dorolle, delinquents destined for Ông Yêm would first be removed from the central prison in Saigon and placed at Chợ Quán Hospital for a period of psychiatric observation. The doctor would be charged with providing the director of the reformatory with "all the useful instructions that touched on the physical and intellectual possibilities of the children."[99] After their transfer, children would continue to receive mental exams every three months by the reformatory's doctor, who also happened to serve as the director of Biên Hòa. In 1934, a psychiatrist was added as a member of the oversight council at Ông Yêm youth reformatory, and he conducted regular psychiatric exams of the detainees.[100] Three years later, in 1938, observation centers for "abnormal delinquent children" were opened in the hospitals of Chợ Quán (Cochinchina) and René Robin (Hanoi).[101]

The second category of reforms called for greater preventive measures, both pre- and postpenitentiary. For the juvenile delinquent, who was nothing but a "future recidivist" in the words of Grinsard, prophylaxis at an early age, before any crime was committed, was imperative.[102] Dorolle therefore recommended the creation of a separate psychiatric service at Chợ Quán Hospital in Saigon for the treatment of nondelinquent children. This service—annexed to the neuropsychiatric clinic for adults but operating with its own personnel—would serve a "double role." The first, "documentary and experimental," related to the study of the mental development of the Vietnamese child. Prolonged observation, combined with intelligence tests used in Europe and America but adapted to the Vietnamese context, would help to establish profiles of different "mental types." A strong understanding of normal childhood development would allow for a more precise study of "mental anomalies," the role of inherited diseases, and that of the "defective conditions" of living. The second, more practical function would provide affluent Vietnamese families plagued by "abnormal difficult children" with recourse to expert advice. Children who presented a "veritable social danger" tended to absorb the bulk of the hospital's resources; the creation of a clinic specifically for children described as "perverted," "unstable," or "retarded" would create new opportunities for the early diagnosis and treatment of a broader population.[103] In 1939, Governor General Jules Brévié authorized the establishment of a service for "abnormal *nondelinquent* children" where "special consultations would be organized for families who wished to receive advice on treatments for abnormal children who were to be conserved under the family roof."[104] Internment in an asylum should be a last resort. To avoid it, the open service would play a preventative role by performing triage and treatment "in freedom" *(en cure libre)*.

These proposals reflect wider efforts of the 1930s, as detailed in chapter 4, to reorient the psychiatric assistance program around the principles of mental hygiene and voluntary care. They also came at a moment of high optimism when the Popular Front, a left-wing coalition that governed France and its empire between 1936 and 1938, relaxed colonial repression and inaugurated a series of social and labor reforms (all while failing to expand representative institutions). In the context of juvenile delinquency, psychiatrists called for a broad-based assault on "social diseases," specifically those with "hereditary repercussions," including syphilis, tuberculosis, alcoholism and opium addiction, the fight against slums and unemployment, the education of mothers, the moral protection of childhood, and the prohibition of gambling.[105]

The extension of psychiatric expertise into the juvenile delinquency establishment was therefore imagined as part of a sweeping vision of social reform: "If the rescue of criminal children begins in the courtroom, it ends in the clinics, the patronages and the penitentiary colonies."[106] The realization of this vision would require not only the funds to support the creation of new institutions but also the availability of specialists to staff them. At the Lanessan and Rene Robin Hospitals in Hanoi, for example, psychiatric services were run without the oversight of a fully trained psychiatrist, the only one available stationed at the Vôi asylum some sixty kilometers away. In 1939, the local director of the health service in Hanoi, De Raymond, described his attempts to recruit a specialist for Voi, which failed because no candidates applied. De Raymond estimated that a full-fledged psychiatric service would run the Tonkin budget 150,000 piasters. This included the funds to support a position for a permanent specialist with benefits similar to those in France, especially as he would be responsible for treating the clientele of the region *and* providing medical expertise for tribunals.[107]

Lacking the cash, infrastructure, and expertise to implement a more comprehensive overhaul of the system, the colonial state instead largely focused its efforts on improving the system already in place, including renaming the reformatory a "house of supervised education."[108] The modesty of these proposals reinforced the more general pessimism that colonial reformatories could ever offer a truly modern form of rehabilitation. Pettelat, the provincial chief of Bắc Giang province, where the Trí Cụ reformatory was located, warned those administrators who naively thought that it could "ever be a house of reeducation in the ideal sense of the word. Whatever title it may carry, it is nothing but a house of correction for minors . . . which can never re-create around the lost child a homelike atmosphere. This ambiance can only be found in a family or charitable institution."[109] The growing consensus over the reformatory's limits—as a site deemed more punishing than protective—only went so far as to signal the need to seek alternatives for abandoned children. As Edouard Marquis warned, "First and foremost, nurseries and orphanages receive thousands of little beings [*petits êtres*] without being too preoccupied about their defects or their degree of degeneration. But it appears, in the course of this rescue operation, that there is a grave danger in mixing these children. The necessity therefore requires public powers to modify the organization of Ông Yêm created for 'little abnormal delinquents' [*petits délinquants anormaux*]."[110] At the same moment that France was abandoning the penitentiary as a site of juvenile rehabilitation, Indochina thus reaffirmed its own commitment to the reformatory.

While children continued to be sent to penal institutions, projects for the regeneration of abandoned youth gained some traction, including the creation of agricultural schools and "vacation colonies" (colonies de vacances), discussed elsewhere in the literature on French policies towards the métis.[111] As early as 1931, the colonial administration had envisioned the eventual proliferation of "separate and smaller groups" of needy children, noting, "The multiplication of small agricultural colonies would be ideal." [112] Efforts to expand the state-run system subsequently included the establishment of a maison de relèvement in Cochinchina specifically for delinquent girls in 1934 and a home for abandoned children in Thủ Dầu Một province, where "little liars and petty thieves" received regular meals, primary education, and professional instruction including carpentry and the tapping of rubber trees.[113] In January of 1938, a "preventorium" opened in Phú Lâm, near the border with Cambodia, supported by the colonial health service and provincial budgets. Described in local news reports as "a prophylactic institution of great humanitarian significance," the establishment housed fifty children between the ages of six and fourteen, described not as seriously ill but rather as "sickly and retarded," the product of poor nutrition and hereditary defects. Unable to engage in normal study, these children were instead sent to the preventorium for a year (or up to two with a doctor's approval), where they received a modified kind of education: three hours of class per day, physical exercise, daily hydrotherapy, light outdoor work and gardening, and attentive medical surveillance. While the preventorium did not tackle the issue of delinquency directly, its appearance nevertheless responded to the wider discussions juvenile crime had generated around physical and mental disability, the importance of prevention, and the need for enhanced forms of medical surveillance of Vietnamese youth.[114]

Colonial officials also reached out to religious and charitable organizations as partners for collaboration, appealing to humanitarian principles in their requests for abandoned children to be granted refuge. Yet even modest attempts to rationalize the system by removing those acquitted and abandoned children from reformatories posed its own set of challenges for the colonial administration. The president of the Society of Annamite Children, for example, informed the resident superior of Tonkin that it would "not be desirable to receive . . . those errant children from the streets of Hanoi who are brought to the institution by the police, having escaped the first time [who] will not be able to adapt themselves to the discipline and regular life of the establishment."[115] He considered them bad examples for the other rural kids (petits campagnards). Still, it's clear that those "abandoned children" previously consigned to the carceral system instead became increasingly integrated into Indochina's growing social welfare network. Between 1936 and 1937, the number of abandoned children sent to Trí Cụ dropped precipitously from twenty-seven to three.[116] Adopting a more protective role by removing the abandoned children from youth penitentiaries, one might argue, ultimately resulted in an even more repressive system for those children convicted of crimes who continued to be sent there.

New Kinds of Threats

On January 21, 1942, the Hanoi municipal police arrested seventeen-year-old Suyen for plastering posters around the city commemorating the thirtieth anniversary of the founding of the Communist Party by the Bolsheviks in Russia.[117] Once detained, Suyen admitted membership in the Hanoi section of Schoolchildren and Youth for the Salvation of the Country (*Secteur des écoliers des jeunesses pour le salut de pays*), a branch of the Indochinese Communist Party that had expanded its activities after the Japanese invasion and occupation of Indochina in 1940. Until the end of the war, the youth population became an important target of propaganda for the Vichy government and the anticolonial resistance alike. Jean Decoux, in charge of the Vichy administration of Indochina between 1940 and 1945, set out to build a network of youth groups—including sports and religious associations and a scouting movement—that would absorb nationalist feelings into Pétain's ultraconservative ideology of "national revolution." Yet attempts to win over children's loyalty—by staging reenactments of the distant Indochinese past and by embracing the Trưng sisters as heroines—backfired badly by instead cultivating the anticolonial sentiments these measures were specifically designed to ward against.[118]

Anti-French elements meanwhile worked to infiltrate these Vichy youth groups and set up youth cells within their own organizations; the files of juvenile delinquents reflect the success of some of these efforts. Much of their political recruitment seemed to have happened at school. An "active group of propaganda revolutionists" reportedly formed at the École Supérieure in Bắc Ninh; many children arrested and sent to Trí Cụ in the early 1940s counted among the school's current or former students. By and large they had been caught distributing communist tracts to their classmates.[119] It was not only the communists who preoccupied colonial authorities. In December 1940, the special police in the far northern reaches of Lạng Sơn province arrested sixteen-year-old Ninh for his affiliation with the League for the

National Restoration of Vietnam (Việt Nam Phục Quốc Đồng Minh Hôi), a pro-Japanese nationalist group that sought the installation of the long term exile Prince Cường Để on the imperial throne.[120] The league joined with the Cao Đài, an important religious movement based in Tây Sơn province in Cochinchina, and expanded its influence into the schools of Saigon.[121] Concerns over juvenile delinquency therefore took on a new valence. Colonial authorities now faced more than a public nuisance problem; they worried about the recruitment of orphaned or abandoned children into subversive political networks, ones that had come to penetrate everyday life.

The arrests of delinquent children offer a revealing portrait of the everyday challenges of late colonial administration. How to address Indochina's crime problem would require new forms of expertise, but the content of that expertise, and how it would be weighed alongside other concerns of colonial governance and finance, proved the source of many struggles both within the psychiatric profession and across the different branches of the colonial government. As this chapter has argued, the history of the medical-legal opinion reveals the production of new forms of psychiatric knowledge while also underscoring the particular challenges doctors faced in extending their expertise into the criminal courts. By forming alliances with the judicial branch and social reform movement, psychiatrists sought expanded markets for their expertise that went beyond individual determinations of mental illness to instead address the social question of crime prevention.

In order to render Indochina's criminal justice system more therapeutic, psychiatrists called for new mechanisms of increased oversight and control and joined with child reformers to advocate the expansion of the legal definition of childhood. In an interesting twist, delinquent children themselves tended to recognize these special provisions, cast in the language of protection and "rehabilitation," as effectively more punitive. This is how the chief prosecutor in Hanoi came to complain that fifteen-year-olds "will pretend to be eighteen with the view of being convicted [as an adult], rather than placed in a penitentiary colony" and thereby reduce the length of their confinement.[122]

The task of preventing crime by addressing the "bad instincts" of children began to take on a different charge with the shift in French political fortunes in the early 1940s. Even as the language of rehabilitation gained traction in child welfare circles, it never replaced the logic of security. Anxieties over mounting anticolonial pressures shaped decision making over whether to approve the release of children from reformatories. By the spring of 1942, the colonial administration found the release of dissident children "inopportune . . . at the moment when the ICP [Indochinese Communist Party] is intensifying its program."[123] The liberation of certain anticolonial youth, like Suyen, in the words of one high-ranking official, would only "irritate" police efforts of suppression.[124] That so many juvenile delinquents faced sentences that extended well into adulthood tests the limits of ideas about the need for a separate justice system to protect the special interests of children. That these sentences projected release dates well into the 1950s reflects both the hubris and the fragility of French colonial rule in Southeast Asia, which would come crashing down in 1954.

Conclusion

Continuities and Change in Postcolonial Vietnam

The epigraph to this book is an inscription left in the guestbook (*livre d'or*) of the Biên Hòa psychiatric hospital on the eve of the collapse of French colonial rule over Indochina. Authored by a fellow colonial administrator and dedicated to the director of the hospital, the poem imagines a traveler pausing on the side of the road to appreciate the elegance of the hospital's buildings complete with "vaulted flowers" and "green foliage mounting high towards the skies," all warmed by the "mellow beauty of the setting sun." This lush, tranquil scene is quickly juxtaposed with the imagined private torments of the hospital's occupants, those patients who know the "worst of Gehenna," a place outside ancient Jerusalem known in the Hebrew Bible as the Valley of the Son of Hinnom and believed to be cursed. Rapidly shifting perspectives from the observer to the observed produces a sense of social distance but also instills in the reader a sense of pity toward those for whom "knowledge, kindness will not ease their pain."

This movement between the worlds inside and outside the colonial asylum—indeed the blurring of boundaries between them and the tensions that result—form the central focus of this book. The stories of patients and their families encountered throughout tend to reinforce Michael Macdonald's observation in *Mystical Bedlam*, his magisterial work on the history of madness and healing in seventeenth-century England: "Madness is the most solitary of afflictions to the people who experience it; but it is the most social of maladies to those who observe its effects."[1] Mental disorders, even more than any other kind of illness, are profoundly anchored in the social conditions and mores of any particular culture. As Michel Foucault famously argued, it is by violating the rules of social life that individuals are pathologized and opened up to expert scrutiny and disciplinary technologies.[2] This process of social exclusion cannot be grasped from the perspective of the asylum alone, leading many historians to situate the development of psychiatry within a wider social context. By adopting perspectives that look beyond the asylum, scholars have demonstrated how values attached to "normal" and "abnormal" behavior are assigned and shift on the basis of extensive negotiations rather than the straightforward application of expert knowledge and how patients and their families experience confinement. And yet these works are almost entirely restricted to North America and Western Europe.[3] Historians of colonial psychiatry have remained focused on a different, narrower set of questions. As long as "colonial" is defined narrowly in terms of racial prejudice or the dynamics of repression and resistance only, the study of colonial psychiatry will invariably lead in one direction.

Throughout this book, I have used a social history of psychiatry and mental illness in colonial Vietnam to open up new avenues for exploring the local dynamics of colonial rule. By examining the relationship between the asylum and the community, I argued that Vietnamese families, French experts, and the colonial state became tied together in unprecedented ways. Psychiatry in the colony developed in response to the many competing and overlapping agendas of different actors that shifted with the massive social and economic changes in the region during the early decades of the twentieth century. These new social arrangements created for the first time the conditions for identifying, quantifying, and treating mental illness as a problem of colonial governance. Debates over the introduction of the legal category of the aliéné tracked shifting perceptions of mental illness as a problem of little interest to colonial administrators to the basis for a far-reaching psychiatric assistance program by the early 1930s. This shift occurred as the result of both international pressures to expand mental health services in the colony and the increasing visibility of "madness," as more and more people poured into urban centers. With the onset of the economic depression in the early 1930s, many families found it increasingly difficult to care for their own, and the burden of care for the sick and indigent increasingly fell to the colonial government. What to do about the sick and unwanted, especially those perceived as mad, would require a complex readjustment in expectations over who should be responsible for their care.

As scholars have widened the scope for inquiry in recent years, we have learned more about the everyday practices of institutions within their social worlds. Yet this move toward more richly textured social histories of prisons and asylums has generally not produced a concomitant shift or revision in thinking about the colonial state. Rather, the state continues to be described in familiar tones—as uneven, fragmented, and decentralized—marked by the absence of any sort of "carceral continuum." These histories tend to reinforce what we already know, the limits of state power, rather than lead us to reconsider how power and resistance are constituted in everyday interactions and in ways that both trouble and overflow our conception of what constitutes the state. In the preceding pages, I have suggested an alternative way of thinking about the colonial state and its institutions in terms of relations of power that cannot be disentangled from the world around them. I proposed that we think about the power of the colonial state as continuous and relational, rather than neat and bounded, and as derived from a series of social interactions that exceeded the formal limits of state institutions.[4] Using patient case files from two colonial-era asylums, I instead traced a kind of colonial micropolitics of psychiatric care in order to insist on the historic permeability of the boundaries between asylum and community. Negotiations over the confinement and release of patients unfolded between French experts, colonial bureaucrats, and Vietnamese families in ways that expanded, rather than limited, the exercise of a new, more diffuse psychiatric power in the colony.

Throughout the 1920s, for example, asylum overcrowding made daily patient management extremely difficult and exerted pressure on asylum directors to release patients from their care. In order to avoid the burdens associated with long-term confinement, colonial psychiatrists increasingly promoted early prevention through the creation of open psychiatric services in major hospitals. These services would require that Vietnamese families share basic understandings about mental illness as something that could be prevented and cured under the proper surveillance of experts. In this way, even with the introduction of a formal asylum system, psychiatrists continued to depend on families and communities for information, care, and surveillance in ways that both expanded and constrained their power as experts. As psychiatric activities diversified and expanded from the treatment of acute mental illness to the early identification of abnormal symptoms, psychiatrists enjoyed a widened scope for their expertise even as they came to rely more than ever on the intervention of the public.

Vietnamese families, meanwhile, motivated by their own concerns over preserving social order and the integrity of kinship networks, often sought or challenged the authority of colonial psychiatrists. French psychiatrists and Vietnamese families debated not only the mental health of the patient but also the capacity of families to assume their care upon release and the asylum itself as the most appropriate site for treatment and rehabilitation. While the categories of normal and abnormal continued to be framed in Western terms, the content of these categories critically relied on the kinds of information Vietnamese were willing or thought relevant to tell French doctors. The arrival of asylums may have marked the beginning of psychiatry as an institutionally based, state-sponsored project in Vietnam, but it was inserted into a preexisting field of knowledge and practice that it never fully succeeded in displacing.

Throughout the interwar period, Vietnamese families continued to pursue their own strategies in ways that both facilitated and constrained the ability of colonial psychiatrists to care for the mentally ill. With the explosive growth in the Vietnamese-language popular press in the 1920s and 1930s, families encountered new ways of learning about mental illness—what it looked like and what could be done about it. By reading scientific articles, medical glossaries, investigative reporting, and fictional works, families learned to recognize unusual behaviors among their own and to subject abnormal individuals to different forms of treatment—whether at an asylum or hospital, the pagoda, or the home. These sources help make sense of family decisions around treatment contained within the pages of patient case files and point to an emerging ethic of self-medication and self-management. They also reveal the extent to which mental illness had entered the public consciousness as both a proxy for social change and a means to criticize both the norms of traditional society and the dangers of the new modern ones taking their place.

We should take these conversations happening outside the official orbit of institutions seriously as an essential aspect of psychiatric power in the colony. Colonial expertise was not only French and not only institutionally sanctioned; it was heterogeneous and produced in exchanges between experts and laypeople. For instance, articles on mental illness took the form of advice columns, which allowed concepts that in scientific language might be too difficult and abstract for the common reader to be recast in the form of confessions and expert responses. By bringing together different understandings of mental illness in a way that was meaningful to the reading public, the Vietnamese popular press played a vital role in making a new kind of localized knowledge possible.

Competing judgments about what makes someone abnormal, in turn, also helped to clarify expectations for normal social life. In a sense, the asylum was a kind of colony within a colony. By simulating the appearance of free-dom and normal life, the asylum as agricultural colony projected a vision of an idealized colonial order, one premised on establishing a kind of continuity between the discipline of institutional order and life in the community. This was reflected in the design of the institution itself—including the explicit racial and spatial segregation of the patient population within the walls of the asylum—but also in the race- and class-based regimes of self-discipline and industry that were taught to patients as an essential aspect of labor ther-apy. Strategies for the "psychiatric reeducation" of the insane emerged as part of a broader network of colonial reform projects that sought to pro-duce a new class of colonial subjects through the disciplinary effects of labor. The form that labor took, cultivating rice paddies and the tapping of rub-ber trees, reflects the particularities of an extractive colonial economy con-cerned about young, mostly Vietnamese men who had escaped absorption into the local labor force.

By the 1930s, psychiatrists in colonial Vietnam argued that their expertise should apply to juvenile delinquents, as a preventive measure, to guard against the development of an adult criminal underclass. Troublesome and trou-bled youth were sent to reformatories, modeled on the famous nineteenth-century French colony of Mettray, where they were set to work and put under medical surveillance. Studying how psychiatric experts reframed the colony's crime problem around the question of abnormal children provides an important opportunity to investigate the continuum of different strate-gies for confinement, a kind of "carceral archipelago" of empire, that linked together the penal and medical services with a growing social assistance pro-gram.[5] Attention to juvenile delinquency allowed colonial psychiatrists to expand their influence outside the medical field and into the criminal courts. Yet it also created the conditions for disagreements to erupt between doc-tors, the police, prosecutors, and judges over who was best poised to make determinations about the fate of delinquents. At stake was fiercely protected jurisdictional territory as well as key philosophical questions about how to compare children across different cultural contexts. Situating the history of psychiatry within a broader social and institutional context yields critical insight into the complex alliances and fractures that characterized the every-day administration of empire.

Postcolonial Developments

While this book concludes before the end of French rule in 1954, the legacy of the French system nevertheless continued to shape the development of psychiatry in the region into the postcolonial era. The psychiatrists who took up the reins were all trained by the French, including Nguyễn Văn Hoài, who studied at the Sorbonne and returned to work at Biên Hòa in 1930. He became its first Vietnamese director in 1950 after the French director abandoned his post. Later accounts—in both Vietnamese and English—describe the experience of Biên Hòa during the First Indochina War (1946–54) as tumultuous and Nguyễn Văn Hoài as a hero who rescued his patients from starvation and neglect. Stories emphasize his fight against Trần Văn Hữu, the prime minister of the state of Vietnam from 1950 to 1952, who cut funding for patient food. One even unmistakably likened him to a modern-day Vietnamese Philippe Pinel, the famous nineteenth-century French alienist who unshackled his patients from the chains of ignorance and superstition. While psychiatric reformers had previously used Pinel's story as a way of asserting the beneficence of French colonial rule in North Africa, here it unfolds in the wake of the French wars of decolonization to assert the moral superiority of a colonized subject.[6] His dedication to patients and staff is evident in one story recounted by a Vietnamese guard at Biên Hòa, who described 1946–47 as the "dark years" (đen tuổi) when French intelligence captured several members of the asylum staff and subjected them to physical torture. French interrogators apparently set out to extract confessions that accused Nguyễn Văn Hoài of diverting hospital resources to the Viet Minh for his own material gain. The guards refused to turn on their beloved leader, "knowing that he would live and die for the hospital."[7] In a 1960 article in *Bách khoa*, the testimonies of those who knew him painted a picture of a life impervious to corruption. After Nguyễn Văn Hoài's death in 1955, the hospital bore his name for several years as a tribute to his service. The creativity of Biên Hòa's various directors, both Vietnamese and French, ensured the institution's survival across multiple regime changes and periods of economic crisis. In fact, 2019 marks the centennial of the opening of the Biên Hòa asylum, now referred to as Central Psychiatric Hospital II. It remains Vietnam's largest psychiatric treatment facility.[8]

The landscape of postwar psychiatry subsequently developed against the backdrop of military conflict and wartime scarcity and the rise of postcolonial nationalism, as well as the growth of international networks of scientific expertise. The World Health Organization's Pacific Regional Office sent mental health consultants to South Vietnam in 1962; their reports reflected a growing interest in mental health care provision as an essential aspect of the region's development.[9] Pierre Dorolle, the committed psychiatric reformer and long-term director of Chợ Quán's neuropsychiatric unit, also incidentally served as the deputy general of the World Health Organization from 1950 to 1973. The Department of Neurology and Psychiatry of Hanoi Medical University was established in 1957; the Association for Neurology, Psychiatry, and Neurosurgery followed in 1962; and the National Psychiatric Hospital (now National Psychiatric Hospital No. 1) opened in 1963.[10] By 1966, the former Biên Hòa asylum housed two thousand beds and employed 143 doctors, nurses, and guards. Meanwhile, the government of the Democratic Republic of Vietnam began building provincial psychiatric hospitals, such as Hai Phong Psychiatric Hospital, which was established in 1960. The Department of Psychiatry established in 1969 at Bạch Mai Hospital became the National Institute of Mental Health in 1991.

The history of mental illness in postcolonial Vietnam—briefly glossed here—still remains to be written. Tracing the connections in mental health practices from the colonial era through the reunification of the country in 1975 and the đổi mới economic reforms of the 1980s would greatly enrich our understanding of contemporary mental health care and Vietnamese society more generally. To combat the growing AIDS epidemic among the injection-drug–using population since the 1990s, technical experts and policy advisers from international organizations and state agencies have poured into Vietnam on the wave of a massive influx of development money.[11] These sorts of international public health efforts in Vietnam originated in the period covered in this book, including the study trips that crisscrossed Southeast Asia during the interwar years, the 1937 conference at Bandoeng, and the creation of a vast new public health infrastructure in the name of colonial development. More recently, gaining steam from the global mental health movement, bilateral and multilateral initiatives have also sought to promote mental health as a priority for the Vietnamese government. They have worked to improve service delivery, increase government spending on community-based mental health care, and promote evidence-based policy and practice as well as strong intersectoral and international collaborations. The current draft of a national mental health strategy includes an explicit commitment to protect the rights of persons with mental disorders. Despite these commitments, there remain insufficient hospital beds and limited availability of both pharmacological and nonpharmacological interventions, fragmented funding, and a critical shortage of psychiatric doctors and nurses.[12]

With the opening of Vietnam to foreign aid, efforts to shift policy perspectives to embrace an evidence-based, human rights approach to public health have met with resistance as Vietnam attempts to maintain national control amid unprecedented levels of foreign investment. In particular, as international public health and human rights organizations have sought to move the needle on policymaking in Vietnam in line with global priorities, they have also faced challenges over what to do about the country's grow-ing network of drug detention centers. In September 2011, Human Rights Watch released a report detailing human rights abuses in drug detention centers in southern Vietnam. Entitled *The Rehab Archipelago*, the report pro-vided an overview of government policies toward drug use while also docu-menting the conditions inside detention centers based on interviews with recently released individuals.[13] The investigation painted a bleak picture of the experience of drug incarceration in Vietnam, marked by the long-term and arbitrary nature of detention in addition to forced detoxification and compulsory labor.[14] The report condemned these practices as clearly at odds with internationally recognized principles of human rights and public health evidence and urged the immediate closure of the centers.

The Human Rights Watch report traces the origins of Vietnam's drug detention centers to the end of the U.S.-Vietnam War in 1975, when drug users, sex workers, and political dissidents were detained in state-run reedu-cation camps. Yet the practice of forced labor, as we have seen, forms part of a long-standing approach to social deviance in the region that dates back to the colonial period. Agricultural colonies for the mentally ill and juve-nile delinquents emerged as part of a global movement in the early twenti-eth century that valorized the countryside as a site of rejuvenation and was geared as much toward affecting a "cure" as toward preparing individuals for reentry into normalized social life. The "colony-asylum" model for recov-ered psychiatric patients, while deemed impractical by French bureaucrats in the late 1930s, was eventually adopted by the government of South Viet-nam in 1964 when the Mental Health Bureau of the Vietnamese Ministry of Health created a rehabilitation village on the periphery of the grounds of the former Biên Hòa psychiatric hospital. It placed seventy patients set to leave the hospital after three or four years of treatment in a kind of halfway institu-tion, where they were left to earn a small living by hiring themselves out to farmers in the surrounding area. Just as with the Dutch experimental model at Lenteng Agung, the objective was to help patients prepare for reintegra-tion into normal life by equipping them with important skills so that they would no longer be a burden on their families or an object of pity in their communities. The Biên Hòa hospital staff deemed the project so successful that the capacity of the village was eventually doubled in 1970.[15]

That the reliance on labor as a form of rehabilitation remained resilient through ideological shifts with the end of French rule, the victory of the communists in the 1970s, and the turn to global capitalism during the mid-1980s, reflects the durability and flexibility of beliefs in the social harms of drug use and the therapeutic value of work. Today, drug use is considered a social evil and is associated with historical forms of Western intervention and oppression, especially linked to the French colonial state's opium monopoly; as a consequence, drug users are subject to forms of moral condemnation and social marginalization. The goals of rehabilitation remain more or less the same—engendering a productive class of laborers who adhere to social norms, however defined—but the political stakes and rationalization for the rehabilitation of drug users have shifted dramatically. What is often taken as a local approach to the rehabilitation of drug addicts is therefore in fact part of a longer and much more global story about forced labor, psychiatric treatment, and the legacies of imperialism.

This book has told the story of the mentally ill in colonial Vietnam from multiple vantage points, from the intimate space of the Vietnamese household to the courtroom spectacle of the murder trial. It has tracked the domestic strategies and institutional arrangements through which certain abnormal individuals were labeled as pathological and therefore unfit for social life. Expert scientific assessments, recorded in the pages of patient case files, nevertheless relied on popular beliefs about mental capacity and responded to anxieties over social order to make their determinations about whether to confine or release patients. Some troubled individuals were abandoned by their families and communities, rendered as anonymous "Xs" in colonial reports, and tested the limits of public assistance and private philanthropy. Others remained jealously guarded by their families at home. Yet the patients who arrived at the colonial asylum were not just the unlucky ones who had simply fallen through the cracks. Rather, their fate is better understood in the context of the penetration of colonial institutions into Vietnamese society, the convergence of multiple systems of medical thought, and a comprehensive shift in the relationship between families and the state. These themes still reverberate in Vietnam, where scientific expertise continues to be negotiated in the clinic and in policy circles and where social stigma remains a major barrier to care. At the same time, it is widely observed that families will often stay with patients at the psychiatric hospital throughout the duration of their treatment, playing the vital role of caretakers even within the walls of the institution. Today, as in the colonial past, these tales of compassion and abandonment bear witness to the lived experience of mental illness and the transformation of Vietnamese society itself.

NOTES

Introduction

1. Trung Tâm Lưu Trữ Quốc Gia II (TTLTQG-II) (Vietnam National Archives Centre II, Hồ Chí Minh City), Fonds du Gouvernement de la Cochinchine (GOU-COCH), IA.8/281(2), Le Procureur Général près la Cour d'Appel de Saigon à Monsieur le Gouverneur de la Cochinchine, June 29, 1925. All patient names used in this book are abbreviated and/or manipulated to protect the privacy of the patients and their families.

2. Here I follow the work of David Wright, who critically reexamines assumptions about the social role of asylums in nineteenth-century Britain. "Getting Out of the Asylum: Understanding the Confinement of the Insane in the Nineteenth Century," *Social History of Medicine* 10, no. 1 (1997): 137–55.

3. For a comprehensive overview of the historical literature on colonial psychiatry see Richard Keller, "Madness and Colonization: Psychiatry in the British and French Empires, 1800–1962," *Journal of Social History* 35, no. 2 (Winter 2001): 295–326.

4. Frantz Fanon, *The Wretched of the Earth*, trans. Constance Farrington (New York: Grove Press, 1963). For a description of Fanon's significance to the history of colonial psychiatry, see also Richard Keller, *Colonial Madness: Psychiatry in French North Africa* (Chicago: University of Chicago Press, 2007), 164–65.

5. In her study of asylums in British India, for example, Waltraud Ernst argues that the maintenance of white privilege was crucial to daily practices of confinement and treatment. Others such as Jonathan Sadowsky and Megan Vaughan have focused on the difficulty of defining insanity across cultures in sub-Saharan Africa and the political uses of psychiatric knowledge to defend against antisocial and especially anticolonial impulses. See Jonathan Sadowsky, *Imperial Bedlam: Institutions of Madness in Colonial Southwest Nigeria* (Berkeley: University of California Press, 1999); Megan Vaughan. *Curing Their Ills: Colonial Power and African Illness* (Palo Alto, CA: Stanford University Press, 1992); Waltraud Ernst, *Mad Tales from the Raj: Colonial Psychiatry in South Asia, 1800–1858* (London: Anthem Press, 2010). For a comprehensive overview of the historical literature on colonial psychiatry see Keller, "Madness and Colonization." See Hans Pols, "The Nature of the Native Mind: Contested Views of Dutch Colonial Psychiatrists in the Former Dutch East Indies," and Jacqui Leckie, "Unsettled Minds: Colonialism, Gender and Settling Madness in Fiji," both in *Psychiatry and Empire*, ed. Sloan Mahone and Megan Vaughan (New York: Palgrave Macmillan 2007), 172–96, 99–123.

6. Richard Keller in his study of colonial psychiatry in Algeria shows how psychiatrists spoke directly to questions about the mental capacity of indigenous populations to assimilate to modernity and French styles of civilization, and so played an

important role in framing debates over the social and political rights of the colonized. Keller, *Colonial Madness*, 8.

7. Sadowsky, *Imperial Bedlam*, 74; Megan Vaughan, introduction to Mahone and Vaughan, *Psychiatry and Empire*, 1–16.

8. John Walton, "Casting Out and Bringing Back in Victorian England," in *The Anatomy of Madness: Essays in the History of Psychiatry*, ed. William Bynum, Roy Porter, and Michael Shepherd (London: Tavistock Books, 1985), 132–47; Akihito Suzuki, *Madness at Home: The Psychiatrist, the Patient, and the Family in England, 1820–1860* (Berkeley: University of California Press, 2006); Joseph Melling and Bill Forsythe, eds., *Insanity, Institutions and Society, 1800–1914: A Social History of Madness in Comparative Perspective*, Studies in the Social History of Medicine (London: Routledge, 1999); Peter Bartlett and David Wright, eds., *Outside the Walls of the Asylum: The History of Care in Community 1750–2000* (New Brunswick, NJ: Athlone Press, 1999); Patricia Prestwich, "Family Strategies and Medical Power: 'Voluntary' Committal in a Parisian Asylum, 1876–1914," in *The Confinement of the Insane, 1800–1965: International Perspectives*, ed. Roy Porter and David Wright (Cambridge: Cambridge University Press, 2003), 79–99.

9. Wright, "Getting Out of the Asylum," 139.

10. See Joseph Melling, "Accommodating Madness: New Research in the Social History of Insanity and Institutions," in Melling and Forsythe, *Insanity, Institutions and Society*, 1–30, 6.

11. Important exceptions for the Asian context include Zhiying Ma, "An Iron Cage of Civilization? Missionary Psychiatry, the Chinese Family and a Colonial Dialect of Enlightenment," in *Psychiatry and Chinese History*, ed. Howard Chiang (London: Pickering and Chatto, 2014), 71–90; Hayang Kim, "Sick at Heart: Mental Illness in Modern Japan" (PhD diss., Columbia University, 2015); Akihito Suzuki, "Between Two Psychiatric Regimes: Migration and Psychiatry in Early Twentieth Century Japan," in *Migration, Ethnicity, and Mental Health: International Perspectives, 1840–2010*, ed. Angela McCarthy and Catharine Coleborne, Routledge Studies in Cultural History (New York: Routledge, 2012), 141–56.

12. On cultural relativism in colonial psychiatric practice, see Jonathan Sadowsky, "The Social World and the Reality of Mental Illness: Lessons from Colonial Psychiatry," *Harvard Review of Psychiatry* 11 (2003): 210–14. See also Sadowsky's brief discussion on the role of families in *Imperial Bedlam*, 54–58. Catherine Coleborne focuses on European families and colonial public hospitals but does not address the interaction of colonial asylums with indigenous families or forms of knowledge. *Madness in the Family: Insanity and Institutions in the Australasian Colonial World, 1860–1914* (New York: Palgrave Macmillan, 2009).

13. Tran-Minh Tung, "The Family and the Management of Mental Health Problems in Vietnam," in *Transcultural Research in Mental Health*, vol. 2 of *Mental Health Research in Asia and the Pacific*, ed. William P. Lebra (Honolulu: University Press of Hawai'i, 1972), 107–14. Michael Nunley, "The Involvement of Families in Indian Psychiatry," *Culture, Medicine and Psychiatry* 22 (1988): 317–53; Robert Franklin et al., "Cultural Response to Mental Illness in Senegal: Reflections through Patient Companions, Part I: Methods and Descriptive Data," *Social Science and Medicine* 42, no. 3 (1996): 325–38; John Elderkin Bell, *The Family in the Hospital: Lessons from Developing Countries* (Washington, DC: National Institutes of Health, 1969).

14. Citing Foucault, one could say that families act as a key "switch point" that assures the passage of individuals from one disciplinary system to another (i.e., from

home to clinic and back again) and therefore play a critical role in the elaboration of psychiatric power. Michel Foucault, *Psychiatric Power: Lectures at the Collège de France, 1973–1974*, trans. Graham Burchell (New York: Palgrave Macmillan, 2006).

15. I borrow the term "micropolitics" from Joseph Melling, whose research focuses on the history of asylum care in New Jersey. See "Accommodating Madness," 1–30.

16. See David Marr, *Vietnamese Tradition on Trial* (Berkeley: University of California Press, 1981); Hue Tam Ho Tai. *Radicalism and the Origins of the Vietnamese Revolution* (Cambridge, MA: Harvard University Press, 1996); Pierre Brocheux and Daniel Hémery, *Indochina: An Ambiguous Colonization* (Berkeley: University of California Press, 2009). There is still very little written on the social history of Vietnam during this period. See Haydon Cherry, *Down and Out in Saigon: A Social History of the Poor in a Colonial City*, (PhD diss., Yale University, 2012)

17. Gerard Sasges, *Imperial Intoxication: Alcohol and the Making of Colonial Indochina* (Honolulu: University of Hawai'i Press, 2017), 52.

18. Christopher Goscha, *Vietnam: A New History* (New York: Basic Books, 2016).

19. See chapter 4 from Keller, *Colonial Madness*, for an extended discussion on the Algiers School and how it figures in the history of psychiatry and the political history of Algeria.

20. On praise of Indochina's mental health program, see H. Aubin, *L'Assistance psychiatrique indigène aux colonies: Rapport de Congrès des Médecins Aliénistes et Neurologistes de France et des Pays de Langue Francaise, XLIIe session—Alger 6–11 Avril 1938* (Paris: Masson et Cie, 1938).

21. Keller, *Colonial Madness*, 9.

22. See introduction in Keller, *Colonial Madness*; Trung Tâm Lưu Trữ Quốc Gia I (TTLTQG-I) (Vietnam National Archives Centre I, Hà Nội), Inspection Générale de l'Hygiène et Santé Publique (IGHSP), 51–01, Hôpital de Chôquan. Rapport sur le fonctionnement du service de psychiatrie de l'Hôpital de Chôquan en 1934.

23. TTLTQG-1, IGHSP, 51–01, Rapport sur le fonctionnement du service de psychiatrie de l'Hôpital de Chô Quan en 1934. Discussed further in chapter 4.

24. Keller, *Colonial Madness*, 7.

25. I prefer the use of the term "spaces of experimentation" rather than "laboratories of modernity" to describe the development of medical science in a colonial context as "locally constituted rather than merely imperially derivative," to quote David Arnold and Erich Dewald, "Cycles of Empowerment? The Bicycle and Everyday Technology in Colonial India and Vietnam," *Comparative Studies in Society and History* 53, no. 4 (October 2011): 971–96.

26. Pierre Brocheux and Daniel Hémery, *Indochine: La colonisation ambiguë, 1858–1954* (Paris: Découverte, 2001).

27. Laurence Monnais, *Médecine et colonisation: L'aventure indochinoise, 1860–1939* (Paris: CNRS Editions, 1999).

28. Laurence Monnais, "In the Shadow of the Colonial Hospital: Developing Health Care in Indochina, 1860–1939," in *Viêt-Nam Exposé: French Scholarship on Twentieth-Century Vietnamese Society*, ed. Gisele L. Bousquet and Pierre Brocheux (Ann Arbor: University of Michigan Press, 2002), 174.

29. Waltraud Ernst, *Mad Tales from the Raj: The European Insane in British India, 1800–1858* (New York: Routledge, 1991).

30. These questions are explored in greater detail in Laurence Monnais, C. Michele Thompson, and Ayo Wahlberg, eds., *Southern Medicine for Southern People:*

Vietnamese Medicine in the Making (Newcastle upon Tyne, UK: Cambridge Scholars Publishing, 2012). See in particular the essays by C. Michele Thompson and Laurence Monnais.

31. Tuong Phan and Derrick Silove, "An Overview of Indigenous Descriptions of Mental Phenomena and the Range of Traditional Healing Practices amongst the Vietnamese, *Transcultural Psychiatry* 36, no. 1 (1999): 79–94.

32. Allan Tran, "A Life of Worry: The Cultural Politics and Phenomenology of Anxiety in Ho Chi Minh City, Vietnam (PhD diss., University of California–San Diego, 2012), 117.

33. Scholars have remarked on the personalized and syncretic nature of most psychiatric treatments in Vietnam and their variation with respect to socioeconomic class and education. See David Craig, *Familiar Medicine: Everyday Health Knowledge and Practice in Today's Vietnam* (Honolulu: University of Hawai'i Press, 2002); Laurence Monnais, C. Michele Thompson, and Ayo Wahlberg, eds., *Southern Medicine for Southern People: Vietnamese Medicine in the Making* (Newcastle upon Tyne, UK: Cambridge Scholars Publishing, 2012); and Tine Gammeltoft, *Women's Bodies, Women's Worries: Health and Family Planning in a Vietnamese Rural Commune* (Copenhagen: Nordic Institute of Asian Studies, 1999).

34. Laurence Monnais and Noémi Tousignant, "The Colonial Life of Pharmaceuticals: Accessibility to Healthcare, Consumption of Medicines, and Medical Pluralism in French Vietnam, 1905–1945," *Journal of Vietnamese Studies* 1, no. 1–2 (2006): 131–66.

35. Sally Swartz, "Colonial Lunatic Asylum Archives: Challenges to Historiography," *Kronos* 34, no. 1 (2008): 285–302; James Mills, "The Mad and the Past: Retrospective Diagnosis, Post-Coloniality, Discourse Analysis and the Asylum Archive," *Journal of Medical Humanities* 21, no. 3 (2000): 141–58.

36. Jonathan Andrews, "Case Notes, Case Histories, and the Patient's Experience of Insanity at Gartnavel Royal Asylum, Glasgow, in the Nineteenth Century," *Social History of Medicine* 11, no. 2 (1998): 255–81; Guenter B. Risse and John Harley Warner, "Reconstructing Clinical Activities: Patient Records in Medical History," *Social History of Medicine* 5, no. 2 (1992): 183–205.

37. Here I draw inspiration from the work of Erica Peters, "Negotiating Power through Everyday Practices in French Vietnam, 1880–1924" (PhD diss., University of Chicago, 2000).

38. Vietnamese diacritic markings are often inconsistent or missing from colonial archival sources. I have elected to use the corrected diacritics for certain institutions, locations, events, and people in the main text of the book when available. I have relied on common English spellings for major cities (Hanoi, Saigon) and colonial territories (Cochinchina, Tonkin, Annam) in order to improve the text's readability. In the endnotes, I use the original spellings as found in archival catalogues and documents so that other researchers may retrace my steps.

1. A Background to Confinement

1. TTLTQG-2, GOUCOCH, IA.8/162(9), Hôpital de Chợ Quán (1886–1887): Au sujet de l'annamite HV Nhut atteint d'alienation mental; TTLTQG-2, GOUCOCH, IA.8/152(1), 1882–1897, Envoi et internement des aliénés à l'hôpital de Chợ Quán, Sochang, September 12, 1884; TTLTQG-2, GOUCOCH, IA.8/162(9), Au sujet des

malades atteints d'alienation mentale (dossiers individuels) à Chợ Quán, Le Médecin de 1er classe charge du service medical de l'hôpital indigène a M. le directeur de l'hôpital, February 6, 1887; TTLTQG-2, GOUCOCH, IA.8/162(9), Au sujet des malades atteints d'aliénation mentale (dossiers individuels) à Chợ Quán, M. André, Directeur de l'hôpital de Chợ Quán à Monsieur le Directeur de l'Intérieur, Saigon, February 8, 1887.

2. Louis Lorion, *Criminalité et médecine judiciare en Cochinchine* (Lyon: A. Storck, 1887), 47.

3. Laurence Monnais, "In the Shadow of the Colonial Hospital: Developing Health Care in Indochina, 1860–1939," in *Viêt-Nam Exposé: French Scholarship on Twentieth-Century Vietnamese Society*, ed. Gisele L. Bousquet and Pierre Brocheux (Ann Arbor: University of Michigan Press, 2002), 174.

4. TTLTQG-2, GOUCOCH, IA.8/152(1), 1882–1897, Le Directeur de l'Intérieur, Beliard à Saigon, May 3, 1882.

5. TTLTQG-2, GOUCOCH, IA.8/152(1), Chợ Quán, April 30, 1882.

6. Lorion, *Criminalité*, 45.

7. Lorion, *Criminalité*, 46.

8. It was Michel Foucault who first introduced the concept of a "surface of emergence" in *The Archaeology of Knowledge* (New York: Pantheon Books, 1972), 41–42.

9. Alexander Woodside, *Vietnam and the Chinese Model* (Cambridge, MA: Harvard University Press, 1971), 43.

10. Ann Bates and A.W. Bates, "Lãn Ông (Lê Hữu Trác, 1720–1791) and the Vietnamese Medical Tradition, *Journal of Medical Biography* 15 (2007): 158–64.

11. French translation by Pierre Huard and Maurice Durand, "Un traité de médecine sino-vietnamienne du XVIIIe siècle: La compréhension intuitive des recettes médicales de Hai-Thuong," *Revue d'histoire des sciences et de leurs applications* 9, no. 2 (1956): 126–49, 142.

12. C. Michele Thompson, "Selections from *Miraculous Drugs of the South* by the Vietnamese Buddhist Monk-Physican Tuệ Tĩnh," in *Buddhism and Medicine: An Anthology of Premodern Sources*, ed. C. Pierce Salguero (New York: Columbia University Press, 2017), 561–68; Leslie E. de Vries, "The Đồng Nhân Pagoda and the Publication of Mister Lazy's Medical Encyclopedia," in Salguero, *Buddhism and Medicine*, 569–74; David Marr, "Vietnamese Attitudes regarding Illness and Healing," in *Death and Disease in Southeast Asia. Explorations in Social, Medical and Demographic History*, ed. Norman G. Owen (Oxford: Oxford University Press, 1987), 162–86.

13. Thompson, "Selections," 563–68.

14. Nguyễn Trần Huân (Docteur en médecine interne des hôpitaux de Hanoi), Contribution à l'Etude de l'Ancienne Thérapeutique Vietnamienne. (Paris: École Française d'Extrême Orient, 1951).

15. See Monnais, Thompson, and Wahlberg, *Southern Medicine for Southern People*, 233; Danielle Groleau and Laurence Kirmayer, "Sociosomatic Theory in Vietnamese Immigrants' Narratives of Distress," *Anthropology & Medicine* 11, no. 2 (2004): 117–33.

16. Gustave Doumoutier, *Essai sur la pharmacie Annamite: Détermination de 300 plantes et produits indigènes, avec leur nom en Annamite, en français, en latin et en chinois et l'indication de leurs qualités thérapeutiques d'après les pharmacopées annamites et chinoises* (Hanoi: F.H. Schneider, 1887).

17. Marr, "Vietnamese Attitudes," 171.

18. Barley Norton, *Songs for the Spirits: Music and Mediums in Modern Vietnam* (Urbana: University of Illinois Press, 2009); Kirsten W. Endres, *Performing the Divine: Mediums, Markets and Modernity in Urban Vietnam* (Copenhagen: Nordic Institute of Asian Studies (NIAS) Press, 2011); Nguyễn Thị Hiền, "Yin Illness: Its Diagnosis and Healing within Len Dong (Spirit Possession) Rituals of the Viet, *Asian Ethnology* 67, no. 2 (2008): 305–21; Tuong Phan and Derrick Silove, "An Overview of Indigenous Descriptions of Mental Phenomena and the Range of Traditional Healing Practices amongst the Vietnamese," *Transcultural Psychiatry* 36, no. 1 (1999): 79–94.

19. For full French translation of the Gia Long Code see Paul Louis Félix Philastre, *Le Code Annamite* (Paris: Ernest Leroux, 1876). For the social implications of the introduction of the Gia Long Code see K. W. Taylor, *A History of the Vietnamese* (Cambridge, UK: Cambridge University Press, 2013); Woodside, *Vietnam and the Chinese Model*, 43.

20. The Lê Dynasty's Hồng Đức Code—which the Gia Long Code replaced—did include certain exemptions for the elderly and disabled but did not specifically cite madness. See Article 665 from Ngọc Huy Nguyễn and Văn Tài Tạ, *The Lê Code: Law in Traditional Vietnam: A Comparative Sino-Vietnamese Legal Study with Historical-Juridical Analysis* (Athens, OH: Ohio University Press, 1987), 278.

21. For the text of Decree 11 of Article 261, see Philastre, *Le Code Annamite*, 226. A discussion of precolonial legal guidelines and sanctions surrounding mental illness can be found in Henri Reboul and Emmanuel Régis, "L'Assistance des aliénés aux colonies" *Rapport au Congrès des Médecins Aliénistes et Neurologistes de France et des Pays de Langue Francaise*, XXIIe session—Tunis, April 1–7, 1912 (Paris: Masson et Cie, 1912): 121–23.

22. For a comprehensive discussion of Qing laws regarding madness, see Fabien Simonis, "Mad Acts, Mad Speech, and Mad People in Late Imperial Chinese Law and Medicine" (PhD diss., Princeton University, 2010). See especially chapters 11 and 12.

23. See Simonis, "Mad Acts," 463.

24. Ng and Simonis adopt different interpretations of what drove the increasingly punitive nature of the legislation. See Vivien Ng, *Madness in Late Imperial China: From Illness to Deviance* (Norman: University of Oklahoma Press, 1990); Simonis, "Mad Acts."

25. For text of Decree 13, Article 261 of the Gia Long Code, see Philastre, *Le Code Annamite*, 227.

26. Simonis, "Mad Acts," 465.

27. John Whitmore, "Social Organization and Confucian Thought," *Journal of Southeast Asian Studies* 15, no. 2 (September 1984): 296–306; Insun Yu, "Law and Family in Seventeenth and Eighteenth Century Vietnam" (PhD diss., University of Michigan, 1978).

28. In the words of the Advisory Committee of Annamite Jurisprudence (Commission Consultatif de Jurisprudence Annamite), referring to the 1883 decree, "All latitude is left to the parents of the aliéné to act in favor of his personal interests." TTLTQG-1, Résidence Supérieur au Tonkin (RST), 73745, Note pour Monsieur l'Administrateur, Chef du 1er Bureau, February 20, 1931.

29. Jeanne Louise Carrière, "Reconstructing the Grounds for Interdiction," *Louisiana Law Review* 54, no. 5 (1994): 1199–1236.

30. Peter Zinoman, *The Colonial Bastille: A History of Imprisonment in Vietnam, 1862–1940* (Berkeley: University of California Press, 2001), 40–41; See also James

David Barnhart, "Violence and the Civilizing Mission: Native Justice in French Colonial Vietnam, 1858–1914" (PhD diss., University of Chicago, 1999).

31. This preoccupation with punishment formed a common point of critique among French officials when referring to the principles of this law and of Vietnamese law more generally. See, for example, F. Pech. "Note sur le régime légal de la Cochinchine," *Journal of the Siam Society* 4 (1907):1–18.

32. A similar development happened in Japan. See Akihito Suzuki, "The State, Family and the Insane in Japan, 1900–1945," in *The Confinement of the Insane: International Perspectives, 1800–1965*, ed. Roy Porter and David Wright (Cambridge: Cambridge University Press, 2003), 193–225.

33. For a broad overview of the 1838 law and projects for its reform in France see Margaret Gwynne Lloyd and Michel Bénézech, "The French Mental Health Legislation of 1838 and Its Reform," *Journal of Forensic Psychiatry* 3, no. 2 (1992): 232–50. The law also served as the model upon which other European countries developed their first legislation around mental illness.

34. Jan Goldstein, *Console and Classify: The French Psychiatric Profession in the Nineteenth Century* (Cambridge: Cambridge University Press, 1987).

35. Between 1870 and 1940, there were some twenty attempts to persuade the National Assemblies to reform the 1838 law, including two major commissions of inquiry in 1870 and 1905. Even into the postwar period there were two major attempts to change the law (first in 1970 and again in 1982). The 1838 law was not finally modified in France until January 1968, when a law passed that strengthened the protection of civil rights of mental patients, particularly those rights related to the administration of their property. See Lloyd and Bénézech, "French Mental Health Legislation." For abuses of the 1838 law, see Arlette Farge and Michel Foucault, eds., *Le Désordre des familles. Lettres de cachet des archives de la Bastille au XVIIIe siècle* (Paris: Gallimard, 1982).

36. Archives Nationales d'Outre Mer (ANOM), Fonds du Gouvernement Général de l'Indochine (GGI), 8317, M. E. Assaud, Procureur Général, Chef du Service judiciaire de la Cochinchine et du Cambodge à Monsieur le Gouverneur Général de l'Indo-Chine à Saigon, September 30, 1897.

37. TTLTQG-1, Fonds de la Résidence Supérieur au Tonkin (RST), 73745, Le Médecin Principal de 1ère classe Collomb, Directeur local de la Santé du Tonkin à Monsieur le Résident Supérieur au Tonkin (3ème Bureau), April 28 1908.

38. TTLTQG-1, RST, 73745, Monsieur Logerot, Administrateur Maire, à Monsieur le Résident Supérieur au Tonkin, Haiphong, May 5, 1908.

39. TTLTQG-1, RST, 73745, L'administrateur Chef du 2ème Bureau Note pour l'Administrateur Chef du 3e Bureau, Hanoi, May 7, 1908.

40. TTLTQG-1, RST, 73745, Résident Supérieur Morel à Monsieur le Gouverneur Général, au sujet de la promulgation de la loi du 30 Juin 1838 sur les aliénés, June 18, 1908.

41. TTLTQG-1, RST, 73745, Le Maire de la Ville de Hanoi, à Monsieur le Résident Supérieur au Tonkin au sujet de la promulgation de la loi du 30 Juin 1838 sur les établissements d'aliénés, May 7, 1908.

42. TTLTQG-1, RST, 73745, Résident Supérieur Morel à Monsieur le Gouverneur Général . . . June 18, 1908.

43. TTLTQG-1, RST, 73745, Le Maire de la Ville de Hanoi, à Monsieur le Résident Supérieur au Tonkin . . . May 7, 1908.

44. Colonial doctors estimated 2.3 cases of mental illness for every 1,000 troops. Reboul and Régis, "L'Assistance des aliénés aux colonies." Information in the text provided in the report by Dr. Rangé, Doctor-Inspector of Sanitary and Medical Services in Indochina, on February 24, 1911.

45. TTLTQG-1, RST, 73745, Le Maire de la Ville de Hanoi, à Monsieur le Résident Supérieur au Tonkin . . . May 7, 1908.

46. TTLTQG-2, GOUCOCH, IA.8/1724(2), Lieutenant Gouverneur à Gouverneur Général, au sujet de la loi du 30 Juin 1838 sur les aliénés, May 7, 1908.

47. For more on colonial republicanism and its Vietnamese variant, see Peter Zinoman, *Vietnamese Colonial Republican: The Political Vision of Vũ Trọng Phụng* (Berkeley: University of California Press, 2014).

48. TTLTQG-1, RST, 73751, La Maire de Haiphong, Gautret, à Monsieur le Résident Supérieur, September 3, 1903.

49. TTLTQG-1, RST, 73745, Résident Supérieur Morel à Monsieur le Gouverneur Général . . . June 18, 1908.

50. TTLTQG-1, RST, 73745, Le Maire de la Ville de Hanoi . . . May 7, 1908.

51. TTLTQG-2, GOUCOCH, IA.8/152(1), Note de Service pour M. le Directeur de Chợ Quán, December 21, 1882.

52. TTLTQG-2, GOUCOCH, IA.8/152(1), Note de Service, Sécretariat Générale—Direction de l'Intérieur pour M. le Directeur de Chợ Quán, 1882.

53. TTLTQG-2, GOUCOCH, IA.8/162(9), M. L. Gudenet, Administrateur de Thudaumot, à Monsieur le Directeur de l'Interieur (3ème Bureau), October 29, 1887.

54. European patients in Tonkin, meanwhile, received treatment at the Hôpital de Hanoi. TTLTQG-2, GOUCOCH, IA.8/085(3), arrêté du Gouverneur General a.s. Construction d'un pavillon pour les aliénés à l'hôpital militaire de Saigon, November 22, 1880.

55. Reboul and Régis, "L'Assistance," 132.

56. Laurence Monnais, "Colonised and Neurasthenic: From the Appropriation of a Word to the Reality of a *Malaise de Civilisation* in Urban French Vietnam," *Health and History* 14, no. 1 (2012): 121–42.

57. TTLTQG-2, GOUCOCH, IA.8/104(1), Le Docteur Henaff, Chef du Service de Santé de la Cochinchine du Cambodge et du Laos, à Monsieur le Lieutenant Gouverneur de la Cochinchine, Saigon, July 15 1903.

58. TTLTQG-2, GOUCOCH, IA.8/104(2), Le Médecin principal de 1ère class Henaff, Sous-Directeur du Service de Santé en Cochinchine, au sujet de "Madame M," à Monsieur le Lieutenant-Gouverneur de la Cochinchine, October 23, 1908.

59. TTLTQG-2, GOUCOCH, IA8/104(4), Le Lieutenant-Gouverneur H. de Lamothe, rapport de la Commission, Saigon, August 30 1902.

60. TTLTQG-2, GOUCOCH, IA.8/097(8), Contrat au sujet de l'hospitalisation des maladies de Cochinchine atteints d'aliénation mentale, November 22, 1902; see also TTLTQG-1, GOUCOCH, IA.9/104(4), Projet de traité avec l'asile public d'aliénés à Marseille, extrait du Conseil Colonial, Séance, September 4, 1902.

61. TTLTQG-2, GOUCOCH, IA.8/104(1), Mesures à prendre lorsqu'un cas d'aliénation de français se produit en Cochinchine, 1903.

62. Reboul and Régis, "L'Assistance," 139.

63. TTLTQG-2, GOUCOCH, IA8/104(4), Rapport de la Commission, August 30, 1902.

64. TTLTQG-1, RST, 73750, L'Administrateur Résident de France à Haiduong à Monsieur le Résident Supérieur (3ème Bureau), October 19, 1903.

65. TTLTQG-1, RST, 73750, L'Administrateur Résident de France à Sontay à Monsieur le Résident Supérieur, October 21, 1903.

66. TTLTQG-1, RST, 73750, L'Administrateur Résident de France à Thu Lang Nhuong à Monsieur le Résident Supérieur, October 17, 1903.

67. TTLTQG-1, RST, 73750, L'Administrateur Résident de France à Truyên-duang à Monsieur le Résident Supérieur, October 19, 1903.

68. TTL1, RST, 73750, L'Administrateur Résident de France à Bac Ran à Monsieur le Résident Supérieur, November 13, 1903.

69. TTLTQG-1, RST, 73750, L'Administrateur Résident de France à Haiduong . . . October 19, 1903.

70. TTLTQG-1, RST, 73750, L'Administrateur Résident de France à Bac Ran . . . November 13, 1903.

71. TTLTQG-1, RST, 73750, L'Administrateur Résident de France à Sontay . . . October 21, 1903.

72. This was especially true for the provinces of Thuy-Ly (letter of November 7) and Ninh Binh (letter of November 4), which counted twenty and eleven aliénés, respectively. See TTLTQG-1, RST, 73750, Avis des Chefs de Province, 1903.

73. TTLTQG-1, RST, 73750, L'Administrateur Résident de France à Phu-Lo à Monsieur le Résident Supérieur, October 19, 1903.

74. This notion of psychiatry as liberating individuals from familial constraint also played out in missionary discourses in China. See Zhiying Ma, "An Iron Cage of Civilization? Missionary Psychiatry, the Chinese Family and a Colonial Dialectic of Enlightenment," in *Psychiatry and Chinese History,* ed. Howard Chiang (New York: Routledge, 2015), 91–110; TTLTQG-1, RST, 73750, L'Administrateur Résident de France à Van Bui à Monsieur le Résident Supérieur, October 27, 1903.

75. TTLTQG-1, RST, 73750, L'Administrateur-Résident de France Duvilliet, à Monsieur le Résident Supérieur au Tonkin, à Hanoi, November, 4, 1903.

76. TTLTQG-1, RST, 73750, L'Administrateur Résident de France à Quang Yen à Monsieur le Résident Supérieur, November 10, 1903.

77. TTLTQG-1, RST, 73750, L'Administrateur Résident de France à Bac Ran . . . November, 13, 1903.

78. TTLTQG-1, RST, 73750, Minute de la lettre no. 248 du 14 Décembre 1903 en Résident Supérieur à M. le Lieutenant Gouverneur de Cochinchine.

79. For a comprehensive overview of public health policy in colonial Indochina see Laurence Monnais, *Médecine et colonisation.*

80. For the French colonial health infrastructure in Cambodia see Sokhieng Au, *Mixed Medicines: Health and Culture in French Colonial Cambodia* (Chicago: University of Chicago Press, 2011).

81. These hospitals and clinics also served as important sites for medical research. Monnais, "In the Shadow," 174.

82. TTLTQG-1, RST, 73751, feuille 107, fait à Bac-Ninh, April 12, 1916.

83. Reboul and Régis, "L'Assistance," 135.

84. By 1912, aliéné had become a category in the official record keeping of Chợ Quán hospital. TTLTQG-2, GOUCOCH, IA.8/096(8), Situation journalière des malades traités à l'Hôpital de Chợ Quán; the Municipal Hospital in Cholon near

Saigon also reported receiving about twenty mentally ill patients per year. TTLTQG-2, GOUCOCH, IA.8/1724(2), Monsieur F. Drouhet, Sécretaire Général des Colonies, Maire de la Ville de Cholon à Monsieur le Lieutenant Gouverneur (3ème Bureau), Saigon, July 31, 1908.

85. TTLTQG-2, GOUCOCH, IA.8/1724(3), Circulaire: Au sujet de l'hospitalisation des aliénés et des incurables sans ressources, Le Gouverneur de 1ère Classes des Colonies Rodier, Lieutenant-Gouverneur de la Cochinchine, a MM. les Administrateurs, Chefs de province de Cochinchine, October 8, 1904.

86. TTLTQG-2, GOUCOCH, IA.8/1724(3). The document is undated but found in a file that spans 1904 to 1908.

87. See TTLTQG-1, RST, 73751, La Maire de Haiphong, Gautret, à Monsieur le Résident Supérieur, September 3, 1903.

88. TTLTQG-1, RST, 73757, L'Inspecteur 3ème classe Sivelle, Commandant la Brigade de Garde Indigène à Haiphong à Monsieur l'Administrateur-Maire de la Ville, April 26, 1916.

89. Andre Augagneur and Le Trung Luong, "Croyances et pratiques pour le traitement des maladies mentales en Indochine," *L'Hygiène Mentale* 23 (1928): 269–76.

90. TTLTQG-1, Mairie de Hanoi (MH), 5882, Résident Supérieur au Tonkin à Monsieur l'Administrateur Maire de la Ville de Hanoi, April 13, 1910.

91. TTLTQG-1, RST, 12879, Lettre de Gouverneur Général au sujet de la création d'un depôt de mendicité à Hanoi, August 1921.

92. TTLTQG-1, RST, 12879, "Lettre de Gouverneur Général . . . August 1921.

93. The colonial state legally defined "vagabonds" as persons who had "no certain domicile" or means of subsistence. See Zinoman, *Colonial Bastille*, 101.

94. Maurice Chautemps, *Vagabondage en pays Annamite* (Paris: Librairie Nouvelle de Droit et de Jurisprudence, 1908).

95. On the effects of demographic growth and economic change in the late seventeenth- and early eighteenth-century countryside, see John K. Whitmore, "Social Organization and Confucian Thought in Vietnam," *Journal of Southeast Asian Studies* 15, no. 2 (September 1984): 296–306, 204. For similar themes from the early nineteenth century, see Masaya Shiraishi, "State, Villagers, and Vagabonds: Vietnamese Rural Society and the Phan Ba Vanh Rebellion," *Senri Ethnological Studies* 13 (1984): 345–400; Goscha, *Vietnam*, 85.

96. TTLTQG-1, RST, 13864, Le Résident Supérieur au Tonkin à Monsieur le Résident Maire Hanoi, December 20, 1919.

97. TTLTQG-1, RST, 13864, "Secours aux indigents," n.d.

98. TTLTQG-1, RST, 12879, Lettre de Gouverneur Général . . . August 1921.

99. Van Nguyen Marshall, "The Moral Economy of Colonialism: Subsistence and Famine Relief in French Indochina, 1906–1917," *International History Review* 27, no. 2 (June 2005): 237–58. (There were also efforts by the Nguyễn imperial court to provide poor relief/charity that predated colonial occupation; these were more concerned with the land and livelihood issues that dominated rural existence than with the kinds of problems cropping up in cities.)

100. TTLTQG-1, MH, 5881, Le Procureur Général, près la Cour d'Appel de Hanoi, à Monsieur l'Administrateur-Maire de la Ville de Hanoi, June 22, 1927.

101. TTLTQG-1, MH, 5886, Organisation et fonctionnement du dépôt de mendicité de la ville de Hanoi, August 31, 1937.

102. A commission was created to discuss the possible establishment of an insane asylum in Cochinchina on November 14, 1907. On May 3, 1908, a decree was issued for the creation of the Biên Hòa asylum. TTLTQG-2, GOUCOCH, IA.8/1724(2), Outrey, Le Lieutenant Gouverneur de Cochinchine au Président du Conseil Colonial au sujet de la commission chargé d'examiner la question de la création en Cochinchine d'un asile d'aliénés, April 16, 1908.

103. Le Courrier saigonnais, Friday, October 14, 1910. As quoted in Reboul and Régis, "L'Assistance," 126–27.

104. As quoted in Reboul and Régis, "L'Assistance," 124.

105. Reboul and Régis, "L'Assistance," 134 (italics in original).

106. As quoted in Reboul and Régis, "L'Assistance," 135.

107. H. Reboul, Médécin Principal des troupes coloniales. "Hospitalisation des aliénés en Indochine," Annales d'hygiene colonial et de médecine coloniales (Oct-Nov-Dec 1913): 1200–1203.

108. Regis and Reboul, "L'Assistance," 9.

109. Keller, Colonial Madness, 29.

110. H. Aubin, "L'Assistance psychiatrique indigène aux colonies," Rapport au Congrès des Médecins Aliénistes et Neurologistes de France et des Pays de Langue Francaise, XLIIe session—Alger 6–11 Avril 1938 (Paris: Masson et Cie, 1938), 147–76.

111. TTLTQG-2, GOUCOCH, IA.8/274(4), Rivet, Gouverneur de l'Indochine à Monsieur le Consul de France, September 21, 1916.

112. See TTLTQG-1, RST, 73747–01, Asile d'Aliénés de Biên Hòa, rapport annuel pour 1928.

113. The budget doubled from 1,527,000 piasters to 3,120,000 piasters. The piastre de commerce was the silver-standard unit used by the French in Indochina between 1885 and 1952. In 1930, the piaster was pegged to the French franc at a rate of 1 piaster to 10 francs.

114. TTLTQG-2, GOUCOCH, IA.8/281(1), Asile d'aliénés de Bienhoa, Rapport annuel de 1923.

115. ANOM, GGI, 65151, Le Gouverneur Général de l'Indochine à Monsieur le Ministre des Colonies, Objet: Projet de décret sur l'assistance psychiatrique en Indochine, February 23, 1928.

116. A second law, promulgated on November 23, 1918, established the rules for the financing and bookkeeping of the institution. See TTLTQG-2, GOUCOCH, IA.8/215(3), Arrêté du Gougal: Création d'un asile d'aliénés à Bienhoa (hospitalisation des personnes atteintes de maladies mentales de l'Indochine), May 3, 1918.

117. Despite the legal regulations that assumed an indigenous patient population, from its earliest days Biên Hòa did receive European patients. By 1928, the constant increases in the European population who remained in Indochina, as well as the increasing number of métis who retained French legal status, drew attention to the critical deficiencies of the 1918 decree. See TTLTQG-1, Inspection Générale de l'Hygiène et Santé Publique (IGHSP), 004, rapport annuel de 1928 sur le fonctionnement de l'Inspection générale des services sanitaires et médicaux de l'Indochine.

118. ANOM, GGI, 65151, Le Gouverneur General de l' Indochine . . . February 23, 1928.

119. ANOM, GGI, 65151, Le Gouverneur General de l' Indochine . . . February 23, 1928.

120. TTLTQG-1, RST, 73745, Résident Supérieur au Tonkin, Poulin, à Directeur Local de Santé, November 2, 1921.

121. TTLTQG-2, GOUCOCH, IA.8/162(9), M. André, Directeur de l'Hôpital de Chợ Quán à Monsieur le Directeur de l'Intérieur à Saigon, February 8, 1887.

122. TTLTQG-1, RST, 73745, Le Ministre des Colonies (Perrier) à Paris à Monsieur le GGI, March 3, 1926.

123. Aubin, *L'Assistance Psychiatrique Indigène*.

124. Indigènes protégés français refers to the natives of "protected" states including Annam, Tonkin, Cambodia, and in Laos, Luang Prabang. Like colonial subjects, they neither were French citizens nor enjoyed the rights associated with French nationality. As for assimilated and "naturalized indigenès,"the same text as the 1838 law applied, but the resident superiors were given the power to manage the affairs of the individual in the colony or to determine his repatriation. ANOM, GGI, 65151, Le Gouverneur General de l' Indochine . . . February 23, 1928.

125. ANOM, GGI, 65151, Le Gouverneur Général de l' Indochine . . . February 23, 1928.

126. TTLTQG-1, RST, 73745, Le Directeur Local de la Santé (Rougier) à Monsieur le Résident Supérieur au Tonkin, January 26, 1928.

127. TTL1, RST, 73745, Le Directeur Local de la Santé (Rougier). . .January 26, 1928.

128. For the full text of the law see TTLTQG-1, RST, 74028, Décret du 18 Juillet 1930 sur le traitement et la garde des malades atteints d'aliénation mentale, 1930.

129. TTLTQG-1, RST, 73750, Note sur l'organisation générale d'un Asile d'Aliénés par le Dr. Augagneur, Médecin Directeur de l'Asile de Biên Hòa, November 30, 1927.

130. TTLTQG-1, IGHSP, 51–01, Rapport sur le fonctionnement du service de psychiatrie de l'Hôpital de Chợ Quán en 1934. Discussed further in chapter 4.

131. Aubin, *L'Assistance Psychiatrique Indigène*.

132. Dr. Lucien-Graux, "La Loi Dubief: Le regime des alienes," *Gazette Médicale de Paris*, February 15, 1907.

133. Pierre Dorolle, *La Législation Indochinoise sur les Aliénés: Exposé et commentaire des dispositions du décret du 18 Juillet 1930* (Saigon: Imprimerie A. Portail, 1941). See also Dr. R. Lefèvre, "L'assistance psychiatrique en Indochine," *Rapport au Congrès des médecins aliénistes et neurologistes de France et des pays de langue française*, XXXVᵉ Session, Bordeaux, April 7–12, 1931 (Paris: Masson et Cie, 1931): 293–97.

134. Dorolle (1941).

135. TTLTQG-1, RST, 73745, Le Directeur Local de la Santé du Tonkin à Monsieur le Médecin Général Inspecteur, Inspecteur Général des Services Sanitaires et Médicaux de l'Indochine, December 3, 1930.

136. TTLTQG-1, RST, 73745, Note du 1er Bureau, October 1930.

137. TTLTQG-1, RST, 73745, Circulaire, Le Résident Supérieur au Tonkin (René Robin), Commandeur de la Légion d'Honneur, à Messieurs les Résidents Chef de province, Commandants de Territoire Militaire, Maires de Hanoi et Haiphong et Directeur local de la Santé, October 20 1930.

138. TTLTQG-1, RST, 73745, Note pour Monsieur l'Administrateur, Chef du 1er Bureau, February 20, 1931; see also TTLTQG-1, RST, 73745, Le Gouverneur des Colonies à Président du Comité Consultatif de Jurisprudence Annamite, March 9, 1931.

139. TTLTQG-1, RST, 73745, Le Gouverneur des Colonies à Président du Comité Consultatif . . . March 9, 1931.

140. TTLTQG-2, GOUCOCH, IA.8/2912(3), Asile d'Aliénés de Bienhoa, rapport annuel de 1927.

141. Monnais, "In the Shadow,"144.

142. TTLTQG-1, RST, 73745, Graffeuil, Le Secrétaire General du Gouvernement General de l'Indochine, à Directeur Local de la Santé au Tonkin à Hanoi, January 11, 1928.

2. Patients, Staff, and the Everyday Challenges of Asylum Administration

1. TTLTQG-2, GOUCOCH, IA.8/2912(3), Rapport annuel de Bienhoa, 1927.

2. TTLTQG-2, GOUCOCH, IA.8/2912(3), Rapport annuel de Bienhoa, 1927.

3. Leslie Topp observes in her study of asylums in late nineteenth-century Germany that the mental hospital's projection of the image of freedom and normality of the familiar outside world was directed as much toward convincing patients as convincing the public. "The Modern Mental Hospital in Late Nineteenth-Century Germany and Austria: Psychiatric Space and Images of Freedom and Control," in *Madness, Architecture and the Built Environment: Psychiatric Spaces in Historical Context*, ed. Leslie Topp, James Moran, and Jonathan Andrews (New York: Routledge, 2007), 241–62.

4. TTLTQG-2, GOUCOCH, IA.8/2912(1), Rapport annuel de Bienhoa, 1926.

5. Ernst, *Mad Tales from the Raj*; James Mills, *Madness, Cannabis, and Colonialism: The "Native-Only" Lunatic Asylums of British India*, 1857–1900 (London: Macmillan, 2000).

6. European prisoners were occasionally held in colonial jails but segregated in separate wards. While there was a limited degree of integration of elite Vietnamese into French schools, in general, the colonial education system remained racially segregated. See Gail P. Kelly, "The Relation Between Colonial and Metropolitan Schools: A Structural Analysis," *Comparative Education* 15, no. 2 (June 1979): 209–15.

7. ANOM, RST, 3750, Compte rendu annuel sur le fonctionnement de l'Asile d'Aliénés de Voi pendant l'annee 1941.

8. ANOM, RST, 3753, Procès-verbal de la commission de Surveillance de l'Asile d'Aliénés de Voi, June 15, 1938.

9. See TTLTQG-1, RST, 18460, Rapport du Directeur de la Santé en Annam sur le régime légal des aliénés en Indochine, 1912. For more on French imperial medical education, see Michael Osbourne, *The Emergence of Tropical Medicine in France* (Chicago: University of Chicago Press, 2014).

10. TTLTQG-1, RST, 73750, Organisation et fonctionnement d'un Asile d'Aliénés à Bien-Hoa (Cochinchine), Note sur l'organisation générale d'un Asile d'Aliénés par le Dr. Augagneur, Médecin Directeur de l'Asile de Bien Hoa, 1927.

11. Lorion, *Criminalité*, 47.

12. H. Aubin, "L'Assistance psychiatrique indigène aux colonies," Rapport au Congrès des Médecins Aliénistes et Neurologistes de France et des Pays de Langue Francaise, XLIIe session—Alger 6–11 Avril 1938.

13. Recueil de notices redigées à l'occasion du Xe congrès de la "Far Eastern Association of Tropical Medicine," Hanoi (Tonkin), November 24–30, 1938 (Hanoi:

Imprimerie G. Taupin, 1938); Laurence Monnais, Médecine et colonisation (1999); Nguyễn Văn Hoài, De l'Organisation de l'Hôpital Psychiatrique du Sud-Vietnam (Saigon: Imprimerie Francaise d'Outre Mer, 1954).

14. TTLTQG-1, RST, 73750, Organisation et fonctionnement d'un Asile d'Aliénés à Bien-Hoa (Cochinchine) . . . 1927.

15. E. L. Peyre, "Les maladies mentales aux colonies," *Journal de Psychiatrie Appliquée* 8 (1934): 185–212.

16. TTLTQG-1, RST, 73750, Organisation et fonctionnement d'un Asile d'Aliénés à Bien-Hoa (Cochinchine) . . . 1927. The director of Bien Hoa proclaimed the floral decorations of patient living quarters a "success." See TTLTQG-1, IGHSP, 50–03, Rapport Annuel de l'Asile d'Aliénés de Bienhoa, 1933.

17. TTLTQG-2, GOUCOCH, IA.8/281(1), Asile d'Aliénés de Bien Hoa, rapport annuel de 1923; TTLTQG-2, GOUCUCH, IA.8/2912(1), Rapport annuel de Bienhoa, 1926.

18. TTLTQG-2, GOUCOCH, IA.8/281(1), Rapport annuel de Bienhoa, 1923.

19. TTLTQG-2, GOUCOCH, IA.8/2912(1), Rapport annuel de Bienhoa, 1926.

20. TTLTQG-2, GOUCOCH, IA.8/2912(3), Rapport annuel de Bienhoa, 1927.

21. TTLTQG-2, GOUCOCH, IA.8/281(1), Asile d'Aliénés de Bien Hoa, rapport annuel de 1923.

22. TTLTQG-1, IGHSP, 48–05, Asile d'Aliénés de Bien Hoa, rapport annuel de 1931.

23. TTLTQG-1, RST, 73744, Monsieur Mourroux, Administrateur des Services civils, Résident Maire de la Ville de Hanoi à Monsieur le Résident Supérieur au Tonkin, November 14, 1921.

24. TTLTQG-1, RST, 73744, Mourroux, Administrateur des Services Civils . . . November 14, 1921.

25. TTLTQG-1, RST, 81330, Le Gouverneur de la Cochinchine à Monsieur le Résident Supérieur au Tonkin, Objet: Au sujet de l'aliéné . . . dit Jean G., September 20, 1927. Also see GOUCOCH, IA.8/2910, 1926–27.

26. TTLTQG-1, IGHSP, 004, Rapport annuel de 1928 sur le fonctionnement de l'Inspection générale des services sanitaires et médicaux de l'Indochine.

27. TTLTQG-2, GOUCOCH, IA.8/281(2), Rapport annuel de Bienhoa, 1925.

28. TTLTQG-2, GOUCOCH, IA.8/2912(3), Rapport annuel de Bienhoa, 1927.

29. TTLTQG-2, GOUCOCH, IA.8/281(2), Rapport annuel de Bienhoa, 1925.

30. TTLTQG-2, GOUCOCH, IA.8/281(2), Rapport annuel de Bienhoa, 1925.

31. TTLTQG-2, GOUCOCH, IA.8/2912(1), Rapport annuel de Bienhoa, 1926.

32. TTLTQG-2, GOUCOCH, IA.8/2912(1), Rapport annuel de Bienhoa, 1926.

33. For more on the financial returns of the Biên Hòa asylum during the 1920s, see Roussy, "Rapport sur le Fonctionnement de l'Asile d'Aliénés de Bienhoa (Cochinchine)," *Annales de Medicine et de Pharmacie Coloniales* 24 (1926): 34–56.

34. TTLTQG-1, IGHSP, 48–05, Asile d'Alienes de Bien Hoa, Rapport annuel de 1931.

35. Roussy, "Rapport sur le fonctionnement de l'Asile d'Aliénés de Bienhoa."

36. TTLTQG-2, GOUCOCH, IA.8/2912(3), Rapport annuel de Bienhoa, 1927.

37. TTLTQG-1, IGHSP, 44–01, Au sujet de la promulgation en Indochine du décret du 21 Novembre 1933 sur le frais d'hospitalisation à l'Asile de Bienhoa, October 22, 1927.

38. TTLTQG-1, IGHSP, 44–01, Au sujet de la promulgation . . . October 22, 1027. See also Leonard Smith, who, in his study of asylum care in Victorian England, similarly points to the commercial imperative to adopt a "mixed economy" of care that integrated pauper lunatics and paying patients into the same institution. "The County Asylum in the Mixed Economy of Care, 1808–1845" in Melling and Forsythe, *Insanity, Institutions and Society,* 33–47.

39. TTLTQG-1, IGHSP, 51–07, Rapport annuel de 1934 sur le fonctionnement du Service de l'Assistance Médicale de Bien Hoa, Sai Gon, Bac Lieu, 1934.

40. TTLTQG-1, Fonds de la Direction des Finances de l'Indochine, 1550, Fixation du prix de remboursement des journées de traitement à l'Asile d'Aliénés de Voi (Bac Giang) par le Résident Supérieur au Tonkin, 1936.

41. TTLTQG-1, Fonds de la Direction des Finances de l'Indochine, 1550, Fixation du prix . . . 1936.

42. TTLTQG-1, IGHSP, 004, Rapport annuel de 1928.

43. I define patient turnover here in terms of length of stay in the asylum and the number of patients released relative to the number admitted. TTLTQG-2, GOUCOCH, IA.8/2912(3), Rapport annuel de Bienhoa, 1927.

44. Centre de Documentation de l'Institut de Médecine Tropicale de la Service de Santé des Armées (PHARO), carton 166, Rapports annuels de la Service de Santé, 1934. In two state asylums in the United States between 1880 and 1910, about half the patients were released after one year, and this proportion rose to 60 percent in private asylums. See Constance M. McGovern, "The Myths of Social Control and Custodial Oppression: Patterns of Psychiatric Medicine in Late Nineteenth-Century Institutions," *Journal of Social History* 20 (1986): 3–23. This is consistent with rates reported from British and Irish asylums in the nineteenth century, with 40–50 percent of the patients admitted to public lunatic asylums staying twelve or fewer months. However, in a departure from what happened in Indochina, those who remained at the asylum tended to stay for much longer. Peter Bartlett and David Wright, "Community Care and Its Antecedents," in *Outside the Walls of the Asylum: The History of Care in Community 1750–2000,* ed. Peter Bartlett and David Wright (London and New Brunswick, NJ: Athlone Press, 1999), 1–18.

45. PHARO, carton 182, Rapport annuel d'ensemble, fonctionnement de l'Asile de Voi, 1934.

46. TTLTQG-2, GOUCOCH, IA.8/2912(3), Rapport annuel de Bienhoa, 1927.

47. This forms an important contrast with French Algeria, where hospitals served far higher proportions of Europeans than North Africans. Keller, *Colonial Madness,* 89.

48. TTLTQG-1, IGHSP, 004, Rapport annuel de 1928.

49. Drs. Gaffiero and P. Dorolle, "Notes de pathologie mentale coloniale (Malades Mentaux observés en deux ans dans un hopital colonial: Hopital de Lanessan à Hanoi)," *Bulletin de la Société Méd-Chirurgicale de l'Indochine* 5 (June 1932): 507–13.

50. TTLTQG-1, IGHSP, 004, Rapport annuel de 1928. Julie Brown, in her study of mental institutions in imperial Russia, argues that the cyclical nature of asylum admittances and departures was linked to the harvesting season. See "Peasant Survival Strategies in Late Imperial Russia: The Social Uses of the Mental Hospital," *Social Problems* 34, no. 4 (1987): 311–29.

51. Ian Dowbiggin, *Inheriting Madness: Professionalization and Psychiatric Knowledge in Nineteenth Century France* (Berkeley: University of California Press, 1991).

52. Roussy, "Rapport sur le fonctionnement de l'asile d'aliénés de Bienhoa"; TTLTQG-1, IGHSP, 004, Rapport annuel de 1928.

53. Dr. Roger Grinsard, "Note sur les principales psychopathies observées à l'asile d'aliénés de Voi en 1936," *Bulletin de la société médico-chirurgicale de l'Indochine* 3 (1936): 392.

54. Syphilis was highly prevalent among the indigenous patient population (227 of the 1,009 patients who ever entered the asylum tested positive for the disease). As of September 1925, all patients routinely underwent a serological examination on the basis of a blood sample and lumbar puncture. The opening of a laboratory at the asylum in 1926 greatly facilitated the expansion of testing. See TTLTQG-2, GOUCOCH, IA.8/2912(1), Rapport annuel de Bienhoa, 1926 TTLTQG-1, IGHSP, 004, Rapport annuel de 1928.

55. TTLTQG-1, IGHSP, 004, Rapport annuel de 1928. Patients suffering from syphilis were treated with sulfarsenol, novarsenobenzol, and Treparsol. By 1934, most syphilis-related psychoses were treated by injections of "stovarsol sodique" using the Sézary and Barbe technique. Because of the "weakness of the constitutions" of their patients, pointing to the poor condition in which they often arrived at the asylum, doctors were forced to reduce the amount of stovarsol administered from 1 gram to 0.50 grams at the beginning of treatment. PHARO, carton 182, Rapport annuel d'ensemble . . . 1934.

56. In 1928, in major hospitals across the colony, among the indigenous population, 707 men were treated for mental illness, followed by 341 women and 68 children. TTLTQG-1, IGHSP, 004, Rapport annuel de 1928.

57. TTLTQG-1, IGHSP, 51–07, Rapport annuel de 1934; PHARO, carton 166, Rapport annuel d'ensemble, Fonctionnement de l'Asile de Voi, 1938.

58. Aude Fauvel "Madness: A 'Female Malady,'" in, *Vulnerability, Social Inequality and Health,* ed. Patrice Bourdelais and John Chircop. (Lisbon: Edições Colibri, 2010), 61–75.

59. See, for example, TTLTQG-1, RST, 73739–01, Certificat Médical de . . . V.V., n.d.

60. TTLTQG-1, IGHSP, 004, Rapport annuel de 1928. On opium addiction in the colonial era see Frank Proschan, "'Syphilia, Opiomania and Pederasty': Colonial Constructions of Vietnamese (and French) Social Diseases," *Journal of the History of Sexuality* 11, no. 4 (October 2002): 610–36.

61. The 1926 Bien Hoa report includes a long discussion on the sale and regulation of alcohol in the colony. See TTLTQG-2, GOUCOCH, IA.8/2912(1), Rapport annuel de Bienhoa, 1926. On the alcohol monopoly in colonial Vietnam see Gerard Sasges, "'Indigenous Representation Is Hostile to All Monopolies': Pham Quynh and the End of the Alcohol Monopoly in Colonial Vietnam," *Journal of Vietnamese Studies* 5, no. 1 (January 2010): 1–36.

62. TTLTQG-2, GOUCOCH, IA.8/281(2), Rapport annuel de Bienhoa, 1925.

63. TTLTQG-1, IGHSP, 004, Rapport annuel de 1928.

64. TTLTQG-1, RST, 73741, Au sujet internement des aliénés classés par ordre alphabétique de nom de C dans des asiles de Voi (Bac Giang) et de Bien Hoa (Cochinchine) en 1925–1935, Rapport d'examen médical de la nommée . . . Can, December 30, 1933.

65. The psychiatric designation of *psychose menstruelle* was first coined by the French alienist Louis Victor Marcé, a student of Esquirol. In an 1862 work, he related menstrual cycles and particularly menstrual psychosis with psychosis immediately following childbirth. Louis Victor Marcé. *Traité de la folie des femmes enceintes: Des nouvelles accouchées et des nourrices* (1858; repr., Paris: Harmattan, 2002).

66. TTLTQG-1, RST, 73742–01, Internement des Aliénés à l'Asile de Voi (Bac Giang) classés par ordre alphabétique des noms de N, 1935. For more on transgressive gender practices in colonial Vietnam, see Quang-Anh Richard Tran, "From Red Lights to Red Flags: A History of Gender in Colonial and Contemporary Vietnam." PhD diss., University of California, Berkeley, 2011.

67. For a breakdown of all injections delivered at Bien Hoa in 1934, see PHARO, carton 182, Rapport annuel d'ensemble . . . 1934.

68. TTLTQG-1, IGHSP, 004, Rapport annuel de 1928.

69. TTLTQG-2, GOUCOCH, IA.8/2912(1), Rapport annuel de Bienhoa, 1926.

70. TTLTQG-1, IGHSP, 004, Rapport annuel de 1928.

71. TTLTQG-2, GOUCOCH, IA.8/2912(1), Rapport annuel de Bienhoa, 1926.

72. Joel T. Braslow, *Mental Ills and Bodily Cures: Psychiatric Treatment in the First Half of the Twentieth Century* (Berkeley: University of California Press, 1997); Jonathan Sadowsky, *Electroconvulsive Therapy in America: The Anatomy of a Medical Controversy* (London: Routledge, 2016). On the global diffusion of shock therapies, especially in Japan, see Akihito Suzuki, "Global Theory, Local Practice: Shock Therapies in Japanese Psychiatry, 1920–1945," in *Transnational Psychiatries: Social and Cultural Histories of Psychiatry in Comparative Perspective, c.1800–2000*, ed. Waltraud Ernst and Thomas Mueller (Newcastle upon Tyne: Cambridge Scholars, 2010), 116–41.

73. See Pierre Dorolle, "Traitement palliatif de l'épilepsie essentielle par la convulsivothérapie électrique (électro-choc) (*Note préliminaire*)," *Revue Médicale Française d'Extrême-Orient* 20 (1942): 835.

74. PHARO, carton 182, Rapport annuel d'ensemble . . . 1934).

75. Dorolle, "Traitement palliatif."

76. Keller, *Colonial Madness*, 104.

77. TTLTQG-2, GOUCOCH, IA.8/2912(3), Asile des aliénés de Bien Hoa: Rapport annuel de 1927.

78. The first serious study of the creation of an asylum to service the north of Annam, Tonkin, and adjacent parts of Laos was pursued in 1913 and again in 1921. The colony's general budget in 1922 dedicated 55,000 piasters to the project, but forward movement stalled. It was even suggested that it was the Vietnamese population who actually demanded the creation of a second psychiatric institution in the colony. See Peyre, "Les maladies mentale."

79. TTLTQG-1, RST, 73757, Le Directeur Local de la Santé à Monsieur le Resident Superieur au Tonkin, August 11, 1927.

80. TTLTQG-1, RST, 73757, Graffeuil, Le Résident Supérieur au Tonkin à Messieurs les Administrateurs Résidents de France à Hàdong, Sontay, Bacninh, Phuc-Yen, Vinh-Yen, Bacgiang, Quang-Yen, Haiduong. December 9, 1927.

81. TTLTQG-1, RST, 73750, Organisation et fonctionnement d'un Asile d'Aliénés à Bien-Hoa (Cochinchine) . . . 1927.

82. TTLTQG-2, GOUCOCH, IA.8/2910, Le Médecin Directeur de l'Asile à Monsieur le Gouverneur de Cochinchine, December 16, 1927.

83. TTLTQG-1, RST, 73750, Organisation et fonctionnement d'un Asile d'Aliénés à Bien-Hoa (Cochinchine) . . . 1927. In addition to the cramped conditions, the enclosures immediately surrounding each pavilion also proved too narrow, making the surveillance of patients difficult. TTLTQG-2, GOUCOCH, IA.9/2910, Le Directeur local de la Santé en Cochinchine à Monsieur le Gouverneur de la Cochinchine, September 24, 1927.

84. TTLTQG-2, GOUCOCH, IA.8/281(2), Rapport annuel de Bienhoa, 1925.

85. TTLTQG-1, RST, 73757, L'Administrateur de 1ère classe Ernest Valette, Résident de France à Quang-Yen à Monsieur le Résident Supérieur au Tonkin, December 12, 1927.

86. TTLTQG-1, RST, 73757, L'architecte principal, Chef du Service des Bâtiments Civils à Monsieur le Résident Supérieur au Tonkin Hanoi, December 22, 1927.

87. TTLTQG-1, RST, 73757, L'architecte principal . . . December 22, 1927.

88. TTLTQG-1, IGHSP, 004, Rapport annuel de 1928.

89. ANOM, RST Nouveau Fonds (RSTNF), 3683, Direction locale de la Santé du Tonkin, rapport annuel de 1931, April 1, 1932.

90. TTLTQG-2, GOUCOCH, IA.8/2912(3), Rapport annuel de Bienhoa, 1927.

91. As a safety precaution, "agitated" patients were not given mosquito nets. TTLTQG-2, GOUCOCH, IA.8/2912(1), Rapport annuel de Bienhoa, 1926.

92. TTLTQG-2, GOUCOCH, IA.8/281(2), Rapport annuel de Bienhoa, 1925.

93. TTLTQG-2, GOUCOCH, IA.8/2912(3), Rapport annuel de Bienhoa, 1927.

94. TTLTQG-1, RST, 73750, Organisation et fonctionnement d'un Asile d'Aliénés à Bien-Hoa (Cochinchine) . . . 1927.

95. TTLTQG-1, IGHSP, 50–03, Rapport annuel de l'Asile d'Aliénés de Bienhoa, 1933.

96. TTLTQG-2, GOUCOCH, IA.8/2912(1), Rapport annuel de Bienhoa, 1926.

97. TTLTQG-1, IGHSP, 50–03, Rapport annuel de l'Asile d'Aliénés de Bienhoa,1933.

98. TTLTQG-1, IGHSP, 48–05, Asile d'Aliénés de Bien Hoa, rapport annuel de 1931.

99. In histories of psychiatry, asylum officials typically take center stage, while attendants generally enter the picture only as a way to illustrate or condemn the abuses of the asylum system. As Lee-Ann Monk observes, the relative neglect of attendants by historians is surprising given the contemporary emphasis on their importance to therapeutic regimes. See "Working in the Asylum: Attendants to the Insane," *Health and History* 11, no. 1 (2009): 83–101. In the colonies, these intermediaries played a vital role in mediating Western and non-Western understandings of health and wellness. Jonathan Saha, " 'Uncivilized Practitioner, Medical Subordinates: Medico-Legal Evidence and Misconduct in Colonial Burma, 1875–1907," *Southeast Asia Research* 20, no. 3 (2012): 423–43; Benjamin N. Lawrence, Emily Lynn Osbourne and Richard L. Roberts, eds., *Intermediaries, Interpreters and Clerks: African Employees in the Making of Colonial Africa* (Madison: University of Wisconsin Press, 2006).

100. The problems of turnover with asylum staff were not unique to Indochina. See, for example, Geertje Boschma, *The Rise of Mental Health Nursing: A History of Psychiatric Care in Dutch Asylums, 1890–1920* (Amsterdam: Amsterdam University Press, 2003); David Wright, "Asylum Nursing and Institutional Service: A Case Study of the South of England, 1861–1881," *Nursing History Review* 7 (1999): 153–69.

101. TTLTQG-2, GOUCOCH, IA.8/2912(1), Rapport annuel de Bienhoa, 1926.

102. TTLTQG-1, IGHSP, 48–05, Asile d'Aliénés de Bien Hoa, rapport annuel de 1931.

103. TTLTQG-2, GOUCOCH, IA.8/2912(3), Rapport annuel de Bienhoa, 1927.

104. TTLTQG-2, GOUCOCH, IA.8/281(1). Asile d'Aliénés de Bien Hoa, rapport annuel de 1923.

105. TTLTQG-1, RST, 73750, Note sur l'organisation générale d'un Asile d'Aliénés par le Dr. Augagneur, Médecin Directeur de l'Asile de Bien Hoa, September 17, 1927.

106. TTLTQG-2, GOUCOCH, IA.8/2912(1), Rapport annuel de Bienhoa, 1926.

107. TTLTQG-2, GOUCOCH, IA.8/2912(3), Rapport annuel de Bienhoa, 1927.

108. TTLTQG-1, IGHSP, 50–03, Rapport annuel de l'Asile d'Aliénés de Bienhoa, 1933.

109. TTLTQG-1, IGHSP, 48–05, Asile d'Aliénés de Bien Hoa, rapport annuel de 1931.

110. TTLTQG-1, IGHSP, 48-05, Asile d'Aliénés de Bien Hoa . . . 1931. For more on the training of nurses, especially female nurses, in colonial Vietnam see Thuy Linh Nguyen, *Childbirth, Maternity and Medical Pluralism in French Colonial Vietnam, 1880–1945* (Rochester, NY: University of Rochester Press, 2016).

111. TTLTQG-2, GOUCOCH, IA.8/2912(3), Rapport annuel de Bienhoa, 1927.

112. TTLTQG-2, GOUCOCH, IA.8/276(2), Asile d'Aliénés de Bien Hoa, rapport annuel de 1924.

113. TTLTQG-2, GOUCOCH, IA.8/2912(3), Rapport annuel de Bienhoa, 1927.

114. TTLTQG-2, GOUCOCH, IA.8/2912(1), Rapport annuel de Bienhoa, 1926.

115. ANOM, BIB 50003, *Journal Officiel de l'Indochine Française*, August 13, 1924.

116. For the role of the prison staff in the daily functioning of the colonial prison, as a point of comparison with the asylum, see "The Regime," chapter 3 of Peter Zinoman's *The Colonial Bastille*.

117. TTLTQG-2, GOUCOCH, IA.8/2912(3), Rapport annuel de Bienhoa, 1927.

118. TTLTQG-2, GOUCOCH, IA.8/2912(1), Rapport annuel de Bienhoa, 1926.

119. TTLTQG-1, RST, 73750, Note sur l'organisation générale d'un Asile d'Aliénés par le Dr. Augagneur, Médecin Directeur de l'Asile de Bien Hoa, September 17, 1927.

120. TTLTQG-1, IGHSP, 48–05, Rapport annuel de 1931 de Bien Hoa.

121. For more on moral treatment see "Moral Treatment," chapter 3 of Anne Digby's *Madness, Morality and Medicine: A Study of the York Retreat, 1796–1914* (London: Cambridge University Press, 1985).

122. TTLTQG-1, RST, 73750, Note sur l'organisation générale d'un Asile d'Aliénés par le Dr. Augagneur, Médecin Directeur de l'Asile de Bien Hoa, September 17, 1927.

123. TTLTQG-1, IGHSP, 51–07, Rapport annuel de 1934.

124. Asylum administrators claimed that the cost of living in Bien Hoa was more expensive than in Saigon because all products arrived via the city, where intermediaries would raise prices. TTLTQG-2, GOUCOCH, IA.8/2912(1), Rapport annuel de Bienhoa, 1926. A significant amount of the asylum staff's salary was apparently spent on transport alone. See TTLTQG-2, GOUCOCH, IA.8/2912(3), Rapport annuel de Bienhoa, 1927.

125. TTLTQG-2, GOUCOCH, IA.8/281(2), Rapport annuel de Bienhoa, 1925.

126. TTLTQG-2, GOUCOCH, IA.8/2912(3), Rapport annuel de Bienhoa, 1927.

127. For an example of proposed indemnities as a means of advancement for personnel, see TTLTQG-1, RST, 73745, Le Directeur Local de la Santé du Tonkin à Monsieur le Résident Supérieur au Tonkin, March 31, 1931.

128. TTLTQG-2, GOUCOCH, IA.8/2912(3), Rapport annuel de Bienhoa, 1927.

129. TTLTQG-2, GOUCOCH, IA.8/2912(3), Rapport annuel de Bienhoa, 1927.

130. TTLTQG-2, GOUCOCH, IA.8/2912(3), Rapport annuel de Bienhoa, 1927.

131. TTLTQG-2, GOUCOCH, IA.8/2912(1), Rapport annuel de Bienhoa, 1926.

132. TTLTQG-2, GOUCOCH, IA.8/2912(3), Rapport annuel de Bienhoa, 1927.

133. TTLTQG-2, GOUCOCH, IA.8/2912(1), Rapport annuel de Bienhoa, 1926. See also Dolly MacKinnon, "'Amusements are Provided': Asylum Entertainment and Recreation in Australia and New Zealand, c 1860–c.1945," in *Permeable Walls: Historical Perspectives on Hospital and Asylum Visiting,* ed. Graham Mooney and Jonathan Reinarz, The Wellcome Series in the History of Medicine (Amsterdam: Editions Rodopi, B.V., 2009), 267–88.

134. TTLTQG-1, IGHSP, 50–03, Rapport annuel de l'Asile d'Aliénés de Bienhoa, 1933.

135. TTLTQG-1, IGHSP, 004, Rapport annuel de 1928. The asylum staff often moved to their new place of employment with their families. In 1925, 360 patients resided at Bien Hoa, plus 130 employees and their families (bringing the number of related staff to 200 people). TTLTQG-2, GOUCOCH, IA.8/281(2), Rapport annuel de Bienhoa, 1925.

136. TTLTQG-1, IGHSP, 51–07, Rapport annuel de 1934.

137. TTLTQG-2, GOUCOCH, 3730, Procès-Verbal de la reunion du 23 Décembre 1935 de la Commission de Surveillance de l'Asile d'Aliénés de Bienhoa, 1935.

138. TTLTQG-1, 73750, RST, Organisation et fonctionnement d'un Asile d'Aliénés à Bien-Hoa (Cochinchine) . . . 1927.

139. TTLTQG-2, GOUCOCH, IA.8/2910, Le Directeur Local de la Santé en Cochinchine à Monsieur le Gouverneur de la Cochinchine, September 24, 1927.

140. TTLTQG-1, IGHSP, 50–03, Rapport annuel de l'Asile d'Aliénés de Bienhoa, 1933.

141. As of 1925, six years after the asylum first opened, Bien Hoa still did not possess a pavilion specifically devoted to their care. See TTLTQG-2, GOUCOCH, IA.8/281(2), Rapport annuel de Bienhoa, 1925.

142. TTLTQG-1, RST, 73752–07, Médecin de l'Assistance Henri Marcel, observation médicale, . . . Huân, April 21, 1938.

143. PHARO, carton 166, Rapport annuel d'ensemble . . . 1938.

144. TTLTQG-1, RST, 73743, . . . Lâm à Monsieur le Directeur de l'Administration de la Justice en Indochine, Chef du Service de la Judstice indigène du Tonkin, June 13, 1932.

145. TTLTQG-1, RST, 73743, Certificat médical, Dr. Naudin, March 23, 1933.

146. TTLTQG-1, RST, 73743, 6613, Lettre de . . . Lâm, June 26, 1933.

147. TTLTQG-1, RST, 73743, 6588, Le Procureur General, Directeur des Services Judiciares de l'Indochine, à Gouverneur Général de l'Indochine, February 2, 1933.

148. TTLTQG-1, RST, 73743, 6613, Lettre de . . . Lâm, June 26, 1933.

149. TTLTQG-1, RST, 73743, 6609, Lettre de . . . Phuc à M. le Résident Supérieur du Tonkin, June 17, 1933.

150. TTLTQG-1, IGHSP, 51–07, Rapport annuel de 1934.

151. TTLTQG-1, IGHSP, 50–03, Rapport annuel de l'Asile d'Aliénés de Bien-hoa,1933.

152. TTLTQG-1, IGHSP, 51–07, Rapport annuel de 1934. In 1936, the colonial administration in Cambodia approved the construction of an asylum at Takhu-mau (in the province of Kandal) near Phnom Penh, provided with credit of one million francs supported by the special budget. See ANOM, Fonds de la commis-sion d'enquête des Territoires d'Outre Mer (Guernut), 22 Bb, Note de la Résidence Supérieure sur Hygiène et Assistance au Cambodge, 1936.

153. PHARO, carton 166, Le Résident Supérieur au Tonkin à Monsieur le Gou-verneur Général de l'Indochine (Direction des Services Economiques et Inspection Générale de l'Hygiène et de la Santé Publiques), November 12, 1937.

154. ANOM, RST, 3753, Le Docteur de Raymond Directeur Local de la Santé à Monsieur le Résident Supérieur au Tonkin (1er Bureau), A.S. Voeux relatifs à l'Asile de Voi, September 21, 1939.

155. Nguyễn Văn Hoài, De l'Organisation de l'Hôpital Psychiatrique, 50.

156. Zinoman, Colonial Bastille, 51.

3. Labor as Therapy

1. Edouard Jeanselme, "La condition des aliénés dans les colonies Françaises, Anglaises et Néerlandaises d'Extrême-Orient," La Presse Médicale, August 9, 1905, 497–98. In 1912, this article was presented to the Conference of French and Franco-phone Alienists and Neurologists in Tunis along with several photographs taken by Jeanselme on his trip. An entire section of the final meeting report of this seminal conference was dedicated to the asylum at Buitenzorg.

2. Jeanselme, "La condition des aliénés."

3. Hans Pols, "The Psychiatrist as Administrator: The Career of W. F. Theunissen in the Dutch East Indies," Health and History 14, no. 1 (2012): 143–64.

4. See Denys Lombard, "Voyageurs Français dans l'Archipel Insulindien, XVIIe, XVIIe, XIXe Siècles," Archipel 1 (1971): 141–68. See also Christian Pelras, "Indonesian Studies in France: Retrospect, Situation and Prospects," Archipel 16 (1978): 7–20. The French restoration of Angkor Wat, for example, relied on techniques developed by the Dutch to preserve their own colonial ruins in Central Java, in particular the Borobudur and the Prambanan temples. Frances Gouda, Dutch Culture Overseas: Colonial Practice in the Netherlands Indies 1900–1942 (Jakarta: Equinox Press, 2008). See page 45 where Gouda discusses the publication of a biweekly magazine by the French Colonial Union, which included a regular feature entitled "The Netherlands Indies." See also G. H. Bos-quet, A French View of the Netherlands Indies (London: Oxford University Press, 1940). Even when critical of the Dutch perspective, Bosquet nevertheless praised the Dutch as a model for French efforts. The Dutch also admired the French opium monopoly in Indochina. See James Rush, Opium to Java: Revenue Farming and Chinese Enterprise in Colonial Indonesia, 1860–191. (Ithaca, NY: Cornell University Press, 1990).

5. J. Chailley Bert, preface to Java et ses habitants (Paris: Armand Colin et Cie, Editeurs, 1900), ix. The book was the third in a series that also included Les Anglais à Hong Kong and Les Anglais en Birmanie.

6. Only recently has this transnational perspective been adopted by colonial his-torians, who have begun to look much more closely at how, in the words of Ann

Stoler and Frederick Cooper, "whole bodies of administrative strategy, ethnographic classification and scientific knowledge were shared and compared in a consolidating imperial world." Stoler and Cooper, introduction to *Tensions of Empire: Colonial Cultures in a Bourgeois World*, ed. Frederick Cooper and Ann Laura Stoler (Berkeley: University of California Press, 1997), 1–56. See also Volker Barth and Roland Cvetkovski, eds., *Imperial Cooperation and Transfer, 1870–1930: Empires and Encounters* (London: Bloomsbury Academic Publishing, 2015).

7. Looking to other parts of world was an important aspect of psychiatric practices at the time; the history of study trips in the history of psychiatry is well documented. See D. I. McDonald, "Frederick Norton Manning 1839–1903," *Journal of the Royal Australian Historical Society* 58, no. 3 (1972): 190–201. The asylum had been based on Thomas S. Kirkbride's *On the Construction, Organization, and General Arrangements of Hospitals for the Insane* (Philadelphia, 1854), which provided a template of the architecture of mental hospitals according to the principles of moral treatment. See Nancy Tomes, *The Art of Asylum Keeping: Thomas Story Kirkbride and the Origins of American Psychiatry* (Philadelphia: University of Pennsylvania Press, 1994).

8. Claire Edington and Hans Pols, "Building Psychiatric Expertise across Southeast Asia: Study Trips, Site Visits and Therapeutic Labor in French Indochina and the Dutch East Indies, 1898–1937," *Comparative Studies in Society and History* 58, no. 3 (July 2016): 636–63. Other recent works exploring interimperial or interregional scientific connections include Deborah Neill, *Networks in Tropical Medicine: Internationalism, Colonialism, and the Rise of a Medical Specialty, 1890–1930* (Stanford: Stanford University Press, 2012); Leida Fernandez Prieto, "Islands of Knowledge: Science and Agriculture in the History of Latin America and the Caribbean," *Isis* 104 (2013): 788–97; Guillaume Lachenal, "Médecine, comparaisons et échanges inter-impériaux dans le Mandat Camerounais: Une histoire croisée Franco-Allemande de la mission Jamot," *Canadian Bulletin of Medical History* 30, no. 2 (2013): 23–45. In the history of psychiatry, increasing numbers of monographs and edited volumes are dedicated to comparative and global perspectives. See Sloane Mahone and Megan Vaughan, eds., *Psychiatry and Empire* (Basingstoke, UK: Palgrave Macmillan, 2007); Roy Porter and David Wright, eds., *The Confinement of the Insane: International Perspectives, 1800–1965* (Cambridge: Cambridge University Press, 2003); Waltraud Ernst and Thomas Müller, eds., *Transnational Psychiatries: Social and Cultural Histories of Psychiatry in Comparative Perspective c. 1800–2000* (Newcastle upon Tyne, UK: Cambridge Scholars, 2010). While much of the focus of comparative work has been across national contexts, scholars have also begun to reach beyond the conceptual confines of single-country case studies in order to explore the transnational movements of institutions, forms, and experts. See Marijke Gijswijt-Hofstra et al., eds., *Psychiatric Cultures Compared: Psychiatry and Mental Health Care in the Twentieth Century* (Amsterdam: Amsterdam University Press); Anne Digby, Waltraud Ernst, and Projit Mukharji, eds., *Crossing Colonial Historiographies: Histories of Colonial and Indigenous Medicines in Transnational Perspectives* (Newcastle upon Tyne, UK: Cambridge Scholars, 2010).

9. While some scholars, such as Ann Stoler, see these projects as part of a global expansion of disciplinary power, others stress the more brutal and punitive aspects of colonial labor regimes attached to prisons, for instance, which paid little lip service to rehabilitative ideals. Stoler, *Along the Archival Grain* (Princeton, NJ: Princeton University Press, 2009); Jeroen Dekker, "Punir, sauver et éduquer: La colonie agricole

"Nederlandsch Mettray" et la rééducation résidentielle aux Pays-Bas, en France, en Allemagne et en Angleterre entre 1814 et 1914," *Le Mouvement Social* 153 (October–December 1990): 63–90; Albert Schrauwers, "The 'Benevolent' Colonies of Johannes van den Bosch: Continuities in the Administration of Poverty in the Netherlands and Indonesia," *Comparative Studies in Society and History* 43, no. 2 (2001): 298–328; Stephen Toth, *Beyond Papillon: The French Overseas Penal Colonies, 1854–1952* (Lincoln: University of Nebraska Press, 2006); Neil Roos, "Work Colonies and South African Historiography," *Journal of Social History* 36, no. 1 (2011): 54–76.

10. See Claude Quétel, *Histoire de la folie: De l'antiquité à nos jours* (Paris: Tallendier, 2009); Ernst and Mueller, *Transnational Psychiatries*; Roy Porter and David Wrights, eds., *The Confinement of the Insane: International Perspectives, 1800–1965*. Cambridge: Cambridge University Press, 2003.

11. Ceri Crossley, "Using and Transforming the French Countryside: The 'Colonies Agricoles' (1820–1850)," *French Studies* 45 (1991): 36–54. See also Laura Lee Downs, *Childhood in the Promised Land: Working-Class Movements and the Colonies de Vacances in France, 1880–1960* (Durham, NC: Duke University Press, 2002). The Mettray agricultural colony for abandoned and delinquent children serves as the most famous example, popularized by Michel Foucault in *Discipline and Punish: The Birth of the Prison*, 2nd ed. (New York: Vintage Press, 1995).

12. For background on "moral treatment," see Anne Digby, *Madness, Morality and Medicine: A Study of the York Retreat, 1796–1914*. London: Cambridge University Press, 1985; Danielle Terbenche, " 'Curative' and 'Custodial': Benefits of Patient Treatment at the Asylum for the Insane, Kingston, 1878–1906," *Canadian Historical Review* 86 (2005): 29–52. An informative edited volume describes the widespread adoption of work as therapy in institutions around the world: Waltraud Ernst, ed., *Work, Psychiatry and Society, c. 1750–2010* (Manchester, UK: Manchester University Press, 2016).

13. For histories of the uses of labor in nineteenth-century prisons, see Rebecca McLennan, *The Crisis of Imprisonment: Protest, Politics, and the Making of the American Penal State, 1776–1941*, The Cambridge History of American Law (Cambridge: Cambridge University Press, 2008); John A. Conely, "Prisons, Production and Profit: Reconsidering the Importance of Prison Industries," *Journal of Social History* 14 (1980): 257–75; Michael Ignatieff, "State, Civil Society and Total Institutions: A Critique of Recent Social Histories of Punishment," *Crime and Justice* 3 (1981): 153–92; Larry Goldsmith, "To Profit by His Skill and to Traffic on His Crime: Prison Labor in Early Nineteenth Century Massachusetts," *Labor History* 4 (1999): 439–57; Michel Foucault, *Madness and Civilization: A History of Insanity in the Age of Reason*, trans. Richard Howard (London: Tavistock, 1967), 59–60. See also Ted McCoy, "The Unproductive Prisoner: Labor and Medicine in Canadian Penitentiaries, 1867–1900," *Labor: Studies in Working-Class History of the Americas* 6, no. 4 (2010): 95–112.

14. As quoted by Firmin Lagardelle, *Étude sur les colonies agricoles d'aliénés* (Moulins: Imprimerie de C. Desrosiers, 1873), 4. For work on agricultural colonies in the history of French psychiatry see Quétel, *Histoire de la folie*.

15. TTLTQG-2, GOUCOCH, IA.8/2912(1), Rapport annuel de Bienhoa, 1926.

16. Ernst, *Work, Psychiatry and Society*; Akira Hashimoto, "Invention of a 'Japanese Gheel': Psychiatric Family Care from a Historical and Transnational Perspective," in Ernst and Mueller, *Transnational Psychiatries*, 142–71; Ana Teresa A. Venancio, "From the Agricultural Colony to the Hospital-Colony: Configurations for Psy-

chiatric Care in Brazil in the First Half of the Twentieth Century," supplement 1, *Historia, Ciencias, Saude—manguinhos* 18 (2011): 35–52.

17. Psychiatrists kept detailed records on all patients who entered the asylum that included their race, age, gender, home province, and criminal background as well as their profession prior to entry. The occupation of "farmer" was, by far, the most commonly cited. See, for example, TTLTQG-2, GOUCOCH, IA.8/2912(1), "Repartition par profession," Rapport annuel de Bienhoa, 1926.

18. TTLTQG-2, GOUCOCH, IA.8/2912(1), Rapport annuel de Bienhoa, 1926.

19. TTLTQG-1, IGHSP, 48–05, Rapport annuel de Bien Hoa de 1931. Geoffrey Reaume discusses how Canadian doctors provided a physiological basis to support their claims about patient work in "Patients at Work: Insane Asylum Inmates' Labour in Ontario, 1841–1900," in *Rethinking Normalcy: A Disability Studies Reader*, Tanya Titchkosky and Rod Michalko, eds. (Toronto: Canadian Scholars' Press, 2009), 158–80.

20. TTLTQG-2, GOUCOCH, IA.8/2912(3), Rapport annuel de Bienhoa, 1927.

21. Charle Ladame and G. Demay, "La thérapeutique des maladies mentales par le travail," in *Congrès des médecins aliénistes et neurologistes de France et des pays de langue française* (Paris: Masson et Cie, 1926), 3–36.

22. TTLTQG-1, IGHSP, 50–03, Rapport annuel de l'Asile d'Aliénés de Bienhoa, 1933.

23. TTLTQG-2, GOUCOCH, IA.8/281(2), Rapport annuel de Bienhoa, 1925.

24. TTLTQG-2, GOUCOCH, IA.8/281(2), Rapport annuel de Bienhoa, 1925.

25. TTLTQG-2, GOUCOCH, IA.8/2912(1), Rapport annuel de Bienhoa, 1926.

26. Laurence Monnais, "Colonised and Neurasthenic: From the Appropriation of a Word to the Reality of a *Malaise de Civilisation* in Urban French Vietnam," *Health and History* 14, no. 1 (2012): 121–42.

27. TTLTQG-2, GOUCOCH, IA.8/281(2), Rapport annuel de Bienhoa, 1925.

28. TTLTQG-2, GOUCOCH, IA.8/281(2), Rapport annuel de Bienhoa, 1925.

29. TTLTQG-2, GOUCOCH, IA.8/2912(3), Rapport annuel de Bienhoa, 1927.

30. TTLTQG-2, GOUCOCH, IA.8/281(2), Rapport annuel de Bienhoa, 1925.

31. ANOM, BIB 12391, Etiologie des psychopathes par Dr. Augagneur, 1931.

32. TTLTQG-2, GOUCOCH, IA.8/2912(1), Rapport annuel de Bienhoa, 1926.

33. ANOM, RST, 3678, Inspection des services sanitaires et médicaux du Tonkin: Rapports, 1936.

34. Laurence Monnais, "'Could Confinement Be Humanised'? A Modern History of Leprosy in Vietnam," in *Public Health in Asia and the Pacific: Historical and Comparative Perspectives*, ed. Milton J. Lewis and Kerrie L. MacPherson (New York: Routledge, 2008).

35. TTLTQG-1, IGHSP, 48–05, Rapport annuel de l'Asile d'Aliénés de Bienhoa, 1931.

36. TTLTQG-2, GOUCOCH, IA.8/2912(1), Rapport annuel de Bienhoa, 1926.

37. TTLTQG-1, IGHSP, 51–07, Rapport annuel de 1934 sur le fonctionnement du Service de l'Assistance Médicale de Bien Hoa, Sai Gon, Bac Lieu, 1934.

38. ANOM, RSTNF, Rapport au sujet de la création d'un asile colonie sur le terrain de l'Asile de Voi par Dr. Grinsard, June 5, 1937. This proposal resulted from Dr. Grinsard's 1937 study trip to the Dutch East Indies, where he witnessed the therapeutic and economic success of a stand-alone agricultural colony installed in Lenteng-Agung, halfway between Batavia and Buitenzorg.

39. The historian Svein Skalevag describes how the pavilion system of asylum architecture, premised on the principle of segregation, reveals the ways in which "socialization was brought to the forefront of psychiatric healing." See Skalevag, "Constructive Curative Instruments: Psychiatric Architecture in Norway, 1820–1920," *History of Psychiatry* 12 (2002): 51–68.

40. TTLTQG-1, IGHSP, 50–03, Rapport annuel de l'Asile d'Aliénés de Bienhoa, 1933. Waltraud Ernst has made similar observations of asylums in British India. Whereas in Britain lower-class patients would be put to work as both a therapeutic and cost-savings measure, in India, Europeans of all social classes, as well as people of mixed race and elite Indian patients, were exempt from asylum labor regimes. See Ernst, "Idioms of Madness and Colonial Boundaries: The Case of the European and 'Native' Mentally Ill in Early Nineteenth-Century British India," *Comparative Studies in Society and History* 39, no. 1 (1997): 153–81.

41. ANOM, RSTNF, 3678, L'Inspecteur Général de l'Hygiène et de la Santé Publique à Monsieur le Gouverneur Général de l'Indochine (Direction des Affaires Economiques et Administratives), June 30, 1936.

42. Christopher Goscha, *Vietnam: A New History* (New York: Basic Books, 2016), 157.

43. Pierre Brocheux and Daniel Hémery, *Indochine: La colonisation ambiguë, 1858–1954* (Paris: Découverte, 2001), 127.

44. Brocheux and Hémery, *Indochine*, 155.

45. On labor regimes in colonial Vietnam see Martin J. Murray, "'White Gold' or 'White Blood'?: The Rubber Plantations of Colonial Indochina, 1910–1940," *Journal of Peasant Studies* 19, no. 3–4 (1992): 41–67; Pierre Brocheux. *The Mekong Delta: Ecology, Economy and Revolution, 1860–1890*, Monograph No. 12, Center for Southeast Asian Studies (Madison: University of Wisconsin, 1995); Mitchitake Aso, "Profits or People? Rubber Plantations and Everyday Technology in Rural Indochina," *Modern Asian Studies* 46, no. 1 (2012): 19–45. In the Dutch East Indies, the emphasis on labor and work in asylums coincided with the gradual transformation of the Indies from a trading empire into an area cultivated and made profitable by indigenous labor on plantations owned and run by Western companies. See Ann Laura Stoler, *Capitalism and Confrontation in Sumatra's Plantation Belt, 1870–1979* (Ann Arbor: University of Michigan Press, 1985); Jan Breman, *Taming the Coolie Beast: Plantation Society and the Colonial Order in Southeast Asia* (Delhi: Oxford University Press, 1989).

46. TTLTQG-1, IGHSP, 004, Rapport annuel de 1928 sur le fonctionnement de l'Inspection générale des services sanitaires et médicaux de l'Indochine.

47. TTLTQG-2, GOUCOCH, IA.8/2910 (1926–1927), Madame de la Souchère, Monsieur l'Administrateur, Chef de la Province de Bienhoa, Asile des aliénés de Bienhoa: Internement des aliénés à l'asile—Frais d'hospitalisation au compte du budget de leur province d'origine, November 4, 1926.

48. TTLTQG-1, IGHSP, 004, Rapport annuel de 1928 sur le fonctionnement de l'Inspection générale des services sanitaires et médicaux de l'Indochine. On the cost of living in Vietnam, see Pierre Brocheux, "The State and the 1930s Depression in French Indochina" in *Weathering the Storm: The Economies of Southeast Asia in the 1930s Depression*, ed. Peter Boomgaard and Ian Brown (Singapore: ISEAS, 2000), 251–70.

49. TTLTQG-1, IGHSP, 44–01, Promulgation en Indochine du décret du 21 Novembre 1933 sur le frais d'hospitalisation à l'Asile de Bienhoa; TTLTQG-1, MH, 5783, Remboursement de l'argent pour le traitement des malades à l'Asile d'Aliénés

de Voi, August 7, 1934; Fixation du prix de remboursement des journées de traite-ment à l'Asile d'Aliénés de Voi (Bac Giang) par le Résuper au Tonkin, Fonds de la Direction des Finances de l'Indochine, 1550, 1936 TTLTQG-1, RST, Procès-verbal de la commission de Surveillance de l'Asile d'Aliénés de Voi, June 15, 1938.

50. Brocheux, "The State and the 1930s Depression in French Indochina", 261.

51. TTLTQG-2, GOUCOCH, IA.8/2912(1), Rapport Annuel de Bienhoa, 1926.

52. TTLTQG-2, GOUCOCH, IA.8/281(2), Asylum report de Bienhoa, 1925.

53. TTLTQG-2, GOUCOCH, IA.8/281(2), Asylum report de Bienhoa, 1925.

54. TTLTQG-2, GOUCOCH, IA.8/2912(3), Rapport annuel de Bienhoa, 1927. See also TTLTQG-2, GOUCOCH, IA.8/281(2), Rapport annuel de Bienhoa, 1925.

55. TTLTQG-1, IGHSP, 48–05, Rapport annuel de Bien Hoa de 1931.

56. TTLTQG-1, IGHSP, 48–05, Rapport annuel de Bien Hoa de 1931.

57. Brocheux and Hémery, *Indochine*, 128.

58. E. L. Peyre, "Les maladies mentales aux colonies," *L'hygiène mentale: journal de psychiatrie appliquée* 29, 8 (September–October 1934): 185–212; R. Lefèvre. "L'assistance psychiatrique en Indochine." *Congrès des médecins aliénistes et neurologistes de France et des pays de langue francaise*, Bordeaux, 1931, 293–97.

59. While historians mention the use of occupational labor in other colonial set-tings, it is typically used to illustrate the abuses of the colonial asylum system rather than in terms of a real tension of practice. See, for example, Lynette Jackson, *Surfacing Up: Psychiatry and Social Order in Colonial Zimbabwe, 1908–1968* (Ithaca, NY: Cornell University Press, 2005), 160–61.

60. TTLTQG-1, IGHSP, 51–07, Rapport annuel de 1934 sur le fonctionnement du Service de l'Assistance Médicale de Bien Hoa, Sai Gon, Bac Lieu.

61. TTLTQG-1, IGHSP, 50–03, Rapport annuel de l'Asile d'Aliénés de Bienhoa, 1933.

62. TTLTQG-2, GOUCOCH, IA.8/2912(1), Rapport annuel de Bienhoa, 1926.

63. TTLTQG-1, RST, 73750, Organisation et fonctionnement d'un Asile d'Aliénés à Bien-Hoa (Cochinchine), Note sur l'organisation générale d'un Asile d'Aliénés par le Dr. Augagneur, Médecin Directeur de l'Asile de Bien Hoa, 1927; GOUCOCH IA.8/2912(1) Rapport annuel de Bien Hoa 1926.

64. TTLTQG-2, GOUCOCH, IA.8/2912(3), Rapport annuel de Bienhoa, 1927.

65. See "Une révolte à la colonie agricole de Chezal Benoit," *Informateur des aliénistes et des neurologistes* 6, no. 25 (June 1911): 140–42.

66. TTLTQG-2, GOUCOCH, IA.8/2912(3), Rapport annuel de Bienhoa, 1927.

67. On prison labor regimes in colonial Vietnam, see Zinoman, *Colonial Bastille*, 84.

68. Hue Tam Ho Tai, *Radicalism and the Origins of the Vietnamese Revolution* (Cambridge, MA: Harvard University Press, 1996); Brocheux and Hémery, *Indochine*; David Del Testa, "Workers, Culture and the Railroads in French Colonial Indochina, 1905–1936," in *French Colonial History*, vol. 2 (2002): 181–98. On the end of forced labor in the French empire see Frederick Cooper, *Decolonization and African Society: The Labor Question in French and British Africa* (Cambridge: Cambridge University Press, 1996), 31.

69. TTLTQG-2, GOUCOCH, 3731, Indemnité allouée aux internés de l'Asile d'Aliénés de Bien Hoa, 1934.

70. TTLTQG-1, IGHSP, 51–07, Rapport annuel de 1934 sur le fonctionnement du Service de l'Assistance Médicale de Bien Hoa, Sai Gon, Bac Lieu.

71. Ladame and Demay, "Thérapeutique des maladies.".

72. TTLTQG-1, IGHSP, 51–07, Rapport annuel de l'Asile d'Aliénés de Bienhoa, 1934.

73. TTLTQG-2, GOUCOCH, IA.8/2912(1), Rapport annuel de Bienhoa, 1926.

74. TTLTQG-2, GOUCOCH, IA.8/2912(3), Rapport annuel de Bienhoa, 1927.

75. TTLTQG-2, GOUCOCH, IA.8/281(1), Rapport annuel de Bienhoa, 1923.

76. TTLTQG-2, GOUCOCH, IA.8/2912(3), Rapport annuel de Bienhoa, 1927.

77. TTLTQG-2, GOUCOCH, IA.8/2912(1), Rapport annuel de Bienhoa, 1926.

78. TTLTQG-2, GOUCOCH, IA.8/281(2), Rapport annuel de Bienhoa, 1925.

79. TTLTQG-2, GOUCOCH, IA.8/274(3), Lettre de Gouverneur Général à Médecin-Directeur de l'Asile de Bienhoa au sujet de . . . Vinh, April 1, 1920.

80. Annick Guénel, "The 1937 Bandung Conference on Rural Hygiene: Toward a New Vision of Healthcare?" in *Global Movements, Local Concerns: Medicine and Health in Southeast Asia*, ed. Laurence Monnais and Harold J. Cook (Singapore: Singapore University Press, 2012), 62–80. See also Socrates Litsios, "Revisiting Bandoeng," *Social Medicine* 8, no. 3 (2014): 113–28.

81. Theodore M. Brown and Elizabeth Fee, "The Bandoeng Conference of 1937: A Milestone in Health and Development," *American Journal of Public Health* 98, no. 1 (2008): 40–43. Brown and Fee note that, following the 1937 conference, and especially after World War II, international health turned to technology-based approaches and vertical programs, which supplanted the older "romantic" vision for rural health.

82. For an overview, see Laurence Monnais and Hans Pols, "Health and Disease in the Colonies: Medicine in the Age of Empire," in *The Routledge History of Western Empires*, ed. Robert Aldrich and Kirsten McKenzie (New York: Routledge, 2014), 270–84.

83. The Far Eastern Association of Tropical Medicine was created through an American initiative in the Philippines. The first congress was held in Manila in 1908, followed by meetings in Hong Kong (1910), Saigon (1913), Batavia (1921), Singapore (1923), Tokyo (1925), Calcutta (1927), Bangkok (1930), Nanking (1934), and Hanoi (1938).

84. John Farley, *To Cast Out Disease: A History of the International Health Division of the Rockefeller Foundation (1913–1951)* (New York: Oxford University Press, 2003).

85. Sunil S. Amrith, *Decolonizing International Health: India and Southeast Asia, 1930–1965* (Basingstoke, UK: Palgrave Macmillan, 2006), 36–42.

86. For an overview of the first two years of Lenteng Agung, see P. M. van Wulff-ten Palthe, "Krankzinnigenverzorging in Nederlandsch-Indië [Care for the insane in the Dutch East Indies]," *Geneeskundig Tijdschrift voor Nederlandsch-Indië* 77 (1937): 1267–80.

87. ANOM, GUERNUT, carton 22, "Note sur la Colonie Agricole d'Aliénés de Lenteng-Agoeng (Java) par le Dr. P. M. Dorolle," October 1937.

88. Annick Guénel describes French missions to the Dutch East Indies to study antimalarial campaigns, in "Malaria, Colonial Economics and Migrations in Vietnam" (paper presented at the Fourth Conference of the European Association of Southeast Asian Studies in Paris, September 1–4, 2004). On comparative studies of

ethnological characteristics, see Madeleien Colani, "Essai d'ethnographie compare," *Bulletin de l'Ecole française d'Extrême Orient* 36 (1936): 197–280. There was also considerable French interest in new techniques for grafting rubber trees and clones, which improved yield and were first developed in the Dutch East Endies. See Aso, "Profits or People?".

89. ANOM, GUERNUT, carton 22, "Note sur la Colonie Agricole d'Aliénés de Lenteng-Agoeng . . . October 1937.

90. ANOM, GUERNUT, carton 22, "Note sur la Colonie Agricole d'Aliénés de Lenteng-Agoeng . . . October 1937.

91. ANOM, GUERNUT, carton 22, "Note sur la Colonie Agricole d'Aliénés de Lenteng-Agoeng . . . October 1937.

92. ANOM, RSTNF, 3752, Rapport au sujet de la création d'un asile colonie sur le terrain de l'Asile de Voi . . . June 5, 1937.

93. ANOM, RST, Lettre du Gouverneur Général de l'Indochine à Monsieur le Resident Superieur au Tonkin, June 7, 1939.

94. ANOM, RST, 3752, Heckenroth, l'Inspecteur Général de l'Hygiène et de la Santé Publiques à Monsieur le Gouverneur Général de l'Indochine, May 9, 1938.

95. ANOM, RST, 3752, Lettre du Gouverneur General de l'Indochine . . . June 7, 1939.

96. ANOM, RSTNF, 3752, Rapport au sujet de la création d'un asile colonie sur le terrain de l'Asile de Voi . . . June 5, 1937.

97. ANOM, RST, 3752, De Raymond, le Directeur Local de la Santé à Monsieur le Résident Supérieur au Tonkin, September 17, 1937.

98. ANOM, RST, 3753, Réunion de la Commission de Surveillance de l'Asile d'Aliénés du Voi, December 5, 1940.

99. See, for example, Jackson, "Surfacing Up," 160–61.

100. Geoffrey Reaume makes a powerful plea for more scholarly attention to the dynamics of patient labor in *Remembrance of Patients Past: Patient Life at the Toronto Hospital for the Insane, 1870–1940* (Toronto: University of Toronto Press, 2000).

4. Going In and Getting Out of the Colonial Asylum

1. TTLTQG-1, IGHSP, 48–05, Rapport annuel de l'Asile d'Aliénés de Bienhoa, 1931.

2. TTLTQG-1, RST, 73744–01, Rapatriement et internement des aliénés indigènes a l'Asile de Voi (Bac Giang), classés par ordre alphabétique de nom de Q à R, au sujet de DV Duong, June 1936.

3. Tran-Minh Tung, "The Family and the Management of Mental Health Problems in Vietnam," in *Transcultural Research in Mental Health*.

4. Here I take cues from Tony Day's use of the family concept in "Ties That (Un) Bind: Families and States in Premodern Southeast Asia," *Journal of Asian Studies* 55, no. 2 (May 1996): 384–409, 387.

5. My thinking about the relationship between care and abandonment is shaped by the work of Sarah Pinto, in particular her article "Crises of Commitment: Ethics of Intimacy, Kin and Confinement in Global Psychiatry," *Medical Anthropology: Cross-Cultural Studies in Health and Illness* 28, no. 1 (2009): 1–10.

6. European and métis patients formed only a small proportion of the total asylum population. In 1926, the Bien Hoa asylum housed 10 European or métis

patients out of a total 379; at the end of 1932, while the total asylum population had grown to 660, only 15 were classified as European or métis. TTLTQG-2, GOU-COCH, IA.8/2912(3), Asile de Bienhoa, rapport annuel 1927; TTLTQG-1, IGHSPI, 50–03, Rapport annuel de 1933 sur le fonctionnement du Service de l'Assistance Médicale de Tan An, Bien Hoa, Rach Gia.

7. TTLTQG-1, RST, 73741, Nguyen Huy Tuong à Monsieur le Résident au sujet renseignements donnés sur . . . Cac, déséquilibré domicilié à Gia-Hoà, huyên de Thach-Thât, April 30, 1928.

8. TTLTQG-1, RST, 73741, Rougier, le Directeur Local de la Santé à Monsieur le Résident Supérieur, May 18, 1928.

9. In 1902, the colonial administration signed a contract with the Asile St. Pierre in Marseille that agreed to receive French patients from Indochina. While patients continued to be repatriated throughout the interwar years, especially those able to pay their own way, the practice was deemed expensive and impractical and formed a major impetus for the decision to build a "mixed" asylum for both European and indigenous patients that opened in 1919. TTLTQG-2, GOUCOCH, IA.8/104(1), Le Docteur Henaff, Chef du Service de Santé de la Cochinchine du Cambodge et du Laos, à Monsieur le Lieutenant Gouverneur de la Cochinchine, Saigon, July 15 1903.

10. TTLTQG-2, GOUCOCH, IA.8/162(9), M. L. Gudenet, administrateur de Thudaumot à Monsieur le Directeur de l'Intérieur (3e Bureau), October 29, 1887.

11. TTLTQG-1, RST, 73751, Le Garde Principal commandant le poste de Dong-Chau à Monsieur l'Administrateur Résident Tuyen Quang, Dong-Chau, June 16, 1912.

12. TTLTQG-1, RST, 73751, M. P. Carlotti, Procureur de la république de Haiphong, à Monsieur le Procureur Général, Chef du Service Judiciaire en Indo-Chine, Hanoi, February 28, 1905.

13. For an analysis of the 1930 law, see Dr. Pierre Dorolle, *La Législation Indo-chinoise sur les aliénés: Exposé et commentaire des dispositions du décret du 18 juillet 1930* (Saigon: Imprimerie A. Portail, 1941).

14. TTLTQG-1, MH, 5782, H. Virgitti à Commissaire Central de Police à Hanoi au sujet . . . Tho, June 11, 1935.

15. TTLTQG-1, RST, 73738–03, Note postale circulaire no. 130 au sujet de l'admission des aliénés à l'asile de Bien-Hoa.

16. These survey forms appear in dozens of patient case files. See, for example, TTLTQG-1, MH, 5782, Le Médecin Directeur de l'Asile d'Aliénés à Monsieur le Chef de Rue Armand Rousseau à Hanoi, au sujet . . . Thanh, May 14, 1935.

17. TTLTQG-1, MH, 5782, Le Médecin Directeur de l'Asile d'Aliénés, à Monsieur le Chef de la Ruelle de Phat-Loc, Hanoi, August 23 1934; Tin, Chef de Rue des Changeurs à Monsieur le Commissaire Central de la Ville de Hanoi, August 1934.

18. TTLTQG-2, GOUCOCH, IA.8/281(20), Le Médecin Directeur de l'Asile à Monsieur le Gouverneur de Cochinchine, August 10, 1926.

19. TTLTQG-2, GOUCOCH, IA.8/275(1), Rapport semestriel de l'Asile de Bien-hoa, December 18, 1919.

20. TTLTQG-1, RST, 73752–01, Rapport médico-légal de . . . Hang, December 30, 1919.

21. TTLTQG-1, RST, 73752–01, Rapport médico-légal de . . . Hang, December 30, 1919.

22. Laurel Kendall and Hien Thi Nguyen, "Dressing Up the Spirits: Costumes, Cross-Dressing, and Incarnation in Korea and Vietnam," in *Women and Indigenous religions,* ed. Sylvia Marcos (New York: Praeger, 2010), 93–114.

23. Dinh Trong Hiêu, "La face, le ventre et autres symboliques du corps chez les Viet," in *La colonization des corps: De l'Indochine au Viet Nam*, ed. François Guillemot et Agathe Larcher-Goscha (Paris: Editions Vendémiaire, 2014), 42.

24. TTLTQG-1, RST, 73746, Internement des aliénés provenant de l'annam a l'Asile d'aliénés à Voi (Bac Giang), Rapport médico-légal du Docteur Cao-Xuan-Cam sur le cas de . . . Nam, August 8, 1934. Italics added by the author.

25. TTLTQG-2, RST, 73743-7, Rapport d'examen médico-légal du nommé . . . Mân, détenu à la Maison Centrale de Hanoi, June 1928.

26. TTLTQG-2, GOUCOCH, IA.8/1724(4), Monsieur C. de Laprade, administrateur de la province de Thudaumot, à Monsieur le Lieutenant-Gouverneur Saigon, February 9, 1909.

27. E. Langlet, *Le peuple annamite: Ses moeurs, croyances et traditions* (Paris: Berger-Levrault 1913).

28. TTLTQG-1, RST, 73750, Note du Chef de Bac Ran, November 13, 1903. See also Reboul and Régis, "L'Assistance des aliénés aux colonies," 124.

29. Shaun Kingsley Malarney, *Culture, Ritual and Revolution in Vietnam* (Honolulu: University of Hawai'i Press, 2002), 95-100.

30. ANOM, BIB 12391, Dr. Gaide, "Les maladies mentales et assistance aux aliénés," 1931.

31. ANOM, BIB 12391, Dr. Gaide, "Les maladies mentales et assistance aux aliénés," 1931. On the international discourse of psychiatric liberation vis-à-vis familial constraint, as seen from China, see Zhiying Ma, "An 'Iron Cage' of Civilization? Missionary Psychiatry and the Making of a 'Chinese Family' at the Turn of the Century," in *Psychiatry and Chinese History*, ed. Howard Chiang (London: Pickering and Chatto), 91-110.

32. TTLTQG-1, RST, 73750, Note du Chef de Bac Ran, November 13, 1903.

33. TTLTQG-1, IGHSPI, 48-05, Rapport annuel de l'Asile d'Aliénés de Bienhoa, 1931.

34. TTLTQG-1, IGHSPI, 48-05, Rapport annuel de l'Asile d'Aliénés de Bienhoa, 1931.

35. TTLTQG-1, IGHSPI, 51-01, Hôpital de Chôquan, Rapport sur le fonctionnement du service de psychiatrie de l'Hôpital de Chôquan en 1934. See also Emily Baum on how Beijing residents saw the psychiatric hospital as a place of last resort and sought out alternative cures. "Spit, Chains, and Hospital Beds: A History of Madness in Republican Beijing, 1912-1938" (PhD diss., University of California, San Diego, 2013).

36. TTLTQG-1, IGHSPI, 48-05, Rapport annuel de l'Asile d'Aliénés de Bienhoa, 1931.

37. In the 1930s, intense media coverage of the overcrowded and unsanitary conditions of prison life, as well as the physical abuse of inmates, generated enough pressure on the colonial administration for it to (partially) enact needed reforms. See Zinoman, *Colonial Bastille*, chap. 8.

38. TTLTQG-1, IGHSP, Rapport mensuel de Janvier à Décembre 1913 sur le fonctionnement du Service de Santé en Annam.

39. ANOM, BIB 12391, Dr. Gaide, "Les maladies mentales et assistance aux aliénés," 1931.

40. TTLTQG-1, IGHSPI, 48-05, Rapport annuel de l'Asile d'Aliénés de Bienhoa, 1931.

41. Andre Augagneur and Le Trung Luong, "Croyances et pratiques pour le traitement des maladies mentales en Indochine," *L'Hygiène Mentale* 23 (1928): 276.

42. PHARO, 182, Rapport annuel d'Ensemble de Service de la Santé, 1934.

43. TTLTQG-1, IGHSPI, 48–05, Rapport annuel de l'Asile d'Aliénés de Bienhoa, 1931.

44. TTLTQG-1, IGHSPI, 51–01, Hôpital de Chôquan . . . 1934.

45. See introduction to Keller, *Colonial Madness*, 1–18; TTLTQG-1, IGHSP, 51–01, Hôpital de Chôquan . . . 1934.

46. See Keller, *Colonial Madness*, 53; Jean-Bernard Wojciechowski, *Hygiène mentale et hygiène sociale* (Paris: Harmattan, 1997); Jean-Christophe Coffin," 'Misery' and 'Revolution': The Organisation of French Psychiatry, 1900–1980," in *Psychiatric Cultures Compared: Psychiatry and Mental Health Care in the Twentieth Century*, ed. M. Gijswit-Hofstra et al. (Amsterdam: Amsterdam University Press, 2005); Hans Pols, "Beyond the Clinical Frontiers: The American Mental Hygiene Movement, 1910–1945," in *International Relations in Psychiatry: Britain, Germany and the United States to World War II*, ed. V. Roelcke, P. Weindling, and L. Westwood (Rochester, NY: University of Rochester Press, 2010).

47. Jessie Rian Hewitt, "Isolating Madness: Doctors, Families and the Gendering of Psychiatric Authority in Nineteenth Century France" (PhD diss., University of California, Davis, 2012).

48. PHARO, carton 182, Rapport annuel d'Ensemble de la Service de Santé, 1934. See also Gaffiero and Dorolle, "Notes de pathologie mentale coloniale."

49. TTLTQG-1, IGHSP, 51–01, Hôpital de Chôquan . . . 1934.

50. TTLTQG-1, IGHSP, 51–01, Hôpital de Chôquan . . . 1934.

51. Aubin, H. "L'Assistance psychiatrique indigène aux colonies." Rapport au Congrès des Médecins Aliénistes et Neurologistes de France et des Pays de Langue Francaise, XLIIe session—Alger 6–11 Avril 1938. Paris: Masson et Cie, 1938.

52. Aubin, "L'Assistance psychiatrique Indigène aux colonies."

53. Aubin, "L'Assistance psychiatrique Indigène aux colonies."

54. PHARO, carton 166, Rapports annuels de la Service de Santé, 1934 and 1939.

55. TTLTQG-1, RST, 78747–01, Asile de Bien Hoa, rapport annuel pour 1928.

56. ANOM, RST, 03749, Lettre à Monsieur le Résident Supérieur au Tonkin, au sujet de l'assistance psychiatrique en faveur de . . . Phien, February 23, 1942.

57. TTLTQG-1, IGHSP, 51–01, Hôpital de Chôquan . . . 1934.

58. Sadowsky, *Electroconvulsive Therapy*.

59. Patricia E. Prestwich.,"Family Strategies and Medical Power: 'Voluntary' Committal in a Parisian Asylum, 1876–1914," in *The Confinement of the Insane, 1800–1965: International Perspectives*, ed. Roy Porter and David Wright (Cambridge: Cambridge University Press, 2003), 79–99.

60. R. Grinsard, "Note sur les principales psychopathies observées à l'asile d'aliénés de Voi en 1936," *Bulletin de la Société Médico-Chirurgicale de l'Indochine*," no. 3 (April 1937): 392.

61. Laurence Monnais and Noémi Tousignant, "The Colonial Life of Pharmaceuticals: Accessibility to Healthcare, Consumption of Medicines, and Medical Pluralism in French Vietnam, 1905–1945," *Journal of Vietnamese Studies* 1, no. 1–2 (2006): 131–66.

62. PHARO, carton 166, Rapports annuels de la Service de Santé, "Fonctionnement de l'Asile d'Aliénés de Voi," 1938.

63. See, for example, TTLTQG-1, RST, 73752–04, Internement à l'Asile de Voi (Bac Giang) des aliénés de 1936, feuille 19, December 16, 1936.

64. Zinoman, *Colonial Bastille*, 282.

65. Dorolle, *La Législation Indochinoise.*

66. David Wright, "The Discharge of Pauper Lunatics from Country Asylums in Mid-Victorian England, the Case of Buckinghamshire, 1853–1872," in Melling and Forsythe, *Insanity, Institutions, and Society*, 106. My attention to family letters also draws inspiration from Farge and Foucault's work on the lettres de cachet of the ancien régime as a window into the politics of family life. See Arlette Farge and Michel Foucault, eds., *Le Désordre des familles: Lettres de cachet des archives de la Bastille au XVIIIe siècle* (Paris: Gallimard, 1982). Natalie Davis examines the formulaic qualities of prisoner narratives in writing to power. See *Fiction in the Archives: Pardon Tales and their Tellers in Sixteenth Century France* (Stanford, CA: Stanford University Press, 1988). For letter writing in the context of asylums see Louise Wannell, "Patients' Relatives and Psychiatric Doctors: Letter Writing in the York Retreat, 1875–1910," *Social History of Medicine* 20, no. 2 (2007): 297–313; Catharine Coleborne. "'His Brain Was Wrong, His Mind Astray': Families and the Language of Insanity in New South Wales, Queensland, and New Zealand, 1880s–1910," *Journal of Family History* 31, no. 1 (2006): 45–65.

67. TTLTQG-2, GOUCOCH, IA.8/162(9), Au sujet de l'annamite . . . Nhut atteint d'aliénation mental, March 7, 1887.

68. TTLTQG-2, RST, 73742, Lettre de Tran-van-Ngoc, Greffier près le tribunal de Ninh-Binh à Monsieur l'Administrateur, Résident à Vinh, July 9, 1930.

69. TTLTQG-2, GOUCOCH, IA.8/275(1), Lettre de . . . Giat au sujet de . . . Phu, December 28, 1919.

70. TTLTQG-2, GOUCOCH, IA.8/274(1), Le Délégué administratif a Monsieur l'Administrateur Chef de la Province de Tra Vinh, November 7, 1922.

71. TTLTQG-2, GOUCOCH, IA.8/2912(2), Lettre à Monsieur le Gouverneur de la Cochinchine, au sujet de . . . Gia, October 26, 1927.

72. TTLTQG-1, RST, 73743, Lettre à Monsieur le Résident Supérieur au Tonkin, June 24, 1933.

73. TTLTQG-2, GOUCOCH, IA.8/2912(2), Lettre à Monsieur le Gouverneur de la Cochinchine . . . October 26, 1927.

74. TTLTQG-2, GOUCOCH, 73743-03, Lettre de . . . Phuc à Monsieur le Résident au Tonkin, July 11, 1963.

75. TTLTQG-1, RST, 73743-7, Lettre de . . . Duyên et . . . Keo à Monsieur le Résident Supérieur au Tonkin, July 27, 1928.

76. TTLTQG-2, GOUCOCH, IA.8/276(2), Le Médecin Directeur de l'Asile à Monsieur le Gouverneur de Cochinchine, September 8, 1927.

77. TTLTQG-2, GOUCOCH, IA.8/281(2), Rapport médico-légal au sujet de l'état mental et de la responsabilité du nommé . . . Sau, June 1925.

78. TTLTQG-2, GOUCOCH, IA.8/276 (2), Le Médecin Directeur de l'Asile de Bienhoa à Monsieur le Gouverneur de la Cochinchine, February 17, 1925.

79. TTLTQG-2, GOUCOCH, IA.8/276(2), Le Médecin Directeur de l'Asile de Bienhoa à Monsieur le Gouverneur de Cochinchine, September 8, 1927.

80. TTLTQG-2, GOUCOCH, IA.8/275(1), Certificat semestriel concernant le nommé . . . Huong, Asile de Bien Hoa, October 1, 1919.

81. TTLTQG-2, GOUCOCH, IA.8/274(3), Lettre de Gouverneur Général à Médecin-Directeur de l'Asile de Bienhoa au sujet de . . . Vinh, April 1, 1920.

82. TTLTQG-2, GOUCOCH, IA.8/274(3), Dr. Mul, Assistance Médicale Province de Mytho, à Monsieur l'Administrateur, Chef de la province de Mytho, March 18, 1920.

83. In her study of asylums in late imperial Russia, Julie Brown makes a similar point about seasonal patterns of asylum utilization coinciding with peak harvest times. Julie V. Brown, "Peasant Survival Strategies in Late Imperial Russia: The Social Uses of the Mental Hospital," *Social Problems* 34, no. 4 (1987): 311–29.

84. TTLTQG-2, GOUCOCH, IA.8/274(3), LT Mai à Monsieur le Gouverneur de la Cochinchine, September 26, 1921.

85. PHARO, carton 182, Rapport annuel d'Ensemble de la Service de Santé, 1934.

86. See Nguyễn Văn Hoài. De l'Organisation de l'Hôpital Psychiatrique du Sud-Vietnam. (Saigon: Imprimerie Française d'Outre Mer, 1954), 148.

87. TTLTQG-2, GOUCOCH, IA.8/274(3), Le Thi Mai à Monsieur le Gouverneur de la Cochinchine, September 26, 1921.

88. TTLTQG-2, GOUCOCH, 73743–03, Lettre de . . . Phuc à Monsieur le Résident au Tonkin, July 11, 1963.

89. TTLTQG-2, GOUCOCH, IA.8/294(2), Le Médecin Directeur de l'Asile d'Aliénés de Bienhoa à Monsieur l'Administrateur, Chef de la Province de Vinhlong, May 27, 1920.

90. TTLTQG-2, GOUCOCH, IA.8/275(1), Le Médecin Directeur de l'Asile des Aliénés à Monsieur le Gouverneur de la Cochinchine, September 7, 1920.

91. TTLTQG-2, GOUCOCH, IA.8/281(2), Le Procureur Général près la Cour d'Appel de Saigon à Monsieur le Gouverneur de la Cochinchine, June 29, 1925.

92. Van Nguyen-Marshall, "The Ethics of Benevolence in French Colonial Vietnam: A Sino-Franco Vietnamese Cultural Borderland," in *The Chinese State at the Borders*, ed. Diana Lary (Vancouver: University of British Columbia Press, 2008), 162–180.

93. Alexander Woodside, "The Development of Social Organizations in Vietnamese Cities in the Late Colonial Period," *Pacific Affairs* 44, no. 1 (Spring 1971): 39–64, 49.

94 ANOM, RSTNF, 3893, Le Résident Supérieur au Tonkin à Monsieur le Gouverneur Général de l'Indochine, August 21, 1930.

95 TTLTQG-1, RST, 73744–02, Le Tri-Huyen de Thanh-Oai à Monsieur le Résident de Hadong, July 26, 1923.

96. TTLTQG-2, GOUCOCH, IA.8/281(2), Le Médecin Directeur de l'Asile à Monsieur le Gouverneur de Cochinchine, August 26, 1926.

97. TTLTQG-2, GOUCOCH, IA.8/2912(2), Le Médecin Directeur de l'Asile à Monsieur le Gouverneur de Cochinchine, December 3, 1927.

98. TTLTQG-2, GOUCOCH, IA.8/2912(2), Le Médecin Directeur de l'Asile à Monsieur le Gouverneur de Cochinchine, December 3, 1927.

99. Ann Laura Stoler, *Carnal Knowledge and Imperial Power: Race and the Intimate in Colonial Rule* (Berkeley: University of California Press, 2001).

100. Hilary Marland, "At Home with Puerparal Mania: The Domestic Treatment of the Insanity of Childbirth in the 19th Century," in Bartlett and Wright, *Outside the Walls of the Asylum*, 45–65.

101. TTLTQG-2, GOUCOCH, IA.8/274(1), Monsieur de Tastes, Administrateur des Services Civils, Président de la Commission municipale de Cholon, à Monsieur le Gouverneur de la Cochinchine, October 6, 1922.

102. TTLTQG-2, GOUCOCH, IA.8/281(1), L'Administrateur des Services Civils Chef de la Province de Vinhong à Monsieur le Gouverneur de la Cochinchine, January 16, 1924.

103. TTLTQG-2, GOUCOCH, IA.8/281(1), Lettre de Commissaire Special Etievant, Monsieur l'Administrateur Chef de la Sureté au sujet de . . . Sau, December 15, 1921.

104. TTLTQG-2, GOUCOCH, IA.8/281(1), Le Procureur de la Republique près le Tribunal de 1ère instance de Saigon à Monsieur le Procureur General à Saigon, May 7, 1925.

105. TTLTQG-2, GOUCOCH, IA.8/276(1), L'Administrateur de Can Tho à Monsieur le Gouverneur de la Cochinchine, September 3, 1923.

106. TTLTQG-2, GOUCOCH, IA.8/276(2), L'Administrateur de Can Tho à Monsieur le Gouvernement de la Cochinchine, February 18, 1925.

107. TTLTQG-2, GOUCOCH, IA.8/294(3), Certificat semestriel de . . . Nham, Asile d'Alienes de Bien Hoa, May 22, 1920.

108. Monnais and Tousignant, "Colonial Life of Pharmaceuticals," 132.

109. TTLTQG-1, IGHSPI, 39–05, Rapport annuel de 1931 sur le fonctionnement des Services Sanitaires et Médicaux à Bien Hoa.

110. Augagneur and Le, "Croyances et pratiques,"269–76. The fact that this piece was coauthored by two practicing doctors—one French, the other Vietnamese—in Inodochina might indicate that it provides a more solid grounding in local understandings and traditions around mental illness than the work of armchair scholars in Paris.

111. Augagneur and Le, "Croyances et pratiques."

112. John Warne Monroe, *Laboratories of Faith Book: Mesmerism, Spiritism, and Occultism in Modern France* (Ithaca, NY: Cornell University Press, 2008). On the relationship between psychiatry and mesmerism in colonial India see Waltraud Ernst, "Colonial Psychiatry, Magic and Religion: The Case of Mesmerism in British India," *History of Psychiatry* 15, no. 1 (2004): 57–71.

113. TTLTQG-1, RST, 73741, Rapport médico-légal [. . .] Cac, February 4, 1938. According to Vietnamese law, sorcerers were subject to harsh recriminations if their practices resulted in the death of the sick individual. See Edouard Jeanselme, "La sorcellerie en extreme Orient," *Journal de Médécine Légal Psychiatrique et Anthropologies Criminelle* 1 (1906): 16–18.

114. TTLTQG-1, IGHSPI, 004, Rapport annuel de 1928.

115. Nguyễn Thị Hiền, "Yin Illness: Its Diagnosis and Healing within Len Dong (Spirit Possession) Rituals of the Viet," *Asian Ethnology* 67, no. 2 (2008): 305–21.

116. Jane Atkinson, "Shamanisms Today," *Annual Review of Anthropology* 21 (1992): 307–30, 313.

117. TTLTQG-1, RST, 73741, Rapport d'examen médical de la nommée . . . Can, December 30, 1933; TTLTQG-2, 155(3), Certificat d'admission du . . . Phan, Asile de Bienhoa, November 3, 1921; TTLTQG-2, 2751(1), Certificat semestriel de . . . Luc, Asile de Bien Hoa, August 2, 1919.

118. TTLTQG-1, 73737, Certificat médical du nommé . . . Thai, June 11, 1936.

119. Paul Sérieux, "Délire mystique," in *Les folies raisonnantes, le délire d'interprétation*, (Paris: Éd. F. Alcan, 1909), 121–28.

120. Jean Quang Trinh Lê, "Croyances et pratiques médicales sino-annamites," Thèse pour obtenir le Grade de Docteur en Médecine, Faculté de Médecine, Université de Montpellier, 1911.

121. TTLTQG-2, RST, 73741, Rapport médical . . . Cac, February 4, 1928.

122. TTLTQG-1, RST, 73752–01, Rapport médico légal . . . Hang, December 30, 1919.

123. ANOM, Haut commissariat de France pour l'Indochine, Service de Protection du Corps expéditionnaire (S.P.C.E.), 385, Notice de renseignments concernant Huynh Phu So, 1942.

124. For more on Huỳnh Phú Sồ, see Pascal Bordeaux, "Emergence et constitution de la communauté du Bouddhisme Hoa Hoa: Contribution à l'histoire sociale du delta du Mékong (1935–1955)" (Thèse de doctorat, École pratique des hautes études, Paris, 2003); Hue Tam Ho Tai, *Millenarianism and Peasant Politics in Vietnam* (Cambridge, MA: Harvard University Press, 1983).

125. R. Grinsard, "Note sur les principales psychopathiesobservées à l'asile d'aliénés de Voi, 392.

126. TTLTQG-2, GOUCOCH, 281(1), Le Médecin Directeur de l'Asile à Monsieur le Gouverneur de la Cochinchine, September 13, 1924.

127. ANOM, RSTNF, Le Resident Supérieur au Tonkin, Yves Châtel, à Gouveneur Général (Direction des Services Economiques et Inspection Générale de l'Hygiène et de la Santé Publique), November 12, 1937.

128. TTLTQG-2, GOUCOCH, IA.8/276(2), Le Médecin Directeur de l'Asile à Monsieur le Directeur local de la Sante en Cochinchine, February 10, 1925.

129. ANOM, RSTNF, Rapport au sujet de la création d'un asile colonie sur le terrain de l'Asile de Voi par Dr. Grinsard, June 5, 1937.

5. Mental Illness and Treatment Advice in the Vietnamese Popular Press

1. "Con Rồ," *Ngọ báo*, March 12, 1932.

2. Peter Zinoman, *Vietnamese Colonial Republican: The Political Vision of Vũ Trọng Phụng*. (Berkeley: University of California Press, 2014); Shaun Kingsley Malarney, introduction to *Lục Xì: Prostitution and Venereal Disease in Colonial Hanoi*, by Vũ Trọng Phụng (Honolulu: University of Hawai'i Press, 2011).

3. For work on the colonial press in Vietnam see Shawn McHale, *Print and Power: Confucianism, Communism and Buddhism in the Making of Modern Vietnam* (Honolulu: University of Hawai'i Press, 2003); Philippe Peycam, *The Birth of Vietnamese Political Journalism* (New York: Columbia University Press, 2012); Marr, *Vietnamese Tradition on Trial*.

4. Sabine Frühstück, "Managing the Truth of Sex in Imperial Japan," *Journal of Asian Studies* 59, no. 2 (May 2000): 332–58.

5. Marr, *Vietnamese Tradition on Trial*, esp. chap. 4, "Language and Literacy," and chap 5, "The Question of Women."

6. Marr, *Vietnamese Tradition on Trial*, 213; Nguyen Thien Tinh, "La médecine française," *Tribune Indigène*, April 6, 1922.

7. Monnais and Tousignant, "Colonial Life of Pharmaceuticals."

8. *The Secret Tale of the Asylum (Bí Mật Trong Nhà Điên)*, translated by Lê Quang Thiệp. Hanoi, 1933.

9. TTLTQG-1, IGHSPI, 48–05, Rapport annuel de l'Asile d'Aliénés de Bienhoa, 1931.

10. TTLTQG-2, GOUCOCH, IA.8/2912(3), Rapport annuel de Bienhoa, 1927.

11. Marr, *Vietnamese Tradition on Trial*, 226.

12. Nguyên-Thi Manh-Manh, "Người điên ở nhà thương Biên-Hòa," *Phụ nữ tân văn*, August 2, 1934.11.

13. "Bác Sĩ Nguyễn Văn Hoài," *Bách khoa*, March 15, 1963, 69–72.

14. Nguyên-Thi Manh-Manh, "*Người* điên ở nhà thương Biên-Hòa," 11.

15. "Bác Sĩ Nguyễn Văn Hoài," 71.

16. "Bác Sĩ Nguyễn Văn Hoài," 71.

17. See Fabien Simonis, "Mad Acts, Mad Speech, and Mad People in Late Imperial Chinese Law and Medicine" (PhD diss., Princeton University, 2010).

18. "Dung hoà y lý của Đông Tây," *Y học tạp chí* 11 (1940): 6.

19. The glossary entries that I refer to in the text are from the medical encyclopedia published in *Bao an y báo* from June 1936 through September 1936 (volumes 32–35), all authored by Nguyễn Văn Luyện.

20. Laurence Monnais, "Colonised and Neurasthenic: From the Appropriation of a Word to the Reality of a Malaise de Civilisation in Urban French Vietnam," *Health and History* 14, no. 1 (2012): 121–42.

21. "Đien," in *Bao an y báo*, June–September 1936.

22. "Dở người," in *Bao an y báo*, June—September 1936.

23. "Cuồng," in *Bao an y báo*, June–September 1936.

24. Allen Tran, "A Life of Worry: The Cultural Politics and Phenomenology of Anxiety in Ho Chi Minh City, Vietnam" (PhD diss., University of California–San Diego, 2012); Tine Gammeltoft, *Women's Bodies, Women's Worries: Health and Family Planning in a Vietnamese Rural Commune* (Copenhagen: Nordic Institute of Asian Studies, 1999), quote on page 211.

25. "Ta nên cẩn-thận đền hộ thần kinh," *Khoa học tạp chí*, July 1, 1938.

26. Gammeltoft, *Women's Bodies*, 144.

27. David Marr, "Concepts of 'Individual' and 'Self' in Twentieth-Century Vietnam," *Modern Asian Studies* 34, no.4 (October 2000): 769–96, 795.

28. "Ta nên cẩn-thận đền hộ thần kinh," *Khoa học tạp chí*, July 1, 1938, 300–302.

29. "Đien," in *Bao an y báo*, June–September 1936.

30. Trinh, "Croyances et pratiques médicales sino-annamites," 58.

31. Nguyễn-đăng-Khanh dit Trân-vĩnh-Ký, "Thuốc gia truyền bệnh loạn óc và suy nhược thần kinh," *Khoa học tạp chí*, Issue 48, June 15, 1933, 14–15.

32. "Ta nên cẩn-thận đền hộ thần kinh," 300–302, 301.

33. "Mách giúp bảo giùm," *Khoa học tạp chí*, Issue 84, October 15, 1934, 22.

34. "Mách giúp bảo giùm," October 15, 1934, 22.

35. Marr, *Vietnamese Tradition on Trial*, 213.

36. Monnais and Tousignant, "Colonial Life of Pharmaceuticals," 144.

37. Monnais and Tousignant, "Colonial Life of Pharmaceuticals," 144.

38. "Hỏi đáp," *Khoa học tạp chí*, Issue 64, February 15, 1934, 20. A number of articles about seizure disorders, especially among children, appear during the press at this time. See, for example, "Các chứng-bệnh của trẻ-con: Kinh-phong" [Convulsion], *Vệ sinh báo*, April 1929, 15–16; "Trẻ con động kinh," *Đàn bà*, Issue 52, 1940, 5.

39. Sabine Frühstück, "Managing the Truth of Sex in Imperial Japan," *Journal of Asian Studies* 59, no. 2 (May 2000): 332–58.

40. Nguyễn Công Tiêu, "Mách Giúp Bào Giùm về khoa học," *Khoa học tạp chí*, November 15, 1932, 1.

41. Nguyễn Công Tiêu, "Mách Giúp Bào Giùm về khoa học," 1.

42. On technologies of the self and neoliberalism in Russia, see Tomas Matza, "Moscow's Echo: Technologies of the Self, Publics, and Politics on the Russian Talk Show," *Cultural Anthropology* 24, no. 3 (2009): 489–522.

43. "Chuyên: Ma làm," *Ngày nay*, July 20, 1940, 4.

44. "Chuyên: Ma làm," 4.

45. George Dutton, "Lý Toét in the City: Coming to Terms with the Modern in 1930s Vietnam," *Journal of Vietnamese Studies* 2, no. 1 (February 2007): 80–108.

46. Marr, *Vietnamese Tradition on Trial*, 344.

47. Laurence Monnais, email correspondence, November 28, 2017.

48. Monnais, "Colonised and Neurasthenic," 132; Nguyễn Văn Ký, *La société vietnamienne face à la modernité: Le Tonkin de la fin du XIXe siècle à la seconde guerre mondiale* (Paris: l'Harmattan, 1995); Vu Cong Hoe, "Du suicide dans la société vietnamienne" (Thèse pour le doctorat en médecine). Hanoi: Imprimerie Tonkinoise, 1937.

49. See Gisèle Blanchette, "Neurasthénie sous influence? L'appropriation d'une maladie 'modern' par les classes moyennes du Viêt Nam colonial (1925–1945)" (MA thesis, University of Montreal, 2015); Monnais, "Colonised and Neurasthenic."

50. Vu Cong Hoe, "Du suicide dans la société vietnamienne," 11.

51. As cited in Nguyễn Văn Ký, *La société vietnamienne face à la modernité*. See also Vu Cong Hoe, "Du suicide dans la société vietnamienne," 339. See, for example, Viet Sinh, "Cac Thu Dich Trong May Nam Nay" [Recent epidemics], *Phong hóa*, September 22, 1933, 4.

52. Lorion, *Criminalité*, 85.

53. Vu Cong Hoe, "Du suicide dans la société vietnamienne," 17.

54. Vu Cong Hoe, "Du suicide dans la société vietnamienne," 20.

55. Vu Cong Hoe, "Du suicide dans la société vietnamienne," 18.

56. Linh Vu, "Drowned in Romance, Tears and Rivers: Young Women's Suicide in Early 20th Century Vietnam," *Explorations: A Graduate Student Journal of Southeast Asian Studies* 9 (Spring 2009): 35–46.

57. Cao Thị Như Quỳnh and John C. Shafer, "From Verse Narrative to Novel: The Development of Prose Fiction in Vietnam," *Journal of Asian Studies* 47, no. 4 (November 1988): 756–77.

58. As quoted by Quỳnh and Shafer, "From Verse Narrative to Novel," 774.

59. As quoted by Quỳnh and Shafer, "From Verse Narrative to Novel," 775.

60. The introduction of the term "individual" (*cá nhân*) into the Vietnamese language in the early twentieth century and the growing use of pronouns like *tôi*—designed to give identity to the self without reference to the "other"—whether high or low, kin or non-kin, male or female—reflects this growing interest in individualism. See Marr, "Concepts of 'Individual' and 'Self.'"

61. Zinoman, *Vietnamese Colonial Republican*, 139.

62. Marr, "Concepts of 'Individual' and 'Self,'" 781.

63. "Tâm lý học" [Psychology] serialized in *Nam phong* from November 1924 to August 1926.

64. Martina T. Nguyen, "The Self-Reliant Literary Group (Tự Lực Văn Đoàn): Colonial Modernism in Vietnam, 1932–1941" (PhD diss., University of California–Berkeley, 2012), 103.

65. Hue Tam Ho Tai, *Radicalism and the Origins of the Vietnamese Revolution* (Cambridge, MA: Harvard University Press, 1996), 72–87; Mark Bradley, "Becoming Van Minh: Civilizational Discourse and Visions of the Self in Twentieth Century Vietnam," *Journal of World History* 15, no. 1 (March 2004): 65–83, 67.

66. "Chuyên: Đien," *Ngày này*, May 25, 1940, 1940, 4.

67. *Dumb Luck: A Novel by Vũ Trọng Phụng*, ed. Peter Zinoman, trans. Nguyễn Nguyệt Cầm and Peter Zinoman (Ann Arbor: University of Michigan Press, 2002), 178.

68. *Dumb Luck*, 179.

69. Tân Thach, "Tôi đã gặp những người điên," *Vịt đực*, September 21, 1938, 6.

70. TTLTQG-1, IGHSP, 004, Rapport annuel de 1928.

71. "Điên vì tình," *Trung bắc tân văn*, June 16, 1940, 4–5.

72. See Hue Tam Ho Tai, *Radicalism*, 88–113 ; Marr, *Vietnamese Tradition on Trial*, 190–251.

73. John Whitmore, "Social Organization and Confucian Thought in Vietnam," *Journal of Southeast Asian Studies* 15, no. 2 (September 1984): 296–306.

74. Marr, *Vietnamese Tradition on Trial*, 214.

75. "Dưới mắt chúng tôi: Cô Vũ thị Cúc điên hay không điên?" *Trung bắc tân văn*, March 24, 1940, 12–13.

76. Zinoman, *Vietnamese Colonial Republican*, 140.

6. Psychiatric Expertise and Indochina's Crime Problem

1. Emmanuelle Saada, *Empire's Children: Race, Filiation and Citizenship in the French Colonies*, trans. Arthur Goldhammer (Chicago: University of Chicago Press, 2012); Christina E. Firpo, *The Uprooted: Race, Children and Imperialism in French Indochina, 1890–1980*. Honolulu: University of Hawai'i Press, 2016; Ann Laura Stoler, "Sexual Affronts and Racial Frontiers: European Identities and the Cultural Politics of Exclusion in Colonial Southeast Asia," *Comparative Studies in Society and History* 34, no. 3 (1992): 514–51; Zinoman, *Colonial Bastille*.

2. My interest here is in the jurisdictional claims between a profession and its work and the kinds of competing claims that drive this boundary making. I take special inspiration from the work of Gil Eyal, who takes up this analysis of jurisdictional struggles by tracing how forms of expertise—analyzed as networks that link together objects, actors, techniques, devices, and institutional and spatial arrangements—are gradually assembled. Eyal, "For a Sociology of Expertise: The Social Origins of the Autism Epidemic," *American Journal of Sociology* 118, no. 4 (January 2013): 863–907. This perspective is a departure from the work of Southeast Asian scholars who have tended to examine the centrality of the criminal to nationalist narratives and the formation of modernity in Southeast Asia. See Vincente Rafael, ed., *Figures of Criminality in Indonesia, the Philippines and Colonial Vietnam* (Ithaca, NY: Cornell Southeast Asia Program, 1999).

3. For examples of indigenous tribunals adjudicating criminal responsibility on the basis of medical opinions according to the Vietnamese legal code, prior to the 1918 regulations, resulting in the sequestering of the accused at home under lock and key, see TTLTQG-1, RST, 73751, Au sujet de . . . Ngôn, April 12, 1916.

4. People could also request their own internment under a *placement volontaire*. See Pierre Dorolle, *La Législation Indochinoise sur les aliénés: Exposé et commentaire des dispositions du décret du 18 juillet 1930* (Saigon: Imprimerie A. Portail, 1941).

5. TTLTQG-1, RST, 73745, État des propositions présentées à l'Inspection Générale des Services Saniatires pour l'application au Tonkin du Décret du 18 Juillet 1930 sur l'assistance psychiatrique; TTLTQG-1, IGHSP, 51–01, Rapport sur le fonctionnement du service de psychiatrie de l'Hôpital de Chôquan en 1934.

6. TTLTQG-1, MH, 5781, Internement des indigènes et européens à l'Asile d'aliénés de Bien Hoa, 1925.

7. See, for example, TTLTQG-1, RST, 73752–01, Rapport médico-légal a.s. du nommé . . . Hang, December 30, 1919.

8. TTLTQG-1, RST, 73741, Rapport médico-légal, d'examen du . . . Cac, 57 ans, cultivateur, détenu, February 4, 1928.

9. TTLTQG-1, RST, 73741, Rapport médico-légal, d'examen du . . . Cac . . . February 4, 1928.

10. Dr. Roussy, "Rapport sur le fonctionnement de l'Asile d'Aliénés de Bienhoa (Cochinchine)," *Annales de médecine et de pharmacie coloniales* 24, 1926: 34–56.

11. TTLTQG-1, IGHSP, 48–05, Rapport annuel de l'Asile d'Aliénés de Bien Hoa, 1931.

12. TTLTQG-1, IGHSP, 51–01, Rapport sur le fonctionnement du service de psychiatrie de l'Hôpital de Chôquan en 1934.

13. Here I follow the work of David Wright, who argues that in nineteenth-century Britain the process of certification assumed a central role as medicine underwent a period of professionalization. Wright, "The Certification of Insanity in Nineteenth-Century England and Wales," *History of Psychiatry* (1998): 267–90, 269.

14. Sloan Mahone,"Psychiatry in the East African Colonies: A Background to Confinement," *International Review of Psychiatry* 18, no. 4 (2006): 327–32.

15. TTLTQG-1, RST, 73748–02, Le Procureur Général, près la Cour d'Appel de Hanoi, à Monsieur le President du Tribunal Provincial, Lang-Son, July 4, 1928.

16. TTLTQG-1, RST, 73748–02, Le Procureur Général, près la Cour d'Appel de Hanoi . . . July 4, 1928.

17. In some cases, once declared cured, former patients would be reintegrated back into prisons; otherwise they would be sent home to families, who would assume responsibility for their care. TTLTQG-2, GOUCOCH, IA.8/276(2), Rapport annuel de Bien Hoa, 1924.

18. TTLTQG-2, GOUCOCH, IA.8/155(2), Le Procureur de la Republique près le Tribunal de 1ère instance de Mytho, à Monsieur le Procureur Général, Chef du Service judiciare de la Cochinchine et du Cambodge à Saigon, June 1, 1898.

19. TTLTQG-1, RST, 7376–02, Note de F. Faugère, Commissaire de Police (Hanoi) pour Monsieur le Contrôleur Général de la Sûreté, Chef des Services de Police au Tonkin, August 10, 1939.

20. Colonial doctors also worried about individuals whom they accused of faking their mental illness so as to avoid prison. See TTLTQG-2, GOUCOCH, IA.8/281(1), Le Médecin Directeur de l'Asile de Bien Hoa à Monsieur le Gouverneur de la Cochinchine, au sujet de . . . Vo, June 15, 1924.

21. TTLTQG-2, GOUCOCH, IA.8/281(2), Rapport Médico-Légal par Dr. Levot, fait à Cantho, May 7, 1925.

22. Roussy, as quoted by Augagneur in TTLTQG-2, IA.8/281(2), GOUCOCH, Médecin Directeur de l'Asile de Bienhoa à Monsieur le Gouverneur de Cochinchine, August 10, 1926.

23. TTLTQG-2, IA.8/281(2), GOUCOCH, Le Médecin Directeur de l'Asile de Bien Hoa . . . August 10, 1926.

24. TTLTQG-2, GOUCOCH, IA.8/281(2), Certificat semestriel de . . . Sau, fait par Robert à Bien Hoa, June 18, 1921.

25. TTLTQG-2, GOUCOCH, IA.8/281(2), Le Procureur Général près la Cour d'Appel de Saigon à Monsieur le Gouverneur de la Cochinchine, June 29, 1925.

26. TTLTQG-2, GOUCOCH, 276(2), Le Médecin Directeur de l'Asile de Bien Hoa à Monsieur le Gouverneur de la Cochinchine, April 22, 1925.

27. TTLTQG-2, GOUCOCH, IA.8/281(2), Le Procureur Général près la Cour d'Appel de Saigon . . . June 29, 1925.

28. TTLTQG-2, GOUCOCH, IA.8/281(2), Le Procureur Général près la Cour d'Appel de Saigon . . . June 29, 1925.

29. TTLTQG-2, GOUCOCH, 1363, Négligence commise par le Parquet de Cantho sur un individu atteint d'aliénation mentale, 1926.

30. ANOM, "Cantho—Anthropophage," in L'opinion, April 20, 1926.

31. TTLTQG-1, 73742, Rapport du Dr. Naudin, médecin traitant au service de psychiatrie, August 5, 1933.

32. TTLTQG-1, 73742, Rapport du Dr. Naudin . . . August 5, 1933.

33. TTLTQG-1, 73742, Le Procureur de la République près le Tribunal de 1ère instance de Hanoi, à Monsieur l'Inspecteur Général de l'Hygiène et de la Santé Publiques, Hanoi, July 24, 1933.

34. TTLTQG-1, 73742, Le Procureur de la République près le Tribunal de 1ère instance de Hanoi . . . July 24, 1933.

35. TTLTQG-1, RST, 73736, Le Docteur Bouisset, Médecin traitant à l'Hôpital René Robin à Monsieur le Directeur Local de la Santé, March 2, 1939.

36. TTLTQG-1, RST, 73736, Le Docteur de Raymond, Directeur Local de la Santé à Monsieur le Résident Supérieur au Tonkin, August 10, 1935.

37. TTLTQG-1, Direction des Finances de l'Indochine, 18460, Rapport du Directeur de la Santé en Annam sur le régime legal des Aliénés en Indochine, 1912.

38. TTLTQG-2, GOUCOCH, IA.8/2910, Le Directeur Local de la Sante en Cochinchine a Monsieur le Gouverneur de la Cochinchine, November 10, 1927.

39. Roger Grinsard, "L'enfance coupable au Tonkin," Revue Médicale Française d'Extrême-Orient, 16, no. 1 (January 1938): 1163–76.

40. TTLTQG-1, Direction des Finances de l'Indochine, 18460, Rapport du Directeur de la Santé en Annam . . . 1912.

41. TTLTQG-1, Direction des Finances de l'Indochine, Rapport du Directeur de la Santé en Annam . . . 1912.

42. See Sarah Fishman, The Battle for Children: World War II, Youth Crime and Juvenile Justice in Twentieth-Century France (Cambridge, MA: Harvard University Press, 2002).

43. Fishman, Battle for Children.

44. As quoted in Grinsard, "L'enfance coupable au Tonkin."

45. Marc Renneville, "La psychiatrie légale dans le projet de réforme du code pénal français (1930–1938)," in Psychiatries dans l'histoire. Actes du 6ème congrès de

l'Association européenne pour l'histoire de la psychiatrie, ed. J. Arveiller (Caen: Presses universitaires de Caen, 2008), 385–405.

46. Paul Schiff, "La prophylaxie criminelle et la collaboration médico-judiciare," *Revue de science criminelle et de droit pénal comparé* 4 (Octobre–Décembre 1936): 479–92.

47. Lê Vân Kim, "La protection légale de l'enfance," in *Semaine de l'enfance du 1er au 7 juillet 1934: Rapports* (Saigon: Imprimerie de l'union, 1934).

48. TTLTQG-1, RST, 72060, Note de M. Habert, Directeur du Service de la Justice en Indochine, sur le régime pénal applicable aux mineurs en Indochine, March 28, 1927.

49. The Trí Cụ reformatory grew out of an earlier penitentiary colony named Nhã Nam. Located in Phủ Lạng Thương, in Bắc Giang province, in 1920 it first received forty prisoners, including seventeen children aged twelve to thirteen, whom it was too expensive and impractical to send to Ông Yêm in Cochinchina. See ANOM, RSTNF, 3684, "Relèvement de l'Enfance (Colonie Agricole de Tri-Cu)," 1934.

50. Monsieur le Président Tran-Van-Ty, 1931 Congrès national de droit pénal colonial, as quoted in Kim, "La protection légale."

51. ANOM, GGI, 65925, Projet de Créations ou de réformes de colonies de rele-vèment moral (filles ou garçons), Monsieur le Directeur des Bureaux du Gouver-nement de la Cochinchine, correspondance privée, Saigon, March 1931; ANOM, RSTNF, 2493, Le Garde Principal Commandant le Poste de Garde Indigene de Tri Cu à Monsieur l'Administrateur Resident de France à Bac Giang, August 25, 1931.

52. TTLTQG-1, RST, 74575–04, Renseignements sur l'organisation de la prévoy-ance et le fonctionnement de l'assistance médicale, sociale, de la société de protec-tion des enfants indigènes, 1937.

53. TTLTQG-1, MH, 3970, Le Commissaire Central de Police à Monsieur l'Administrateur Maire de la Ville de Hanoi, October 6, 1926.

54. TTLTQG-1, MH, 3971–03, Interrogatoire de . . . Lan, Police Municipale de Hanoi, September 9, 1935; TTLTQG-1, MH, 3971–03, Interrogatoire de . . . Sen, Police Municipale de Hanoi, May 18, 1935.

55. TTLTQG-1, RST, 56151, Le Commissaire Central de Police à Monsieur le Résident Maire de la Ville, au sujet de l'internement de . . . Thuon à la colonie agri-cole de Tri Cu (Bac Giang), January 14, 1929.

56. TTLTQG-1, MH, 3971–03, Interrogatoire de . . . Đât, Police Municipale de Hanoi, February 12, 1935.

57. TTLTQG-1, MH, 3971–03, Interrogatoire de . . . Sen . . . May 18, 1935.

58. In fact, delinquents at Trí Cụ who proved well behaved could subsequently find themselves farmed out to the neighboring Anloc and Courtenay plantations, where they made a small salary. ANOM, GGI, 65925, Rapport de M. G. Boyer Judge de Paix à compétence étendue Bienhoa à Monsieur le Procureur Général à Saigon, sur la visite des jeunes détenus d'Ong-Yêm detaches à la Plantation d'Anlôc, 1927.

59. ANOM, GGI, 65925, Le Procureur Général près la Cour d'Appel de Saigon à Monsieur le Procureur Général, Directeur des Services judiciaires de l'Indochine à Hanoi, Saigon, February 15, 1939.

60. Zinoman, *Colonial Bastille*, 206.

61. Zinoman, *Colonial Bastille*, 206.

62. *Rapports au Conseil de Gouverment Général de l'Indochine, Deuxième Partie* (Hanoi: Imprimerie d'Extrême Orient, 1927), 274; ANOM, GGI, 65925, Gouverneur

General de l'Indochine à Monsieur le Directeur de l'Agence Economique de l'Indochine, Situation des mineurs coupables en Indochine, August 24, 1931.

63. Zinoman, *Colonial Bastille*, 208.

64. TTLTQG-2, GOUCOCH, 1261, Le Directeur de la Colonie Pénitentiaire d'Ong-Yem a Monsieur le Gouverneur de la Cochinchine, June 3, 1931.

65. See, for example, ANOM, RST, 2493, Le Chef Local de Police à Monsieur le Résident Supérieur au Tonkin, au sujet. . . . Hoa, February 1, 1943.

66. ANOM, GGI, 65925, Le Resident Superieur au Tonkin à Monsieur le Premier Président, Chef de l'Administration de la Justice en Indochine, November 19, 1924.

67. ANOM, GGI, 65925, Note de M. Habert . . . March 28, 1927.

68. See, for example, ANOM, 65603, GGI, Le Procureur Général près la Cour d'Appel de Hanoi à Monsieur le Directeur de l'Administration de la Justice en Indochine, November 9, 1926.

69. ANOM, RSTNF, 2493, Note pour Monsieur le Résident Supérieur a/s . . . Nuôi, August 6, 1934.

70. Between 1929 and 1943 women made up 5 percent of the inmate population in provincial prisons (9,589 out of 163,686), and 13 percent of the inmate population in central prisons (4,253 out of 29,450). See Zinoman, *Colonial Bastille*, 105. See also ANOM, GGI, 65925, Le Gouverneur de la Cochinchine, à Monsieur le Directeur de l'Administration Judiciaire en Indochine, April 9, 1927.

71. ANOM, RSTNF, 2493, Le Résident Supérieur au Tonkin à Monsieur le Président de la Société de Protection des enfants annamites et a Madame la Directrice de l'Asile des Incurables à Thai-Ha-Ap, August 14, 1924.

72. Laurence Monnais, "Preventive Medicine and 'Mission Civilisatrice': Uses of the BCG Vaccine in French Colonial Vietnam between the Two World Wars," *International Journal of Asia Pacific Studies* 2, no. 1 (2006): 41–68.

73. Monnais, "Preventive Medicine."

74. ANOM, GGI, 65925, Projet de Créations ou de réformes de colonies . . . March 1931.

75. As quoted in David M. Pomfret, *Youth and Empire: Trans-Colonial Childhoods in British and French Asia* (Stanford, CA: Stanford University Press, 2015), 144.

76. For the history of maternal and child health care in colonial Vietnam, including a discussion of healthy baby contests, see Thuy Linh Nguyen, *Childbirth, Maternity and Medical Pluralism in French Colonial Vietnam, 1880–1945* (Rochester, NY: University of Rochester Press, 2016).

77. Fishman, *Battle for Children*, 26.

78. Attempts to make uniform the age of majority across Indochina (in Cochinchina it was shifted upwards to eighteen in accordance with French law, while in Tonkin it remained at sixteen, a relic of the Gia Long Code), as well as to align juvenile justice regimes across Indochina and France, predate the 1934 meeting. See ANOM, GGI, 65603, Le Procureur Général près la Cour d'appel de Saigon, à Monsieur le Directeur de l'Administration de la Justice à Hanoi, February 28, 1927; TTLTQG-1, RST, 72060, Note de M. Habert . . . March 28, 1927.

79. ANOM, GGI, 65925, Le Résident Supérieur au Tonkin à Monsieur le Directeur de l'Administration Judiciare en Indochine au sujet création colonie agricole de Tri-Cu, August 29, 1925. For data on increasing numbers of children sentenced to youth reformatories, see ANOM, GGI, 65925, Etats des mineurs justiciables du Tribunal

de 1er Instance de Hanoi pendant les années 1926, 1927, 1928, 1929, and 1930. The number drops again in 1931, for unknown reasons.

80. Kim, "La protection légale," 26.

81. Grinsard, "L'enfance coupable au Tonkin, " 1163.

82. ANOM, 65925, GGI, Note de M. Habert . . . March 28, 1927.

83. ANOM, 65603, GGI, Le Résident Supérieur au Tonkin à Monsieur le Gouverneur General de l'Indochine au sujet de l'extension à l'Indochine de la législation sur l'enfance coupable, February 9, 1924.

84. Grinsard, "L'enfance coupable au Tonkin," 1172.

85. TTLTQG-1, RST, 3753, Procès-verbal de la commission de surveillance de l'Asile d'Aliénés de Voi, June 15, 1938.

86. TTLTQG-1, RST, 3753, Procès-verbal de la commission de surveillance de l'Asile d'Aliénés de Voi, June 15, 1938.

87. TTLTQG-2, GOUCOCH, IA.8/281(2), Rapport médico-légal de André G., fait à Can Tho par le Dr. Levot, May 7, 1925.

88. Grinsard, "L'enfance coupable du Tonkin," 1167–72.

89. Grinsard, "L'enfance coupable du Tonkin," 1175.

90. ANOM, RSTNF, 3907, Le Gouverneur Général de l'Indochine Jules Brévié à Monsieur le Ministre des Colonies (Inspection Générale du Service de Santé des Colonies 2ème Section), July 1, 1938.

91. ANOM, RSTNF, 3907, Le Gouverneur Général de l'Indochine Jules Brévié . . . July 1, 1938.

92. Kim, "La protection légale."

93. Kim, "La protection légale."

94. Trân Van Ty address at the 1931 meeting of the Congrès national de droit pénal colonial, as quoted in Kim, "La protection légale."

95. *Rapport au Conseil Supérieur (Gouvernement générale de l'Indochine)*, (Hanoi: Imprimerie d'Extrême Orient, 1927), 260.

96. ANOM, RST, 03749, Le Directeur Local de la Santé à Monsieur l'Inspecteur Général de l'Hygiène et de la Santé Publiques en Indochine, August 24, 1938.

97. Pierre Dorolle, as quoted in Edouard Marquis, "La protection de l'enfance en Cochinchine," *Revue médico-sociale et de protection de l'enfance* 5 (1937): 369–81, 379.

98 Dorolle as quoted in Edouard Marquis, *L'oeuvre humaine de la France en cochinchine* (Saigon: Imprimerie du Théâtre, 1956), 59.

99. ANOM, RST, 3907, Jules Brévié, le Gouverneur Général de l'Indochine à Monsieur le Résident Supérieur au Tonkin, January 10, 1939.

100. ANOM, 65926, Le Gouverneur Général de l'Indochine à Monsieur le Gouverneur de la Cochinchine au sujet "voeu du Conseil de perfectionnement de la colonie agricole de Ong-Yêm," March 9, 1935.

101. ANOM, Agence économique de la France d'outre mer (AGEFOM), 238, "En faveur de l'enfance malheureuse et déficiente," *Bulletin quotidien*, October 4, 1939.

102. Grinsard, "L'enfance coupable du Tonkin," 1174.

103. Dr. Pierre Dorolle in 1934, as quoted by Marquis, *L'oeuvre humaine de la France,* 58.

104. ANOM, RSTNF, 3907, Jules Brévié, le Gouverneur Général de l'Indochina . . . January 10, 1939 (emphasis added by author). See also ANOM, AGEFOM, 238, "En faveur de l'enfance malheureuse et déficiente."

105. Grinsard, "L'enfance coupable du Tonkin," 1175.

106. Kim, "La protection légale."

107. ANOM, RST, 3753, Le Docteur de Raymond Directeur Local de la Santé à Monsieur le Résident Supérieur au Tonkin (1er Bureau), Hanoi, September 21, 1939.

108. ANOM, GGI, 65925, Projet de Créations ou de réformes de colonies . . . March 1931; ANOM, RST, 2493, L'Administrateur de 2ème classe Pettelat Résident de France à Bac-Giang à Monsieur le Résident Supérieur au Tonkin (Cabinet), August 17, 1937.

109. ANOM, RST, 3907, L'Administrateur de 2ème classe Pettelat, Résident de France a Bacgiang à Monsieur le Résident Supérieur au Tonkin, March 30, 1938.

110. Marquis, *L'oeuvre humaine de la France*, 46.

111. See various newspaper clippings related to the "colonies de vacances" for children in ANOM, AGEFOM, 238, Santé: Enfance et jeunesse.

112. ANOM, 65925, Projet de Créations ou de réformes de colonies . . . March 1931.

113. Marquis, *L'oeuvre humaine de la France*, 55.

114. ANOM, AGEFOM, 237, "Informations Coloniales: Cochinchine: Pour l'enfance déficient," April 19, 1939.

115. ANOM, RST, 3907, Lettre de Yves Châtel à Inspecteur Général du Travail en Indochine, March 10, 1938.

116. TTLTQG-1, RST, 74575–04, Renseignements sur l'organisation de la prévoyance et le fonctionnement de l'assistance médicale, sociale, de la société de protection des enfants indigènes, 1937.

117. ANOM, RST, 2493, Note pour Monsieur le Résident Supérieur au sujet. . . . Suyen, July 23, 1943.

118. For more on youth and Vichy in Indochina, see Paul Sager, "Youth and Nationalism in Vichy Indochina," *Journal of Vietnamese Studies* 3, no. 3 (Fall 2008): 291–301; Micheline Lessard, "Tradition for Rebellion: Vietnamese Students and Teachers and Anti-colonial Resistance, 1888–1931" (PhD diss., Cornell University, 1995); Anne Raffin, "The Causes and Consequences of Patriotic Youth Mobilization in Vichy France and Indochina during and after World War II" (PhD diss., New School, 2000); Marr, *Vietnamese Tradition on Trial*; see Eric Jennings, "Conservative Confluences, 'Nativist' Synergy: Reinscribing Vichy's National Revolution in Indochina, 1940–1945," *French Historical Studies* 27, no. 3 (2004): 601–35; also David Marr, *Vietnam 1945: The Quest for Power*. Berkeley: University of California Press, 1997.

119. ANOM, RST, 2493, P. Pujol Controleur Général de la Sûreté à Monsieur le Résident Supérieur au Tonkin a.s. . . . Chuyen, February 10, 1942.

120. ANOM, RST, 2493, Hanoi, le 24 Avril 1942 Le Chef des Services de Police au Tonkin à Monsieur le Résident Supérieur au Tonkin, au sujet mésures de clémence (. . . Ninh), April 24, 1942.

121. Jacques Cantier and Eric Jennings, *Empire colonial sous Vichy* (Paris: Odile Jacob, 2004), 47.

122. ANOM, GGI, 65603, Le Procureur Général à Monsieur le Directeur de l'Administration de la Justice en Indochine, Feburary 26, 1927.

123. ANOM, RST, 2493, Note de Chef du 1er Bureau pour Monsieur le Résident Supérieur, May, 7, 1942.

124. ANOM, RST, 2493, Le Commissaire du Gouvernement à Monsieur le Général de Corps d'Armée, Commandant Supérieur des Troupes du Groupes de l'Indochine, au sujet . . . Suyen, July 15, 1943.

Conclusion

1. Michael Macdonald, *Mystical Bedlam: Madness, Anxiety and Healing in Seventeenth-century England* (Cambridge: Cambridge University Press, 1981).

2. See Michel Foucault, *Madness and Civilization: A History of Insanity in the Age of Reason.* (New York: Penguin Random House, 1988).

3. Important exceptions for the Asian context include Zhiying Ma, "An Iron Cage of Civilization? Missionary Psychiatry, the Chinese Family and a Colonial Dialect of Enlightenment," in *Psychiatry and Chinese History*, ed. Howard Chiang (London: Pickering and Chatto, 2014), 71–90; Hayang Kim, "Sick at Heart: Mental Illness in Modern Japan" (PhD diss., Columbia University, 2015); Akihito Suzuki, "Between Two Psychiatric Regimes: Migration and Psychiatry in Early Twentieth Century Japan," in *Migration, Ethnicity and Health*, ed. Angela McCarthy and Catharine Coleborne (New York: Taylor and Francis, 2001), 141–56.

4. In *Psychiatric Power*, which immediately precedes *Discipline and Punish*, Foucault offers a view of power that is continuous and relational, as evidenced in the interactions between patients and doctors, the family and the asylum. Discipline does not substitute for repression, but together they exist in a larger equation in which the relation of power is fundamental.

5. On the "carceral archipelago" of empire see Ann Laura Stoler, *Along the Archival Grain.*

6. Robert A. McKinley, "Psychiatry in Vietnam—1966," *American Journal of Psychiatry* 123, no. 4 (October 1966): 421; Richard C. Keller, "Pinel in the Maghreb: Liberation, Confinement and Psychiatric Reform in French North Africa," *Bulletin of the History of Medicine* 79, no. 3 (Fall 2005): 459–99.

7. "Bác Sĩ Nguyễn Văn Hoài," *Bách Khoa* 149 (March 15, 1963): 69–72, 72.

8. For more on Central Psychiatric Hospital II, formerly Biên Hòa, see the work of the medical anthropologist Allen Tran, "A Life of Worry: The Cultural Politics and Phenomenology of Anxiety in Ho Chi Minh City, Vietnam" (PhD diss., University of California–San Diego, 2012).

9. *Work of WHO in the Western Pacific Region*, Twelfth Annual Report of the Regional Director to the Regional Committee for the Western Pacific (1962), WP/RC13/2 (available online: http://apps.who.int/iris/handle/10665/207377).

10. Harry Minas et al., "Mental Health in Vietnam," in *Mental Health in Asia and the Pacific: Historical and Comparative Perspectives*, ed. Harry Minas and Milton Lewis (New York: Springer, 2017), 145–62.

11. The sum of $266.6 million was used to fund HIV treatment in Vietnam from 2009 to 2010, of which almost three-fourths came from international donors. See Ahmed Tanvir et al., "HIV and Injecting Drug Users in Vietnam: An Overview of Policies and Responses," *World Medical and Health PoliWorld Medical and Health Policy* 6, no. 4 (2014): 395–418.

12. Harry Minas et al., "Mental Health in Vietnam," in *Mental Health in Asia and the Pacific: Historical and Comparative Perspectives*, ed. Harry Minas and Milton Lewis (New York: Springer, 2017), 145–62.

13. Human Rights Watch, *The Rehab Archipelago: Forced Labor and Other Abuses in Drug Detention Centers in Vietnam*, 2011, https://www.hrw.org/sites/default/files/reports/vietnam0911ToPost.pdf.

14. Claire Edington, "Drug Detention and Human Rights in Post-Đổi Mới Vietnam," in *The Postcolonial World*, ed. David Kim and Jyotsna Singh (London: Routledge, 2016), 325–42.

15. Tran-Minh Tung, "The Family and the Management of Mental Health Problems in Vietnam."

Bibliography

Unpublished Archival Sources

Vietnam

Trung Tâm Lưu Trữ Quốc Gia I (TTLTQG-I) (Vietnam National Archives Centre I), Hà Nội
Fonds de la Direction des Finances de l'Indochine
Fonds du Gouvernement Général de l'Indochine (GGI)
Fonds la Mairie de Hanoi (MH)
Fonds de la Résidence de Bac Giang
Fonds de la Résidence de Ha Dong
Fonds de la Résidence de Nam Dinh
Fonds de la Résidence Supérieur au Tonkin (RST)
Fonds de la Service Local de la Santé du Tonkin
Inspection Générale de l'Hygiène et Santé Publique (IGHSP)
Trung Tâm Lưu Trữ Quốc Gia II (TTLTQG-II) (Vietnam National Archives Centre II), Hồ Chí Minh City
Fonds du Gouvernement de la Cochinchine (GOUCOCH)

Cambodia

National Archives of Cambodia (NAC), Phnom Penh
Résidence Supérieur au Cambodge (RSC)

France

Archives Nationales d'Outre Mer (ANOM), Aix-en-Provence
Affaires politiques (AFF POL)
Agence économique de la France d'outre mer (AGEFOM)
Commission d'Enquête des Territoires d'Outre Mer (Guernut)
Fonds du Gouvernement General de l'Indochine (GGI)
Iconothèque (ICO)
Fonds de la Résidence Supérieur au Tonkin, Nouveau Fonds (RSTNF)
Gouvernement Général de l'Indochine, Service économique (SE)
Haut commissariat de France pour l'Indochine, Service de Protection du Corps expéditionnaire (S.P.C.E.)

Indochine, Ancien fonds (INDO AF)
Indochine, Nouveau fonds (INDO NF)
Ministère des colonies, Service de liaison avec les originaires des territoires
    français d'outre-mer (SLOTFOM)
Centre de Documentation de l'Institut de Médecine Tropicale de la Service de
    Santé des Armées (PHARO), Marseille

Libraries

Bibliothèque Inter-Universitaire de Médecine, Paris
Bibliothèque Nationale de France, Paris
Butler Library, Columbia University, New York
New York Academy of Medicine, New York
Thư Viện Quốc Gia Việt Nam (Vietnam National Library), Hà Nội

Published Sources
Periodicals

FRANCE

Annales d'hygiene et de médecine coloniales, Paris, 1898–1914
Annales de médecine et de pharmacie coloniales, Paris, 1920–1940
Gazette médicale de Paris: journal de médecine et des sciences accessoires, Paris, 1830–
    1915
Informateur des alienistes et des neurologists, Paris, 1906–1925
L'hygiène mentale: journal de psychiatrie appliquée, Paris, 1925–1973
Journal de médécine légal psychiatrique et d'anthropologie criminelle, Paris, 1906
La presse médicale, Paris, 1893–1945
Revue médico-sociale et de protection de l'enfance, Paris, 1933–1939
Revue de science criminelle et de droit pénal comparé, Paris, 1936–1959

VIETNAM

Bách khoa, Saigon, 1957–1975
Bao an y báo. Revue de vulgarisation médicale, Hanoi, 1934–1938
Bulletin de l'Ecole française d'Extrême Orient, Hanoi, 1901–2004; Paris, 2005–2015
Bulletin de la société médico-chirurgicale de l'Indochine, Hanoi, 1908–1937; later:
    Revue médicale française d'Extrême-Orient, Hanoi, 1938–1944
Khoa học tạp chí. Revue de vulgarisation scientifique, Saigon, 1923–1926
Nam phong, Hanoi, 1917–1934
Ngày nay, Hanoi, 1935–1940
Ngọ Báo, Hanoi, 1927–1952
Phụ nữ tân văn, Saigon, 1929–1934
Tribune indigène, Saigon, 1917–1925

Trung bắc tân văn, Hanoi, 1940–1945
Vệ sinh báo. Journal de vulgarisation d'hygiène, Hanoi, 1926–1933
Vịt đực, Hanoi, 1938–1939
Y học tạp chí. Revue de médecine, Hanoi, 1937–1941

Articles and Books

Amrith, Sunil S. *Decolonizing International Health: India and Southeast Asia, 1930–1965.* Basingstoke, UK: Palgrave MacMillan, 2006.

Anderson, Warwick. *Colonial Pathologies: American Tropical Medicine, Race and Hygiene in the Philippines.* Durham, NC: Duke University Press, 2006.

——. "Making Global Health History: The Postcolonial Worldliness of Biomedicine." *Social History of Medicine* 27, no. 2 (May 2014): 372–84.

Anderson, Warwick, Deborah Jenson, and Richard Keller. *Unconscious Dominions: Psychoanalysis, Colonial Trauma, and Global Sovereignties.* Durham, NC: Duke University Press, 2011.

Andrews, Jonathan. "Case Notes, Case Histories, and the Patient's Experience of Insanity at Gartnavel Royal Asylum, Glasgow, in the Nineteenth Century." *Social History of Medicine* 11, no. 2 (1998): 255–81.

Arnold, David, and Erich Dewald, "Cycles of Empowerment? The Bicycle and Everyday Technology in Colonial India and Vietnam." *Comparative Studies in Society and History* 53, no. 4 (October 2011): 971–96.

Aso, Mitchitake. "Profit or People? Rubber Plantations and Everyday Technology in Rural Indochina." *Modern Asian Studies* 46, no. 1 (2012): 19–45.

Atkinson, Jane. "Shamanisms Today." *Annual Review of Anthropology* 21 (1992): 307–30.

Au, Sokhieng. *Mixed Medicines: Health and Culture in French Colonial Cambodia.* Chicago: University of Chicago Press, 2011.

Aubin, H. "L'Assistance psychiatrique indigène aux colonies." *Rapport au Congrès des Médecins Aliénistes et Neurologistes de France et des Pays de Langue Française, XLIIe session—Alger 6–11 Avril 1938.* Paris: Masson et Cie, 1938.

Barnhart, James David. "Violence and the Civilizing Mission: Native Justice in French Colonial Vietnam, 1858–1914" PhD diss., University of Chicago, 1999.

Barth, Volker, and Roland Cvetkovski, eds. *Imperial Cooperation and Transfer, 1870–1930: Empires and Encounters.* London: Bloomsbury Academic Publishing, 2015.

Bartlett, Peter, and David Wright, eds. *Outside the Walls of the Asylum: The History of Care in Community 1750–2000.* London: Athlone Press, 1999.

Bates, Ann, and A. W. Bates. "Lãn Ông (Lê Hữu Trác, 1720–1791) and the Vietnamese Medical Tradition." *Journal of Medical Biography* 15 (2007): 158–64.

Baum, Emily. *Spit, Chains and Hospital Beds: A History of Madness in Republican Beijing.* PhD diss, University of California, San Diego, 2013.

Bell, John Elderkin. *The Family in the Hospital: Lessons from Developing Countries.* Washington, DC: National Institutes of Health, 1969.

Biehl, João. *Vita: Life in a Zone of Social Abandonment.* Berkeley: University of California Press, 2005.

Blanchette, Gisèle. "Neurasthénie sous influence? L'appropriation d'une maladie 'moderne' par les classes moyennes du Việt Nam colonial (1925–1945)." PhD diss., University of Montreal, 2015.

Boomgaard, Peter, and Ian Brown, eds. *Weathering the Storm: The Economies of Southeast Asia in the 1930s Depression*. Singapore: ISEAS, 2000.

Bordeaux, Pascal. "Emergence et constitution de la communauté du Bouddhisme Hoa Hoa: Contribution à l'histoire sociale du delta du Mékong (1935–1955)." Thèse du doctorat, École pratique des hautes études, Paris, 2003.

Boschma, Geertje. *The Rise of Mental Health Nursing: A History of Psychiatric Care in Dutch Asylums, 1890–1920*. Amsterdam: Amsterdam University Press, 2003.

Bosquet, G. H. *A French View of the Netherlands Indies*. London: Oxford University Press, 1940.

Bradley, Mark. "Becoming Van Minh: Civilizational Discourse and Visions of the Self in Twentieth Century Vietnam." *Journal of World History* 15, no. 1 (March 2004): 65–83.

Breman, Jan. *Taming the Coolie Beast: Plantation Society and the Colonial Order in Southeast Asia*. Delhi: Oxford University Press, 1989.

Brocheux, Pierre. *The Mekong Delta: Ecology, Economy and Revolution, 1860–1890* Monograph No. 12. Madison: Center for Southeast Asian Studies, University of Wisconsin, 1995.

Brocheux, Pierre, and Daniel Hémery. *Indochine: La colonisation ambiguë, 1858–1954*. Paris: Découverte, 2001.

Brown, Julie V. "Peasant Survival Strategies in Late Imperial Russia: The Social Uses of the Mental Hospital." *Social Problems* 34, no. 4 (1987): 311–29.

Brown, Theodore M., and Elizabeth Fee. "The Bandoeng Conference of 1937: A Milestone in Health and Development." *American Journal of Public Health* 98, no. 1 (2008): 40–43.

Campbell, Chloe. "Juvenile Delinquency in Colonial Kenya, 1900–1939." *Historical Journal* 45, no. 1 (2002): 129–51.

Cantier, Jacques, and Eric Jennings, *Empire colonial sous Vichy*. Paris: Odile Jacob, 2004.

Carrière, Jeanne Louise. "Reconstructing the Grounds for Interdiction." *Louisiana Law Review* 54, no. 5 (1994): 1199–1236.

Chailley Bert, J. *Java et ses habitants*. Paris: Armand Colin et Cie, Editeurs, 1900.

Chautemps, Maurice. *Le Vagabondage en Pays Annamite*. Paris: Librarie Nouvelle de Droit et de Jurisprudence, 1908.

Cherry, Haydon. "Down and Out in Saigon: A Social History of the Poor in a Colonial City, 1860–1940." PhD diss. Yale University, 2012.

Chiang, Howard, ed. *Psychiatry and Chinese History*. New York: Routledge, 2015.

Coleborne, Catherine. "'His Brain Was Wrong, His Mind Astray': Families and the Language of Insanity in New South Wales, Queensland, and New Zealand, 1880s–1910." *Journal of Family History* 31, no. 1 (2006): 45–65.

——. "Insanity, Gender and Empire: Women Living a 'Loose Kind of Life' on the Colonial Institutional Margins, 1870–1910." *Health and History* 14 (2012): 77–99.

——. *Madness in the Family: Insanity and Institutions in the Australasian Colonial World, 1860–1914*. New York: Palgrave Macmillan, 2009.

Collignon, René. Pour une histoire de la psychiatrie colonial francaise. A partir de l'exemple du Sénégal. *L'Autre* 3 (2002): 455–80.

Conley, John A. "Prisons, Production and Profit: Reconsidering the Importance of Prison Industries." *Journal of Social History* 14 (1980): 257–75.

Cooper, Frederick. *Decolonization and African Society: The Labor Question in French and British Africa*. Cambridge: Cambridge University Press, 1996.

Cooper, Frederick, and Ann Laura Stoler, eds. *Tensions of Empire: Colonial Cultures in a Bourgeois World*. Berkeley: University of California Press, 1997.

Craig, David. *Familiar Medicine: Everyday Health Knowledge and Practice in Today's Vietnam*. Honolulu: University of Hawai'i Press, 2002.

Crossley, Ceri. "Using and Transforming the French Countryside: The *'Colonies Agricoles'* (1820–1850)." *French Studies* 45 (January 1991): 36–54.

Davis, Natalie Zemon. *Fiction in the Archives: Pardon Tales and their Tellers in Sixteenth Century France*. Stanford, CA: Stanford University Press, 1988.

Day, Tony. "Ties That (Un)Bind: Families and States in Premodern Southeast Asia," *Journal of Asian Studies* 55, no. 2 (May 1996): 384–409.

Dekker, Jeroen. "Punir, sauver et éduquer: La colonie agricole 'Nederlandsch Mettray' et la rééducation résidentielle aux Pays-Bas, en France, en Allemagne et en Angleterre entre 1814 et 1914." *Le Mouvement Social* 153 (October–December 1990): 63–90.

Del Testa, David. "Workers, Culture and the Railroads in French Colonial Indochina, 1905–1936," *French Colonial History* 2 (2002): 181–98.

de Vries, Leslie E. "The Dong Nhan Pagoda and the Publication of Mister Lazy's Medical Encyclopedia." In *Buddhism and Medicine: An Anthology of Premodern Sources*, edited by C. Pierce Salguero, 569–74. New York: Columbia University Press, 2017.

Digby, Anne. *Madness, Morality and Medicine: A Study of the York Retreat, 1796–1914*. Cambridge, UK: Cambridge University Press, 1985.

Digby, Anne, Waltraud Ernst, and Projit Mukharji, eds. Crossing Colonial Historiographies: Histories of Colonial and Indigenous Medicines in Transnational Perspectives. Newcastle upon Tyne, UK: Cambridge Scholars, 2010.

Dorolle, Pierre. *Histoire de vie*. Paris: Factuel, 2002.

——. *La Législation Indochinoise sur les Aliénés: Exposé et commentaire des dispositions du décret du 18 juillet 1930*. Saigon: Imprimerie A. Portail, 1941.

Dowbiggin, Ian. *Inheriting Madness: Professionalization and Psychiatric Knowledge in Nineteenth Century France*. Berkeley: University of California Press, 1991.

Downs, Laura Lee. *Childhood in the Promised Land: Working-Class Movements and the Colonies de Vacances in France, 1880–1960*. Durham, NC: Duke University Press, 2002.

Doumoutier, Gustave. *Essai sur la pharamcie Annamite: Determination de 300 plantes et produits indigènes, avec leur nom en Annamite, en français, en latin et en chinois et l'indication de leurs qualités thérapeutiques d'après les pharmacopées annamites et chinoises*. Hanoi: F.H. Schneider 1887.

Dumb Luck: A Novel by Vũ Trọng Phụng, edited by Peter Zinoman, translated by Nguyễn Nguyệt Cầm and Peter Zinoman. Ann Arbor: University of Michigan Press, 2002.

Dutton, George. "Lý Toét in the City: Coming to Terms with the Modern in 1930s Vietnam." *Journal of Vietnamese Studies* 2, no. 1 (February 2007): 80–108.

Edington, Claire. "Drug Detention and Human Rights in Post–Đổi Mới Vietnam." In *The Postcolonial World*, edited by David Kim and Jyotsna Singh, 325–42. London: Routledge, 2016.

——. "Going In and Getting Out of the Colonial Asylum: Families and Psychiatric Care in French Indochina." *Comparative Studies in Society and History* 55, no. 3 (2013): 725–55.

Edington, Claire, and Hans Pols. "Building Psychiatric Expertise across Southeast Asia: Study Trips, Site Visits and Therapeutic Labor in French Indochina and the Dutch East Indies, 1898–1937." *Comparative Studies in Society and History* 58, no. 3 (July 2016): 636–63.

Endres, Kirsten W. *Performing the Divine: Mediums, Markets and Modernity in Urban Vietnam.* Copenhagen: Nordic Institute of Asian Studies (NIAS) Press, 2011.

Ernst, Waltraud. "Colonial Psychiatry, Magic and Religion: The Case of Mesmerism in British India." *History of Psychiatry* 15, no. 1 (2004): 57–71.

——. "Idioms of Madness and Colonial Boundaries: The Case of the European and 'Native' Mentally Ill in Early Nineteenth Century British India." *Comparative Studies in Society and History* 39, no. 1 (1997): 153–81.

——. *Mad Tales from the Raj: The European Insane in British India, 1800–1858.* New York: Routledge, 1991.

——, ed. *Work, Psychiatry, and Society, 1750–2015.* Manchester, UK: Manchester University Press, 2016.

Ernst, Waltraud, and Thomas Mueller, eds. *Transnational Psychiatries: Social and Cultural Histories of Psychiatry in Comparative Perspective, c. 1800–2000.* Cambridge: Cambridge University Press, 2010.

Eyal, Gil. "For a Sociology of Expertise: The Social Origins of the Autism Epidemic." *American Journal of Sociology* 118, no. 4 (2013): 863–907.

Fanon, Frantz. *The Wretched of the Earth.* Translated by Constance Farrington. New York: Grove, 1963.

Farge, Arlette, and Michel Foucault, eds. *Le Désordre des familles. Lettres de cachet des archives de la Bastille au XVIIIe siècle.* Paris: Gallimard, 1982.

Farley, John. *To Cast Out Disease: A History of the International Health Division of the Rockefeller Foundation (1913–1951).* New York: Oxford University Press, 2003.

Fauvel, Aude. "Madness: A 'Female Malady.'" In *Vulnerability, Social Inequality and Health,* edited by Patrice Bourdelais and John Chircop, 61–75. Lisbon: Edições Colibri, 2010.

Firpo, Christina E. "Lost Boys: 'Abandoned' Eurasian Children and the Management of the Racial Topography in Colonial Indochina, 1938–1945," *French Colonial History* 8 (2007): 203–21

——. *The Uprooted: Race, Children and Imperialism in French Indochina, 1890–1980.* Honolulu: University of Hawai'i Press, 2016.

Fishman, Sara. *The Battle for Children: World War II, Youth Crime and Juvenile Justice in Twentieth-Century France.* Cambridge, MA: Harvard University Press, 2002.

Foucault, Michel. *Abnormal: Lectures at the College de France, 1974–1975.* New York: Picador, 2003.

——. *The Archaeology of Knowledge.* New York: Pantheon Books, 1972.

——. *Discipline and Punish: The Birth of the Prison.* 2nd ed. New York: Vintage Press, 1995.

——. *Madness and Civilization: A History of Insanity in the Age of Reason.* New York: Penguin Random House, 1988.

——. *Psychiatric Power: Lectures at the Collège de France, 1973–1974.* Translated by Graham Burchell. New York: Palgrave Macmillan, 2006.

Franklin, Robert R., Doudou Sarr, Momar Gueye, Omar Sylla, and René Collignon. "Cultural Response to Mental Illness in Senegal: Reflections through Patient Companions, Part I: Methods and Descriptive Data." *Social Science and Medicine* 42, no. 3 (1996): 325–38.

Frühstück, Sabine. *Managing the Truth of Sex in Imperial Japan. Journal of Asian Studies* 59, no. 2 (May 2000): 332–58.

Gammeltoft, Tine. *Women's Bodies, Women's Worries: Health and Family Planning in a Vietnamese Rural Commune.* Copenhagen: Nordic Institute of Asian Studies, 1999.

Gijswijt-Hofstra, Marijke, et al., eds. *Psychiatric Cultures Compared: Psychiatry and Mental Health Care in the Twentieth Century.* Amsterdam: Amsterdam University Press, 2005.

Goldsmith, Larry. "To Profit by His Skill and to Traffic on His Crime: Prison Labor in Early Nineteenth Century Massachusetts." *Labor History* 4 (1999): 439–57.

Goldstein, Jan. *Console and Classify: The French Psychiatric Profession in the Nineteenth Century.* Cambridge: Cambridge University Press, 1987.

Good, Mary-Jo DelVecchio, Sandra Teresa Hyde, Sarah Pinto, and Byron J. Good, eds. *Postcolonial Disorders.* Berkeley: University of California Press, 2008.

Goscha, Christopher. "'The Modern Barbarian': Nguyen Van Vinh and the Complexity of Colonial Modernity in Vietnam." *European Journal of East Asian Studies* 3, no. 1 (2004): 135–69.

——. *Vietnam: A New History.* New York: Basic Books, 2016.

Gouda, Frances. *Dutch Culture Overseas: Colonial Practice in the Netherlands Indies 1900–1942.* Jakarta: Equinox Press, 2008.

Groleau, Danielle, and Laurence Kirmayer. "Sociosomatic Theory in Vietnamese Immigrants' Narratives of Distress," *Anthropology & Medicine* 11, no. 2 (2004): 117–33.

Guillemot, François, and Agathe Larcher-Goscha. *La colonisation des corps: De l'Indochine au Viet Nam.* Paris: Éditions Vendémiaire, 2014.

Heaton, Matthew. *Black Skin, White Coats: Nigerian Psychiatrists, Decolonization, and the Globalization of Psychiatry.* Athens: Ohio University Press, 2013.

Hewitt, Jessica Rian. "Isolating Madness: Doctors, Families and the Gendering of Psychiatric Authority in Nineteenth-Century France." PhD diss., University of California, Davis, 2012.

Ho Tai, Hue Tam. *Millenarianism and Peasant Politics in Vietnam.* Cambridge, MA: Harvard University Press, 1983.

——. *Radicalism and the Origins of the Vietnamese Revolution.* Cambridge, MA: Harvard University Press, 1996.

Huard, Pierre and Maurice Durand. "Un traité de médecine sino-vietnamienne du XVIIIe siècle: La compréhension intuitive des recettes médicales de Hai-Thuong." *Revue d'histoire des sciences et de leurs applications* 9, no. 2 (1956): 126–49.

Human Rights Watch. *The Rehab Archipelago: Forced Labor and Other Abuses in Drug Detention Centers in Vietnam,* 2011. https://www.hrw.org/sites/default/files/reports/vietnam0911ToPost.pdf.

Ignatieff, Michael. "State, Civil Society and Total Institutions: A Critique of Recent Social Histories of Punishment," *Crime and Justice* 3 (1981): 153–92.

Jackson, Lynette. *Surfacing Up: Psychiatry and Social Order in Colonial Zimbabwe, 1908–1968.* Ithaca, NY: Cornell University Press, 2005.

Jennings, Eric. "Conservative Confluences, 'Nativist' Synergy: Reinscribing Vichy's National Revolution in Indochina, 1940–1945." *French Historical Studies* 27, no. 3 (2004): 601–35.

Keith, Charles P. *Catholic Vietnam: A Church from Empire to Nation.* Berkeley: University of California Press, 2012.

Keller, Richard C. *Colonial Madness: Psychiatry in French North Africa.* Chicago: University of Chicago Press, 2007.

——. "Madness and Colonization: Psychiatry in the British and French Empires, 1800–1962." *Journal of Social History* 35, no. 2 (Winter 2001): 295–326.

——. "Pinel in the Maghreb: Liberation, Confinement and Psychiatric Reform in French North Africa." *Bulletin of the History of Medicine* 79, no. 3 (Fall 2005): 459–99.

Kelly, Gail P. "The Relation Between Colonial and Metropolitan Schools: A Structural Analysis." *Comparative Education* 15, no. 2 (June 1979): 209–15.

Kendall, Laurel, and Hien Thi Nguyen. "Dressing Up the Spirits: Costumes, Cross-Dressing, and Incarnation in Korea and Vietnam." In *Women and Indigenous religions,* edited by Sylvia Marcos, 93–114. New York: Praeger, 2010.

Kim, Hayang. "Sick at Heart: Mental Illness in Modern Japan." PhD diss., Columbia University, 2015.

Kleinman, Arthur. *Patients and Healers in the Context of Culture: An Exploration of the Borderland between Anthropology, Medicine and Psychiatry.* Berkeley: University of California Press, 1981.

Lachenal, Guillaume. "Médecine, comparaisons et échanges inter-impériaux dans le Mandat Camerounais: Une histoire croisée Franco-Allemande de la mission Jamot." *Canadian Bulletin of Medical History* 30, no. 2 (2013): 23–45.

Ladame, Charles, and G. Demay. "La thérapeutique des maladies mentales par le travail." *Rapport au Congrès des médecins aliénistes et neurologistes de France et des pays de langue française.* Paris: Masson et Cie, 1926.

Lagardelle, Firmin. *Étude sur les colonies agricoles d'aliénés.* Moulins: Imprimerie de C. Desrosiers, 1873.

Langlet, E. *Le peuple annamite: Ses moeurs, croyances et traditions.* Paris: Berger-Levrault, 1913.

Lawrence, Benjamin N., Emily Lynn Osbourne, and Richard L. Roberts, eds. *Intermediaries, Interpreters and Clerks: African Employees in the Making of Colonial Africa.* Madison: University of Wisconsin Press, 2006.

Lê, Jean Quang Trinh. "Croyances et pratiques médicales sino-annamites." Thèse (Docteur en médecine), Université de Montpellier Faculté de Médecine, 1911.

Lefèvre, R. "L'assistance psychiatrique en Indochine." *Congrès des médecins aliénistes et neurologistes de France et des pays de langue française, XXXVe Session, Bordeaux, April 7–12, 1931.* Paris: Masson et Cie.

Lessard, Micheline. "Tradition for Rebellion: Vietnamese Students and Teachers and Anti-colonial Resistance, 1888–1931." PhD diss., Cornell University, 1995.

Lê Vân Kim. "La protection légale de l'enfance." In *Semaine de l'enfance du 1er au 7 juillet 1934: Rapports.* Saigon: Imprimerie de l'union, 1934.

Litsios, Socrates. "Revisiting Bandoeng," *Social Medicine* 8, no. 3 (2014): 113–28.

Lloyd, Margaret Gwynne, and Michel Bénézech "The French Mental Health Legislation of 1838 and Its Reform." *Journal of Forensic Psychiatry* 3, no. 2 (1992): 232–50.

Lombard, Denys. "Voyageurs Français dans l'Archipel Insulindien, XVIIe, XVIIe, XIXe Siècles." *Archipel* 1 (1971): 141–68.

Lorion, Louis. *Criminalité et médecine judiciare en Cochinchine.* Lyon: A. Storck, 1887.

Ma, Zhiying. "An Iron Cage of Civilization? Missionary Psychiatry, the Chinese Family and a Colonial Dialect of Enlightenment." In *Psychiatry and Chinese History,* edited by Howard Chiang, 71–90. London: Pickering and Chatto, 2014.

Macdonald, Michael. *Mystical Bedlam. Madness, Anxiety and Healing in Seventeenth-Century England.* Cambridge: Cambridge University Press, 1981.

Mahone, Sloane. "Psychiatry in the East African Colonies: A Background to Confinement." *International Review of Psychiatry* 18, no. 4 (2006): 327–32.

Mahone, Sloane, and Megan Vaughan, eds. *Psychiatry and Empire.* New York: Palgrave Macmillan, 2007.

Malarney, Shaun Kingsley. *Culture, Ritual and Revolution in Vietnam.* Honolulu: University of Hawai'i Press, 2002.

——. Introduction to *Lục Xì: Prostitution and Venereal Disease in Colonial Hanoi,* by Vũ Trọng Phụng. Honolulu: University of Hawai'i Press, 2011.

Marcé, Louis Victor. *Traité de la folie des femmes enceintes: Des nouvelles accouchées et des nourrices.* Paris: L'Harmattan, 2002. First published 1858.

Marquis, Edouard. *L'oeuvre humaine de la France en Cochinchine.* Saigon: Imprimerie du Théâtre, 1956.

Marr, David. "Concepts of 'Individual' and 'Self' in Twentieth-Century Vietnam." *Modern Asian Studies* 34, no. 4 (October 2000): 769–96.

——. *Vietnam 1945: The Quest for Power.* Berkeley: University of California Press, 1997.

——. "Vietnamese Attitudes Regarding Illness and Healing." In *Death and Disease in Southeast Asia.* Explorations in Social, Medical and Demographic History, edited by Norman G. Owen, 162–86. Oxford: Oxford University Press, 1987.

——. *Vietnamese Tradition on Trial: 1920–1945.* Berkeley: University of California Press, 1981.

Marshall, Van Nguyen. "The Ethics of Benevolence in French Colonial Vietnam: A Sino-Franco Vietnamese Cultural Borderland." In *The Chinese State at the Borders,* edited by Diana Lary, 162–80. Vancouver: University of British Columbia Press, 2008.

——. *In Search of Moral Authority: The Discourse on Poverty, Poor Relief, and Charity in French Colonial Vietnam.* New York: Peter Lang, 2008.

——. "The Moral Economy of Colonialism: Subsistence and Famine Relief in French Indochina, 1906–1917." *International History Review* 27, no. 2 (June 2005): 237–58.

Matza, Thomas. "Moscow's Echo: Technologies of the Self, Publics, and Politics on the Russian Talk Show." *Cultural Anthropology* 24, no. 3 (2009): 489–522.

McCoy, Ted. "The Unproductive Prisoner: Labor and Medicine in Canadian Penitentiaries, 1867–1900." *Labor: Studies in Working-Class History of the Americas* 6, no. 4 (2010): 95–112.

McDonald, D. I. "Frederick Norton Manning 1839–1903." *Journal of the Royal Australian Historical Society* 58, no. 3 (1972): 190–201.

McGovern, Constance C. "The Myths of Social Control and Custodial Oppression: Patterns of Psychiatric Medicine in Late Nineteenth-Century Institutions." *Journal of Social History* 20 (1986): 3–23.

McHale, Shawn. *Print and Power: Confucianism, Communism and Buddhism in the Making of Modern Vietnam.* Honolulu: University of Hawai'i Press, 2003.

McKinley, Robert A. "Psychiatry in Vietnam—1966." *American Journal of Psychiatry* 123, no. 4 (October 1966): 420–26.

McLennan, Rebecca. *The Crisis of Imprisonment: Protest, Politics, and the Making of the American Penal State, 1776–1941.* Cambridge: Cambridge University Press, 2008.

Melling, Joseph, and Bill Forsythe, eds. *Insanity, Institutions and Society, 1800–1914.* Studies in the Social History of Medicine. London: Routledge, 1999.

Mills, James. "The Mad and the Past: Retrospective Diagnosis, Post-Coloniality, Discourse Analysis and the Asylum Archive." *Journal of Medical Humanities* 21, no. 3 (2000): 141–58.

——. *Madness, Cannabis, and Colonialism: The "Native-Only" Lunatic Asylums of British India, 1857–1900.* London: Macmillan, 2000.

Minas, Harry, Claire Edington, Nhan La, and Ritsuko Kakuma. "Mental Health in Vietnam." In *Mental Health in Asia and the Pacific: Historical and Comparative Perspectives,* edited by Harry Minas and Milton Lewis, 145–62. New York: Springer, 2017.

Monk, Lee-Ann. "Working in the Asylum: Attendants to the Insane." *Health and History* 11, no. 1 (2009): 83–101.

Monnais, Laurence. "Colonised and Neurasthenic: From the Appropriation of a Word to the Reality of a *Malaise de Civilisation* in Urban French Vietnam." *Health and History* 14, no. 1 (2012): 121–42.

——. "'Could Confinement Be Humanised'? A Modern History of Leprosy in Vietnam." In *Public Health in Asia and the Pacific: Historical and Comparative Perspectives,* edited by Milton J. Lewis and Kerrie L. MacPherson, 122–38. New York: Routledge, 2008.

——. "In the Shadow of the Colonial Hospital: Developing Health Care in Indochina, 1860–1939." In *Viêt-Nam Exposé: French Scholarship on Twentieth-Century Vietnamese Society,* edited by Gisele L. Bousquet and Pierre Brocheux, 140–84. Ann Arbor: University of Michigan Press, 2002.

——. *Médecine et colonisation: L'aventure indochinoise, 1860–1939.* Paris: CNRS Editions, 1999.

——. "Preventive Medicine and 'Mission Civilisatrice': Uses of the BCG Vaccine in French Colonial Vietnam between the Two World Wars." *International Journal of Asia Pacific Studies* 2, no. 1 (2006): 41–68.

Monnais, Laurence, and Harold J. Cook, eds. *Global Movements, Local Concerns: Medicine and Health in Southeast Asia.* Singapore: Singapore University Press, 2012.

Monnais, Laurence, and Hans Pols. "Health and Disease in the Colonies: Medicine in the Age of Empire." In *The Routledge History of Western Empires*, edited by Robert Aldrich and Kirsten McKenzie, 270–84. New York: Routledge, 2014.

Monnais, Laurence, C. Michele Thompson, and Ayo Wahlberg, eds. *Southern Medicine for Southern People: Vietnamese Medicine in the Making*. Newcastle upon Tyne, UK: Cambridge Scholars Publishing, 2012.

Monnais, Laurence, and Noémi Tousignant. "The Colonial Life of Pharmaceuticals: Accessibility to Healthcare, Consumption of Medicines, and Medical Pluralism in French Vietnam, 1905–1945." *Journal of Vietnamese Studies* 1, no. 1–2 (2006): 131–66.

Monroe, John Warne. *Laboratories of Faith: Mesmerism, Spiritism, and Occultism in Modern France*. Ithaca, NY: Cornell University Press, 2008.

Mooney, Graham, and Jonathan Reinarz, eds. *Permeable Walls: Historical Perspectives on Hospital and Asylum Visiting*. The Wellcome Series in the History of Medicine. Amsterdam: Editions Rodopi, B.V., 2009.

Moran, James, Leslie Topp, and Jonathan Andrews, eds. *Madness, Architecture and the Built Environment: Psychiatric Spaces in Historical Context*. New York: Routledge, 2007.

Morlat, Patrice. *La repression coloniale au Vietnam (1908–1940)*. Paris: L'Harmattan, 1990.

Murray, Martin J. " 'White Gold' or 'White Blood'?: The Rubber Plantations of Colonial Indochina, 1910–1940." *Journal of Peasant Studies* 19, no. 3–4 (1992): 41–67.

Neill, Deborah. *Networks in Tropical Medicine: Internationalism, Colonialism, and the Rise of a Medical Specialty, 1890–1930*. Stanford, CA: Stanford University Press, 2012.

Ng, Vivien. *Madness in Late Imperial China: From Illness to Deviance*. Norman: University of Oklahoma Press, 1990.

Nguyễn, Martina T. "The Self-Reliant Literary Group (Tự Lực Văn Đoàn): Colonial Modernism in Vietnam, 1932–1941." PhD diss., University of California, Berkeley, 2012.

Nguyêñ, Ngọc Huy, and Văn Tài Tạ. *The Le Code: Law in Traditional Vietnam: A Comparative Sino-Vietnamese Legal Study with Historical-Juridical Analysis*. Athens: Ohio University Press, 1987.

Nguyễn, Thị Hiền. "Yin Illness: Its Diagnosis and Healing within Len Dong (Spirit Possession) Rituals of the Viet." *Asian Ethnology* 67, no. 2 (2008): 305–21.

Nguyễn, Thuy Linh. *Childbirth, Maternity and Medical Pluralism in French Colonial Vietnam, 1880–1945*. Rochester, NY: University of Rochester Press, 2016.

Nguyễn, Trần Huân. *Contribution à l'Etude de l'Ancienne Therapeutique Vietnamienne*. Hanoi: Ecole Francaise d'Extreme Orient, 1951.

Nguyễn, Văn Hoài. *De l'organisation de l'Hôpital Psychiatrique du Sud-Vietnam*. Saigon: Imprimerie Française d'Outre Mer, 1954.

Nguyêñ, Văn Ký. *La société vietnamienne face à la modernité: Le Tonkin de la fin du XIXe siecle à la seconde guerre mondiale*. Paris: l'Harmattan, 1995

Norton, Barley. *Songs for the Spirits: Music and Mediums in Modern Vietnam*. Urbana: University of Illinois Press, 2009.

Nunley, Michael. "The Involvement of Families in Indian Psychiatry." *Culture, Medicine and Psychiatry* 22 (1988): 317–53.

Nye, Robert A. *Crime, Madness and Politics in Modern France: The Medical Conception of National Decline.* Princeton, NJ: Princeton University Press, 1984.

O'Brien, Patricia. *The Promise of Punishment: Prisons in Nineteenth-Century France.* Princeton, NJ: Princeton University Press, 1982.

Osbourne, Michael. *The Emergence of Tropical Medicine in France.* Chicago: University of Chicago Press, 2014.

Parle, Julie. *States of Mind: Searching for Mental Health in Natal and Zululand, 1868–1918.* Scottsville, South Africa: University of KwaZulu-Natal Press, 2007.

Pech, F. "Note sur le régime légal de la Cochinchine." *Journal of the Siam Society* 4 (1907): 1–18.

Pelras, Christian. "Indonesian Studies in France: Retrospect, Situation and Prospects," *Archipel* 16 (1978): 7–20.

Peycam, Philippe. *The Birth of Vietnamese Political Journalism.* New York: Columbia University Press, 2012.

Peters, Erica. "Negotiating Power through Everyday Practices in French Vietnam, 1880–1924." PhD diss., University of Chicago, 2000.

Phan, Tuong, and Derrick Silove. "An Overview of Indigenous Descriptions of Mental Phenomena and the Range of Traditional Healing Practices amongst the Vietnamese." *Transcultural Psychiatry* 36, no. 1 (1999): 79–94.

Pinto, Sarah. "Crises of Commitment: Ethics of Intimacy, Kin and Confinement in Global Psychiatry." *Medical Anthropology: Cross-Cultural Studies in Health and Illness* 28, no. 1 (2009): 1–10.

Philastre, Paul Louis Félix. *Le Code Annamite.* Paris: Ernest Leroux, 1876.

Pols, Hans. "Beyond the Clinical Frontiers: The American Mental Hygiene Movement, 1910–1945." In *International Relations in Psychiatry: Britain, Germany and the United States to World War II,* edited by V. Roelcke, P. Weindling, and L. Westwood. Rochester, NY: University of Rochester Press, 2010.

——. The Development of Psychiatry in Indonesia: From Colonial to Modern Times." *International Review of Psychiatry* 18, no. 4 (2006): 363–70.

——. "The Psychiatrist as Administrator: The Career of W. F. Theunissen in the Dutch East Indies." *Health & History* 14 (2012): 143–64.

——. "Psychological Knowledge in a Colonial Context: Theories on the Nature of the 'Native Mind' in the Former Dutch East Indies." *History of Psychology* 10 (2007): 111–31.

Pomfret, David M. *Youth and Empire: Trans-Colonial Childhoods in British and French Asia.* Stanford, CA: Stanford University Press, 2015.

Porter, Roy. *A Social History of Madness: The World through the Eyes of the Insane.* New York: Weidenfeld and Nicolson, 1988.

Porter, Roy, and David Wright, eds. *The Confinement of the Insane, 1800–1965: International Perspectives.* Cambridge: Cambridge University Press, 2003.

Prieto, Leida Fernandez. "Islands of Knowledge: Science and Agriculture in the History of Latin America and the Caribbean," *Isis* 104 (2013): 788–97.

Proschan, Frank. "'Syphilia, Opiomania and Pederasty': Colonial Constructions of Vietnamese (and French) Social Diseases." *Journal of the History of Sexuality* 11, no. 4 (October 2002): 610–36.

Quétel, Claude. *Histoire de la folie: De l'antiquité à nos jours.* Paris: Tallendier, 2009.

Quỳnh, Cao Thị Như, and John C. Shafer. "From Verse Narrative to Novel: The Development of Prose Fiction in Vietnam." *Journal of Asian Studies* 47, no. 4 (November 1988): 756–77.

Rafael, Vicente L., ed. *Figures of Criminality in Indonesia, the Philippines, and Colonial Vietnam.* Ithaca, NY: Cornell Southeast Asia Program, 1999.

Raffin, Anne. "The Causes and Consequences of Patriotic Youth Mobilization in Vichy France and Indochina during and after World War II." PhD diss., New School, 2000.

Reaume, Geoffrey. "Patients at Work: Insane Asylum Inmates' Labour in Ontario, 1841–1900." In *Rethinking Normalcy: A Disability Studies Reader*, edited by Tanya Titchkosky and Rod Michalko, 158–80. Toronto: Canadian Scholars' Press, 2009.

——. *Remembrance of Patients Past: Patient Life at the Toronto Hospital for the Insane, 1870–1940.* Toronto: University of Toronto Press, 2000.

Reboul, Henri, and Emmanuel Régis. "L'Assistance des aliénés aux colonies" *Rapport au Congrès des médecins aliénistes et neurologistes de France et des pays de langue française, XXIIe session. Tunis, 1–7 April 1912.* Paris: Masson et Cie, 1912.

Recueil de notices redigées à l'occasion du Xe congrès de la "Far Eastern Association of Tropical Medicine," Hanoi (Tonkin), November 24–30, 1938. Hanoi: Imprimerie G. Taupin, 1938.

Renneville, Marc. "La psychiatrie légale dans le projet de réforme du code pénal français (1930–1938)." In *Psychiatries dans l'histoire. Actes du 6ème congrès de l'Association européenne pour l'histoire de la psychiatrie*, edited by J. Arveiller, 385–405. Caen: Presses universitaires de Caen, 2008.

Risse, Guenter B. and John Harley Warner. "Reconstructing Clinical Activities: Patient Records in Medical History." *Social History of Medicine* 5, no. 2 (1992): 183–205.

Roos, Neil. "Work Colonies and South African Historiography." *Journal of Social History* 36, no. 1 (2011): 54–76.

Rothman, David. *The Discovery of the Asylum: Social Order and Disorder in the New Republic.* Boston: Little, Brown, 1971.

Roussy. "Rapport sur le fonctionnement de l'Asile d'Aliénés de Bienhoa (Cochinchine)."*Annales de médecine et de pharmacie coloniales* 24 (1926): 34–56.

Rush, James. *Opium to Java: Revenue Farming and Chinese Enterprise in Colonial Indonesia, 1860–191.* Ithaca, NY: Cornell University Press, 1990.

Saada, Emmanuelle. *Empire's Children: Race, Filiation and Citizenship in the French Colonies.* Translated by Arthur Goldhammer. Chicago: University of Chicago Press, 2012.

Sadowsky, Jonathan. *Electroconvulsive Therapy in America: The Anatomy of a Medical Controversy.* London: Routledge, 2016.

——. *Imperial Bedlam: Institutions of Madness in Colonial Southwest Nigeria.* Berkeley: University of California Press, 1999.

——. "The Social World and the Reality of Mental Illness: Lessons from Colonial Psychiatry." *Harvard Review of Psychiatry* 11 (2003): 210–14.

Sager, Paul. "Youth and Nationalism in Vichy Indochina," *Journal of Vietnamese Studies* 3, no. 3 (Fall 2008): 291–301.

Saha, Jonathan. "Madness and the Making of a Colonial Order in Burma." *Modern Asian Studies* 47, no. 2 (March 2013): 406–35.

—— "'Uncivilized Practitioners': Medical Subordinates, Medico-Legal Evidence and Misconduct in Colonial Burma, 1875–1907." *Southeast Asia Research* 20, no. 3 (2012): 423–43.

Sasges, Gerard. *Imperial Intoxication: Alcohol and the Making of Colonial Indochina.* Honolulu: University of Hawai'i Press, 2017.

——. "'Indigenous Representation Is Hostile to All Monopolies': Pham Quynh and the End of the Alcohol Monopoly in Colonial Vietnam." *Journal of Vietnamese Studies* 5, no. 1 (January 2010): 1–36.

Schrauwers, Albert. "The 'Benevolent' Colonies of Johannes van den Bosch: Continuities in the Administration of Poverty in the Netherlands and Indonesia." *Comparative Studies in Society and History* 43, no. 2 (2001): 298–328.

Scull, Andrew. *The Most Solitary of Afflictions: Madness and Society in Britain, 1700–1900.* New Haven: Yale University Press, 1993.

—— *Museums of Madness: The Social Organization of Insanity in 19th Century England.* New York: Penguin Books, 1979.

Sen, Satadru. *Colonial Childhoods: The Juvenile Periphery of India, 1850–1945.* London: Anthem, 2005.

Shiraishi, Masaya. "State, Villagers, and Vagabonds: Vietnamese Rural Society and the Phan Ba Vanh Rebellion," *Senri Ethnological Studies* 13 (1984): 345–400.

Shorter, Edward, and David Healy, eds. *Shock Therapy: A History of Electroconvulsive Treatment in Mental Illness.* New Brunswick, NJ: Rutgers University Press, 2013.

Simonis, Fabien. "Mad Acts, Mad Speech, and Mad People in Late Imperial Chinese law and Medicine." PhD diss., Princeton University, 2010.

Skalevag, Svein. "Constructive Curative Instruments: Psychiatric Architecture in Norway, 1820–1920." *History of Psychiatry* 12 (2002): 51–68.

Stoler, Ann Laura. *Along the Archival Grain.* Princeton, NJ: Princeton University Press, 2009.

——. *Capitalism and Confrontation in Sumatra's Plantation Belt, 1870–1979.* Ann Arbor: University of Michigan Press, 1985.

——. *Carnal Knowledge and Imperial Power: Race and the Intimate in Colonial Rule.* Berkeley: University of California Press, 2001.

——. "Sexual Affronts and Racial Frontiers: European Identities and the Cultural Politics of Exclusion in Colonial Southeast Asia." *Comparative Studies in Society and History* 34, no. 3 (1992): 514–51.

Suzuki, Akihito. "Between Two Psychiatric Regimes: Migration and Psychiatry in Early Twentieth Century Japan." In *Migration, Ethnicity, and Mental Health: International Perspectives, 1840–2010*, edited by Angela McCarthy and Catharine Coleborne, 141–56. Routledge Studies in Cultural History. New York: Routledge, 2012.

——. *Madness at Home: The Psychiatrist, the Patient, and the Family in England, 1820–1860.* Berkeley: University of California Press, 2006.

Swartz, Sally. "Colonial Lunatic Asylum Archives: Challenges to Historiography." *Kronos* 34, no. 1 (2008): 285–302.

Tanvir, Ahmed, Nguyen Thanh Long, Phan Thi Thu Huong, and Donald Edwin Stewart. "HIV and Injecting Drug Users in Vietnam: An Overview of Policies and Responses," *World Medical and Health PoliWorld Medical and Health Policy* 6, no. 4 (2014): 395–418.

Taylor, K. W. *A History of the Vietnamese.* Cambridge, UK: Cambridge University Press, 2013.

Terbenche, Danielle. "'Curative' and 'Custodial': Benefits of Patient Treatment at the Asylum for the Insane, Kingston, 1878–1906." *Canadian Historical Review* 86 (2005): 29–52.

Thompson, C. Michele. "Selections from *Miraculous Drugs of the South* by the Vietnamese Buddhist Monk-Physican Tuệ Tĩnh." In *Buddhism and Medicine: An Anthology of Premodern Sources,* edited by C. Pierce Salguero, 561–68. New York: Columbia University Press, 2017.

———. *Vietnamese Traditional Medicine: A Social History.* Singapore: National University of Singapore Press, 2015.

Tomes, Nancy. *The Art of Asylum Keeping: Thomas Story Kirkbride and the Origins of American Psychiatry.* Philadelphia: University of Pennsylvania Press, 1994.

Topp, Leslie, James Moran, and Jonathan Andrews, eds. *Madness, Architecture and the Built Environment: Psychiatric Spaces in Historical Context.* New York: Routledge, 2007.

Toth, Stephen. *Beyond Papillon: The French Overseas Penal Colonies, 1854–1952.* Lincoln: University of Nebraska Press, 2006.

Tran, Allen. "A Life of Worry: The Cultural Politics and Phenomenology of Anxiety in Ho Chi Minh City, Vietnam." PhD diss., University of California–San Diego, 2012.

———. "Neurasthenia, Generalized Anxiety Disorder, and the Medicalization of Worry in a Vietnamese Psychiatric Hospital." *Medical Anthropology Quarterly* 31, no. 2 (2017): 198–217.

Tran, Quang-Anh Richard. "From Red Lights to Red Flags: A History of Gender in Colonial and Contemporary Vietnam." PhD diss., University of California, Berkeley, 2011.

Tran Minh Tung, "The Family and the Management of Mental Health Problems in Vietnam." In *Transcultural Research in Mental Health,* vol. 2 of *Mental Health Research in Asia and the Pacific,* edited by William P. Lebra, 107–14. Honolulu: University Press of Hawai'i, 1972.

Trong Tuan Luu. "Building Vietnamese Medical Terminology via Language Contact." *Australian Journal of Linguistics.* 29, no. 3 (September 2009): 315–36.

Tuong Phan, and Derrick Silove. "An Overview of Indigenous Descriptions of Mental Phenomena and the Range of Traditional Healing Practices Amongst the Vietnamese." *Transcultural Psychiatry* 36, no. 1 (1999): 79–94.

Vaughan, Megan. *Curing Their Ills: Colonial Power and African Illness.* Palo Alto, CA: Stanford University Press, 1992.

Venancio, Ana Teresa A. "From the Agricultural Colony to the Hospital-Colony: Configurations for Psychiatric Care in Brazil in the First Half of the Twentieth Century." *Historia, Ciencias, Saude—manguinhos,* Rio de Janeiro, v. 18, supl.1, December 2011. Available at http://www.scielo.br/pdf/hcsm/v18s1/en_03.pdf.

Vu, Cong Hoe. "Du suicide dans la société vietnamienne." Thèse pour le doctorat en médecine. Hanoi: Imprimerie Tonkinoise, 1937.

Vu, Linh. "Drowned in Romance, Tears and Rivers: Young Women's Suicide in Early 20th Century Vietnam." *Explorations: A Graduate Student Journal of Southeast Asian Studies* 9 (Spring 2009): 35–46.

Walton, John. "Casting Out and Bringing Back in Victorian England." In *The Anatomy of Madness: Essays in the History of Psychiatry*, edited by William Bynum, Roy Porter, and Michael Shepherd, 132–46. London: Tavistock Books, 1985.

Wannell, Louise. "Patients' Relatives and Psychiatric Doctors: Letter Writing in the York Retreat, 1875–1910." *Social History of Medicine* 20, no. 2 (2007): 297–313.

Whitmore, John. "Social Organization and Confucian Thought in Vietnam." *Journal of Southeast Asian Studies* 15, no. 2 (September 1984): 296–306.

Wojciechowski, Jean-Bernard. *Hygiène mentale et hygiène sociale.* Paris: Harmattan, 1997.

Woodside, Alexander. "The Development of Social Organizations in Vietnamese Cities in the Late Colonial Period." *Pacific Affairs* 44, no. 1 (Spring 1971): 39–64, 49.

——. *Vietnam and the Chinese* Model. Cambridge, MA: Harvard University Press, 1971.

Work of WHO in the Western Pacific Region, Twelfth Annual Report of the Regional Director to the Regional Committee for the Western Pacific (1962), WP/RC13/2. Available at http://apps.who.int/iris/handle/10665/207377.

Wright, David. "Asylum Nursing and Institutional Service: A Case Study of the South of England, 1861–1881." *Nursing History Review* 7 (1999): 153–69.

——. "The Certification of Insanity in Nineteenth-Century England and Wales." *History of Psychiatry* 9 (1998): 267–90.

——. "The Discharge of Pauper Lunatics from Country Asylums in Mid-Victorian England, the Case of Buckinghamshire, 1853–1872." In Melling and Forsythe, *Insanity, Institutions and Society*, 93–12.

——. "Getting Out of the Asylum: Understanding the Confinement of the Insane in the Nineteenth Century." *Social History of Medicine* 10, no. 1 (1997): 137–55.

Wu, H., and Wen-Ji Wang. "Making and Mapping Psy Sciences in East and Southeast Asia." *East Asian Science, Technology and Society: An International Journal* 10 (2016): 1–12.

Yu, Insun. "Law and Family in Seventeenth and Eighteenth Century Vietnam" PhD diss., University of Michigan, 1978.

Zinoman, Peter. *The Colonial Bastille: A History of Imprisonment in Vietnam, 1862–1940.* Berkeley: University of California Press, 2001.

——. *Vietnamese Colonial Republican: The Political Vision of Vũ Trọng Phụng.* Berkeley: University of California Press, 2014.

INDEX

admissions, 123–136, 183; at Biên Hòa asylum, 56–59, 66–69, 67, 68, 77, 185; criteria for, 125–126, 184; family requests for, 129–132; at Vôi asylum, 136
agricultural colonies, 55–56, 96–102, 114–115, 218; economics of, 103–109, 106–109; patient reeducation at, 100–102, 118–120
AIDS, 217
alcohol abuse, 9, 34, 36, 70, 71, 166; as hereditary disorder, 205; legal responsibility and, 189; mental illness with, 100, 159, 184
Algeria: colonial psychiatry in, 221n4, 221n6; medical experimentation in, 73
Algiers School of French Psychiatry, 10
aliénés, 43–47, 162, 176, 191, 192; definitions of, 19, 22, 31–32, 51; suicide and, 171–172
allure anormale, 126
Alzheimer's disease, 25
Amrith, Sunil, 114
Angkor Wat, restoration of, 95, 241n4
antisocial behavior, 50, 86, 164; diagnosis of, 128, 188, 191, 221n5; Heuyer on, 194; juvenile delinquency and, 182, 194, 203; voluntary confinement for, 133
arson, 126, 144, 185
asile colonie ("colony asylum"), 115–119, 116, 151, 218
Assaud, M. E., 30–31
Assistance Médicale Indigène, 12
asylum(s), 4–9, 56; abuses in, 156–157, 168; budget difficulties at, 64–66, 142; at Buitenzorg, 93–96, 94; for criminally insane, 86–87, 134, 178, 183–189; Fanon on, 4; Foucault on, 5; at Hà Đông, 150–151; Indian, 13, 57, 62, 221n5, 245n40; legislation on, 22–23, 30–34, 46–53, 183, 247n35; at Lenteng Agung, 114–118, 116; at Marseille, 35, 249n9; open services at, 132–136; outpatient clinics of, 132–133;

overcrowding at, 40, 142, 151; popular perceptions of, 130–132, 156–160, 158, 175–176; at Takhumau, 241n152. *See also* Biên Hòa asylum
Atkinson, Jane, 148
Augagneur, André, 74, 78–79, 188; on labor therapy, 97–99; on traditional medicine, 146

Bạch Mai Hospital, 217
Ballet, Gilbert, 66
Beau, Paul, 12
beriberi, 40, 93, 114, 148
beta asterone, 25
Biên Hòa asylum, 46–47, 55–73, 204, 216; admissions at, 56–59, 66–69, 67, 68, 77, 185; agricultural output from, 106–109; budgetary constraints at, 64–66, 78–79, 86; criminally insane at, 86–87, 184–185; daily routine at, 60–62; deaths at, 69; diagnostic practices at, 70–72; Dutch influences on, 94–95, 218; electrical outages at, 79; entrance gate of, 55, 56; European patients at, 57, 59–66, 60, 79, 85–86; family cooperation at, 131; family discharge request at, 139; isolation cells at, 59, 63; layout design of, 55–56, 59, 61, 77–78; meals at, 59–60, 64; as model for Vôi asylum, 73–79; overcrowding at, 64, 86; patient labor at, 103, 106, 107, 111; pavilion design at, 62; rehabilitation village at, 218; staff concerns at, 79–86; treatment regimens at, 58, 72–74, 160
Bosquet, G. H., 241n4
Bourget, Paul, 173
Brévié, Jules, 203, 205
Brocheux, Pierre, 12, 106
Brown, Theodore, 113–114
Buddhism, 139, 160, 164; health beliefs of, 15, 24, 25; millenarian traditions of, 149–150

283

Studies of the
Weatherhead East Asian Institute
Columbia University

Selected Titles

(Complete list at http://weai.columbia.edu/publications/studies-weai/)

Statebuilding by Imposition: Resistance and Control in Colonial Taiwan and the Philippines, by Reo Matsuzaki. Cornell University Press, 2019.

Nation-Empire: Ideology and Rural Youth Mobilization in Japan and Its Colonies, by Sayaka Chatani. Cornell University Press, 2019.

The Invention of Madness: State, Society, and the Insane in Modern China, by Emily Baum. University of Chicago Press, 2018.

Fixing Landscape: A Techno-Poetic History of China's Three Gorges, by Corey Byrnes. Columbia University Press, 2018.

Japan's Imperial Underworlds: Intimate Encounters at the Borders of Empire, by David Ambaras. Cambridge University Press, 2018.

Heroes and Toilers: Work as Life in Postwar North Korea, 1953–1961, by Cheehyung Harrison Kim. Columbia University Press, 2018.

Electrified Voices: How the Telephone, Phonograph, and Radio Shaped Modern Japan, 1868–1945, by Kerim Yasar. Columbia University Press, 2018.

Making Two Vietnams: War and Youth Identities, 1965–1975, by Olga Dror. Cambridge University Press, 2018.

A Misunderstood Friendship: Mao Zedong, Kim Il-sung, and Sino–North Korean Relations, 1949–1976, by Zhihua Shen and Yafeng Xia. Columbia University Press, 2018.

Raising China's Revolutionaries: Modernizing Childhood for Cosmopolitan Nationalists and Liberated Comrades, by Margaret Mih Tillman. Columbia University Press, 2018.

Buddhas and Ancestors: Religion and Wealth in Fourteenth-Century Korea, by Juhn Y. Ahn. University of Washington Press, 2018.

Idly Scribbling Rhymers: Poetry, Print, and Community in Nineteenth Century Japan, by Robert Tuck. Columbia University Press, 2018.

China's War on Smuggling: Law, Economic Life, and the Making of the Modern State, 1842–1965, by Philip Thai. Columbia University Press, 2018.

Forging the Golden Urn: The Qing Empire and the Politics of Reincarnation in Tibet, by Max Oidtmann. Columbia University Press, 2018.

The Battle for Fortune: State-Led Development, Personhood, and Power among Tibetans in China, by Charlene Makley. Cornell University Press, 2018.

Aesthetic Life: Beauty and Art in Modern Japan, by Miya Elise Mizuta Lippit. Harvard University Asia Center, 2018.

Where the Party Rules: The Rank and File of China's Communist State, by Daniel Koss. Cambridge University Press, 2018.

Resurrecting Nagasaki: Reconstruction and the Formation of Atomic Narratives, by Chad R. Diehl. Cornell University Press, 2018.

China's Philological Turn: Scholars, Textualism, and the Dao in the Eighteenth Century, by Ori Sela. Columbia University Press, 2018.

Making Time: Astronomical Time Measurement in Tokugawa Japan, by Yulia Frumer. University of Chicago Press, 2018.

Mobilizing Without the Masses: Control and Contention in China, by Diana Fu. Cambridge University Press, 2018.

Post-Fascist Japan: Political Culture in Kamakura after the Second World War, by Laura Hein. Bloomsbury, 2018.

China's Conservative Revolution: The Quest for a New Order, 1927–1949, by Brian Tsui. Cambridge University Press, 2018.

Promiscuous Media: Film and Visual Culture in Imperial Japan, 1926–1945, by Hikari Hori. Cornell University Press, 2018.

The End of Japanese Cinema: Industrial Genres, National Times, and Media Ecologies, by Alexander Zahlten. Duke University Press, 2017.

The Chinese Typewriter: A History, by Thomas S. Mullaney. The MIT Press, 2017.

Forgotten Disease: Illnesses Transformed in Chinese Medicine, by Hilary A. Smith. Stanford University Press, 2017.

Borrowing Together: Microfinance and Cultivating Social Ties, by Becky Yang Hsu. Cambridge University Press, 2017.

Food of Sinful Demons: Meat, Vegetarianism, and the Limits of Buddhism in Tibet, by Geoffrey Barstow. Columbia University Press, 2017.

Youth For Nation: Culture and Protest in Cold War South Korea, by Charles R. Kim. University of Hawaii Press, 2017.

Socialist Cosmopolitanism: The Chinese Literary Universe, 1945–1965, by Nicolai Volland. Columbia University Press, 2017.

The Social Life of Inkstones: Artisans and Scholars in Early Qing China, by Dorothy Ko. University of Washington Press, 2017.

Darwin, Dharma, and the Divine: Evolutionary Theory and Religion in Modern Japan, by G. Clinton Godart. University of Hawaii Press, 2017.

Dictators and Their Secret Police: Coercive Institutions and State Violence, by Sheena Chestnut Greitens. Cambridge University Press, 2016.

The Cultural Revolution on Trial: Mao and the Gang of Four, by Alexander C. Cook. Cambridge University Press, 2016.

Inheritance of Loss: China, Japan, and the Political Economy of Redemption After Empire, by Yukiko Koga. University of Chicago Press, 2016.

Homecomings: The Belated Return of Japan's Lost Soldiers, by Yoshikuni Igarashi. Columbia University Press, 2016.

Samurai to Soldier: Remaking Military Service in Nineteenth-Century Japan, by D. Colin Jaundrill. Cornell University Press, 2016.

The Red Guard Generation and Political Activism in China, by Guobin Yang. Columbia University Press, 2016.

Accidental Activists: Victim Movements and Government Accountability in Japan and South Korea, by Celeste L. Arrington. Cornell University Press, 2016.

Ming China and Vietnam: Negotiating Borders in Early Modern Asia, by Kathlene Baldanza. Cambridge University Press, 2016.

CPSIA information can be obtained
at www.ICGtesting.com
Printed in the USA
LVHW111741270319
612039LV00007B/65/P